How Did They Die?

Volume 3

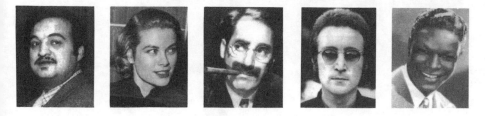

How Did They Die?

V o l u m e 3

■

Norman Donaldson

St. Martin's Press ■ *New York*

Production Editor: David Stanford Burr

Design: Judith Stagnitto

Library of Congress Cataloging-in-Publication Data
(Revised for v. 3)

Donaldson, Norman.
        How did they die?

        1. Biography.   2. Death—Causes.   I. Donaldson, Betty,
joint author.   II. Title.
CT105.D6   920   79-22871
ISBN 0-312-39488-8 (vol. 1)
ISBN 0-312-11000-6 (vol. 3)

First Edition: July 1994

10 9 8 7 6 5 4 3 2 1

For Rachel

Table of Contents

Acknowledgments

The original *How Did They Die?*, by my late wife Betty and myself, was published in 1980. Its 320-odd articles were later divided between two paperbacks, titled *How Did They Die? Vol. 1* and *Vol. 2*. Several more articles, written by both of us before Betty's death in 1988, are included in the present volume, which also covers more recent deaths and those, like Anne Frank's and Charles Lindbergh's, that had for one reason or another been left out of the original work. It was the offer of a new friend, Carol Mathews, to transform my barely legible scribble into a manuscript fit for the publishers that encouraged me to complete this book. She also made numerous astute suggestions for improving the final text.

Another good friend, John H. Dirckx, M.D., director of the Student Health Center at the University of Dayton, has again been kind enough to look over the manuscript, paying particular attention to my medical and technical terminology. I particularly appreciate his forbearance in overlooking certain acceptable popularisms, so long as they have not introduced error or ambiguity, which he would eschew in his own writing on medical subjects. Dr. Dirckx has protected me from many serious errors in chronology, Latin quotations, etc., and has sometimes felt it necessary to question my appraisal of a subject's character. But of course I, not he, must bear responsibility for any errors that remain.

I am grateful to the authors of the innumerable biographies I have used for most of the details in this book. Where one biography was especially valuable, I have noted the author's name at the end of my account, and the date of the biography. In other cases I have made use of two or more sources, including press reports and obituaries.

For help with Rudyard Kipling's correspondence I wish to thank Lisa Lewis of the Kipling Society (London). Rachel Stewart supplied valuable help with Dame Margot Fonteyn. Anne Sayer, biographer of the unfortunate Rosalind E. Franklin, offered valuable unpublished information. Dr. Eric A. Gordon, whose excellent 1989 biography of Marc Blitzstein shed light for the first time on the U.S. composer's mysterious murder, also took time to look over my articles on many other musicians and suggest several improvements.

Abbott, William *(Bud)* (1895-1974)

The tall straight man of the Abbott-Costello partnership suffered frequent epileptic seizures. In their early days in burlesque, Lou Costello (q.v.) would bring him out of on-stage attacks by hitting him hard in the solar plexus. The duo was split up at Costello's insistence in 1956.

Deep in debt to the tax authorities, Abbott in his last decade was plagued by strokes and hip and leg fractures. He died quietly at his modest home in Woodland Hills, California, 24 April 1974, and his ashes were scattered over the ocean.

Agee, James (1909-1955)

In his posthumous Pulitzer Prize–winning novel *A Death in the Family* (1957), the U.S. writer exploited much autobiographical material, notably the death of his father in a car crash in 1916 and his adoption of a surrogate father, the Episcopal priest James Harold Flye, whom he met two years later. This was when, as an eight-year-old at boarding school in Tennessee, he was forbidden by his mother, who lived a few yards away, to see her more than once a week. Agee's obsession with death (it "figures," wrote one critic, "in sixteen of his twenty-one known pieces of fiction") no doubt led to his disorderly, self-destructive life, with three marriages, countless affairs, and gross overindulgence in tobacco and alcohol.

His first heart attack occurred in January 1951 while he was in California writing the screenplay for *The African Queen,* which was to win him an Oscar nomination. Back in New York and unable to climb stairs, Agee and his wife Mia found a first-floor apartment at 17 King Street in Greenwich Village. In January 1955 he was reporting to Father Flye that his periods of cardiac fibrillation (irregular heartbeat) numbered as many as eight a day. He was by now disgusted with the "mess" he had made of his life and freely admitted he was a hopeless alcoholic. Needing money while trying to complete *A Death in the Family,* he worked on a film script about Colonial Williamsburg and sought out similar work. But to the last he was "incapable of moderation" as Mia told Agee's biographer Mark A. Doty, and his motto was "a little bit too much is just enough for me."

On the morning of 16 May 1955 he took a taxicab to keep an appointment with his doctor, Arthur Sutherland. On the way he suffered chest pains, the worst angina he had ever experienced. As he lost consciousness the cabbie, never identified, raced him to Roosevelt Hospital, where he was found dead on arrival. Father Flye flew in from Kansas and concluded a funeral service at St. Luke's Chapel in New York. The same afternoon Flye and several others drove with the casket two hundred miles north to Hillsdale, New York, where, a hundred yards from Agee's farmhouse, he was buried in a simple grave. He left no will or insurance policy; he had $450 in his bank account. *See* Laurence Bergreen (1984).

Allen, Gracie (1906-1964)

She was only five feet tall and weighed a hundred pounds, but her energy was boundless and she was the chief talent in one of the century's greatest comedy twosomes. Her husband and partner George Burns wrote, "for forty years my act consisted of only one joke. And then she died." Her greatest wish was to wear a strapless evening gown, but after she pulled a pot of scalding tea over herself when eighteen months old her left shoulder and arm were "terribly scarred" and amputation was threatened; thereafter she wore only long sleeves. A second childhood accident with a broken storm lamp threw glass shards into her eye, after which one eye was blue, the other green. And she suffered lifelong migraine headaches.

Her long career in vaudeville, radio, and television ended in 1958 when, after years of delay for George's sake, she finally retired. For several years she had experienced mild angina attacks, or "episodes," as she preferred to call them. The first was in the early 1950s during a railroad trip; "Nattie," she whispered from the lower berth, "I have pains in my chest." (His real name is Nathan Birnbaum; he called her "Googie.") Thereafter she depended on nitroglycerin tablets; she would place one under her tongue and George would hold her until the pains were gone.

In retirement matters went along happily for a few years, but in 1961 a serious "episode" of angina sent her to the hospital and from then on she hired a nurse companion, Claribel Crewell. She could still leave her house and go shopping with Claribel or out to lunch at the Beverly Hills Hotel, but she had to pace herself carefully. Very gradually her condition worsened; often Burns would lie awake listening to her breathing. But she never fussed; if she could not greet guests with her usual cheerfulness, she stayed in her room.

On the evening of 27 August 1964, Burns was downstairs working on a script. Gracie was in bed, watching an old Spencer Tracy movie, when she called him, complaining of breathing difficulties. "I'll be okay; just give me a pill." But the pill didn't help. As he held her the pain increased and she started sweating. The doctor was called and he phoned for an ambulance. As she was laid on a stretcher, she apologized: "I'm sorry, boys, I'm all wet." At Cedars of Lebanon Hospital, Burns waited anxiously for a short time with their two adopted children, Sandy and Ronnie, and two friends. When the doctor returned, he said simply, "I'm sorry, George. Gracie's gone. We couldn't save her."

There were thirteen hundred at the funeral; Burns was on the verge of collapse and Jack Benny broke down twice while reading a eulogy in the Church of the Recessional at Forest Lawn in Glendale, California. Though a Catholic, Gracie's service was Episcopalian. A family friend explained to the press: "George wants to be buried with Gracie. Since he is Jewish, he cannot be buried in Catholic consecrated ground. So he figures that Episcopal rites would be . . . the closest thing to a Catholic ceremony." Well into his nineties, Burns still went regularly to Gracie's tomb to talk to his "Googie." *See* George Burns, *Gracie: A Love Story* (1988).

Amundsen, Roald (1872-1928)

The Norwegian explorer's greatest achievement, the discovery of the South Pole in December 1911, was dimmed, at least in British eyes, by the deaths of Captain R. F. Scott and his homeward-bound party, who were beaten to the target by only thirty-four days. In 1926, he flew over the North Pole with Umberto Nobile, in the dirigible *Norge*. Though he quarreled with the Italian later, it was in a search for him that he lost his life. Determined to be the first to reach the doomed Nobile, whose dirigible *Italia* had crashed on an ice floe in Arctic waters, he set off with two companions in an overloaded Latham 47 seaplane from Tromsø, Norway, on 18 June 1928. Months later a fuel tank and float were found; they showed clear signs of having been used as life rafts.

Anastasia (1901-1984)

The mystery woman who may well have been the youngest of the four daughters of the assassinated Tsar Nicholas II married a former professor of the University of Virginia, John E. Manahan, in 1968. They lived on University Circle in Charlottesville, Virginia, during her remaining years. In 1977 a prominent West German forensic specialist, Dr. Moritz Furtmayr, bolstered her claim to be a Russian grand duchess when, working from photographs of the tsar's daughter and Mrs. Manahan and comparing details of ear convolutions, he found seventeen points of agreement (he had much earlier found good facial and cranial matches). But by then her claims had long since been dismissed by courts in Hamburg as unproven, and anyway, she would say, "What does it matter?"

She had a puzzling and well-established predilection for living in squalor; beginning in 1978 the Charlottesville authorities repeatedly hauled the Manahans into court and ordered them to clean up the house and yard. "We haven't used a vacuum in six years," said Jack, "and now it's too late." Though nineteen years younger than his wife, he found her, increasingly lame and disoriented, difficult to care for.

When she celebrated her putative eightieth birthday on 18 June 1981 on her front lawn, surrounded by seventy-five guests, she announced that her longtime champion Prince Frederick Ernest of Saxe-Altenburg, who had rescued her from East Germany in 1946, had sent greetings. In 1983 a court-appointed guardian, William C. Preston, sent in nurses to take care of her, but the Manahans would hide or escape to their farm at Scottsville, twenty miles to the south. In November 1983 Anastasia was brought to the psychiatric ward of Blue Ridge Hospital, but on the twenty-ninth Dr. Manahan made off with her and for three days police in thirteen states were put on the alert. Tracked down by gun-toting officers near Amherst, Virginia, she was entrusted to a small adult-care facility in Charlottesville. There, she began to fail rapidly and may have suffered a stroke two months later. Her husband was with her when she died peacefully on 12 February 1984. Her body was cremated the same afternoon. Her ashes, in accordance with her wishes, were returned to Castle Seeon, ancestral home of the dukes of Leuchtenberg in Bavaria, where she had spent many months as an honored guest in 1927. *See* "Afterword" (1986) in Peter Kurth, *Anastasia* (1983, 1986).

Anderson, Sherwood (1876-1941)

At the end of February 1941, the U.S. writer set off with his fourth wife Eleanor on a South American goodwill trip sponsored by the State Department. He was unaware that he had swallowed a toothpick fragment at a farewell cocktail party. He fell ill with peritonitis on 2 March, the third day out, and the ship, the *Santa Lucia*, was met by an ambulance at Cristóbal. For a man who succumbed to a punctured intestine, the location of the military hospital where he died on 8 March 1941 was fitting: Colón in the Panama Canal Zone. He is buried in the hilltop cemetery at Marion, Virginia. *See* J. Schevill (1951).

Armstrong, Louis (1900-1971)

For over half a century "Satchmo" Armstrong dominated the American jazz scene with his powerful lungs, his gravelly voice, and his golden trumpet. He was in hospital often in his last years and for his final engagement, at the Empire Room in New York's Waldorf-Astoria Hotel in March 1971, he had to be helped onto the stage. On the fifteenth he suffered a heart attack and spent several weeks in Beth Israel Hospital. Back home in his modest house on 107th Street in the Corona District of Queens, New York, with his fourth wife Lucille, he planned late summer appearances "as soon as my treaders get in as good shape as my chops."

Early on 6 July 1971 he suddenly succumbed to a heart attack in his sleep. Thousands viewed the open casket in Corona and later in Manhattan, and observed the worn spot on his upper lip produced by decades of trumpet playing. The funeral service at the Corona Congregational Church was attended by many dignitaries, including Governor Rockefeller and the mayors of New York and his native city, New Orleans. He was buried in Flushing Cemetery, New York.

Arnold, Benedict (1741-1801)

The most notorious traitor of the American Revolution had earlier been a national hero. He had been wounded in the left leg during the assault on Quebec in 1775 and led his forces to victory against the British in the second battle of Saratoga, turning point of the Revolutionary War. But in 1779, already affronted by what he saw as a lack of recognition of his military exploits, he reacted angrily to an investigation into his financial dealings. Shortly after his marriage in April of that year to the daughter of Loyalist parents he made secret overtures to the enemy. His planned betrayal of the West Point Military Academy led to the capture and execution of John André. His treachery won him £6,000, and the rank of British cavalry colonel.

Crippled by gout and dropsy in his last years in London, he called just before his death for his Continental major-general's uniform, complete with the sword knots and epaulets General Washington had given him. "Let me die in my old uniform," he gasped with difficulty, for asthma also afflicted him. "God forgive me for ever putting on any other." He died at 6:30 A.M. on 14 June 1801; one of the mourners who followed his coffin to St. Mary's Church in Battersea on the south bank of the Thames was Lord Cornwallis. "If you are ever captured by your old comrades," he had once been warned by a prisoner of the British, "your left leg will be given a military burial and the rest of you summarily hanged." His only monument, at Saratoga, New York, depicts the image of a left leg in a Colonial boot surmounted by a laurel wreath; it bears no name.

Astaire, Fred (1899-1987)

George Balanchine once called him "the greatest dancer in the world." His first movie musical was *Dancing Lady* (in 1933 with Joan Crawford); his last major appearance was in *That's Entertainment Part II* (1976), which he cohosted with Gene Kelly. In ten of his more than thirty musicals his partner was Ginger Rogers.

In his eighties Astaire continued his lifelong abstemious lifestyle, eating lightly and drinking rarely and maintaining his dapper frame at 135 pounds. His first wife Phyllis died of lung cancer in September 1954, just as he began work on *Daddy Long Legs,* and another marriage always seemed out of the question. But in 1980 he met the young jockey Robyn Smith at Blue Valley Ranch, his horse-breeding farm in the San Fernando Valley; going against the strongly expressed wishes of his family, including his sister and first dancing partner Adele, the couple were married on 24 June. He was eighty-one, she was thirty-seven, but they were a devoted pair. Concerned with her safety, he begged her to quit the saddle and she reluctantly agreed. "I loved riding," she said. "But I loved Fred more. And I couldn't have both." They visited Adele at Christmas 1981, a month before she died of a stroke.

Because his lingering cold worried her, Robyn had Fred admitted to Century City Hospital, Los Angeles, on 12 June 1987 under an assumed name, Fred Giles. Tests indicated pneumonia. On 22 June 1987 he died in his wife's arms. Though the family declined to reveal the location of his grave, a mourner said he was buried next to Phyllis and Adele.

Auden, Wystan Hugh (1907-1973)

The British-born poet became a U.S. citizen in 1946 and lived on New York's Lower East Side for twenty-two years. Yet, spending his last year in an Oxford cottage, he found that city noisier than his former home—and it was in England that he was robbed for the first time.

On the evening of 28 September 1973 the sixty-six-year-old poet gave a reading in Vienna to the Austrian Literary Society and afterward, complaining of tiredness, was driven back to his hotel, the Altenburgerhof on Walfischgasse. Next morning his companion (since 1939), Chester Kallman (1921–1975), knocked on his bedroom door and received no response. The management were summoned to gain entry and Auden was found to have been dead for several hours. "He was lying on the wrong side," Kallman reported. "He never lay on his left side; he thought it was bad for his heart. He was cold when I touched him."

His last poem was a haiku: "He still loves life / But O O O O how he wishes / The good Lord would take him." It was written at the summer home the two men shared in the Austrian village of Kirchstetten. After Kallman objected to the death wish, Auden seems to have discarded the manuscript; at any rate, it has never been found and existed only in his friend's memory.

W. H. Auden, an Anglican, was buried at the Catholic church in Kirchstetten by priests of the two faiths reciting words of the service alternately in English and German. His will left everything to Kallman. A year later a memorial stone was laid for him in Westminster Abbey's Poets' Corner. *See* Humphrey Carpenter (1981).

Balanchine, George (1904-1983)

The Soviet-American choreographer came to the United States in 1933 and cofounded the New York City Ballet in 1948. He had good health until the late 1970s, when severe angina led to coronary bypass surgery in 1980. The first sign of his fatal malady was an almost imperceptible one: early in 1982 he found himself unable to demonstrate a pirouette to the right while standing on the left foot without losing his balance. The neurological disability quickly worsened, but doctors were unable to reach a conclusive diagnosis, merely agreeing that there was degeneration of the cerebellum, the portion of the brain where the sense of balance is located. By November 1982 Balanchine was profoundly confused and falling frequently at his Manhattan home, despite around-the-clock care, and he was admitted to Roosevelt Hospital for observation. He never left the hospital; quickly his legs and then his hands lost their powers and his memory quite failed him. He would talk Russian when American friends visited him. At last he had difficulty swallowing and this led to his death from pneumonia on 30 April 1983.

Microscopic study of Balanchine's brain, slice by slice, showed that the number of nerve cells was greatly reduced. Astrocytes, star-shaped support cells that help in brain repair, were increased in size and number, evidence of some kind of injury. The really telltale signs were the spongy state of the brain, which displayed numerous empty spaces, and, most significant of all, pink circles with threadlike projections called kuru plaques.

Kuru is one of the "slow infections," so called because of their very lengthy incubation periods. Some of these infections are caused by viruses, but kuru is suspected of being transmitted by mysterious particles that, unlike all other forms of life, including viruses, appear to contain no nucleic acids (DNA or RNA) and therefore must reproduce by a totally different method, so far unelucidated. They are proteinaceous infectious particles, dubbed (because life is short) "prions." Prions cause four neurological diseases in animals, including scrapie in sheep and goats, and three in humans. One of the latter is kuru; another is Creutzfeldt-Jakob Syndrome, named for the physicians who, separately, first described it in 1920–21. It is this disease that was finally diagnosed as causing Balanchine's death. How he contracted it is unknown. It is rare, with perhaps two hundred cases each year reported in the United States. Prions are resistant to some conventional methods used for sterilizing surgical instruments, and this is one possible source. The suggestion has even been made that Balanchine was infected by "rejuvenating" animal extracts with which he was injected many years earlier.

Even if the correct diagnosis had been reached during Balanchine's lifetime, nothing could have been done to save him. There is no known cure for the Creutzfeldt-Jakob Syndrome.

The great ballet master was honored at crowded services in New York's small Russian Orthodox cathedral. He was buried in Sag Harbor, a small town on Long Island whose attractions he had only recently discovered.

Balanchine's will left most of his estate to Barbara Horgan, his longtime personal assistant, and Karin von Aroldingen Gerwitz, a principal dancer at the City Ballet who, with her husband, had been the dead man's closest friends.

Belushi, John (1949-1982)

The Chicago-born comedian and mimic, star of NBC Television's *Saturday Night Live,* broke into movies with the tremendously successful *National Lampoon's Animal House* (1978). But later films were not such big money-makers, and his manager was gently insistent that Belushi come to terms with Paramount's president, Michael D. Eisner, to make *The Joy of Sex* rather than the star's own rewrite of a romantic comedy titled *Sweet Deception.* The new script, titled *Noble Rot,* was hopelessly bad, too-evidently conceived in a drug-crazed atmosphere.

Belushi, in February 1982, was in the midst of one of his periodic "binges": a snort of cocaine to bring him up, Quaaludes to bring him down, help him sleep. His wife Judy in New York was increasingly worried. He was spending around $50,000 a month, much of it on drugs. When sober he was bright, talented, enormously energetic; at other times he was sloppy, undisciplined, unreliable—just a "big kid." He needed a "lift" to perform properly, he would say when he went so far as to admit to a "habit." Judy looked back on it later as peer pressure, "to be *that* for people . . . He would refuse and they would say 'come on' . . . like he was letting them down." She called John's former "antidrug enforcer," Richard "Smokey" Wendell on 4 March, asking him to fly to Los Angeles, where her husband had returned for meetings four days earlier. By now she was desperate enough to have him committed, threaten divorce. His partner Dan Aykroyd was also prepared to fly to the rescue: "We'll handcuff him if necessary."

Immediately upon arrival in Hollywood, Belushi sought out Cathy Smith, a thirty-five-year-old heroin addict and drug supplier. She "shot him up" with a "speedball," a mixture of cocaine and heroin, and he enjoyed the new experience. Next day he wandered around with Smith and a writer friend, Nelson Lyon, being shot up several times; on 3 March he slept for nearly twenty-four hours; the fourth was a repetition of the second. In the early hours of 5 March, Smith drove Belushi to his place, Bungalow No. 3 at the Chateau Malmont Hotel on Sunset Boulevard at Monteel. Two actor friends dropped by: the comedian Robin Williams, who was discomfited by Smith's "crusty," frightening appearance; and Robert De Niro. They left; so did Lyon, leaving Belushi alone with Smith. Belushi felt cold and turned up the heat. Smith mixed a speedball for each of them ("half a tenth each of cocaine and heroin"). Belushi showered and went to bed; she tucked him in and turned the heat up further. He slept; she wrote a letter to a friend. Belushi coughed and wheezed; his lungs were congested, he said. She gave him a glass of water. "Don't leave," he begged—perhaps his last words. When she drove off in his car at 10:15 A.M. he was snoring loudly.

Bull "Superfoot" Wallace, a karate champion who acted as Belushi's trainer and bodyguard, had been out of town. He called at the bungalow around noon and found the place hot, dry, and eerily silent. Belushi was under the covers on his right side in a fetal position with his head under a pillow; his tongue was halfway out, his lips were purple. "John, time to get up," said Wallace, shaking his shoulder. Shocked, he flipped the body onto its back and began mouth-to-mouth resuscitation: No response. "Oh, you dumb son of a bitch," he wailed, over and over again.

Paramedics pronounced thirty-three-year-old, 222-pound John Belushi dead at 12:45 P.M., 5 March 1982. The postmortem found the brain swollen, the heart enlarged; there was more than enough cocaine and heroin present to account for respiratory failure. The funeral procession, at Abel's Hill Cemetery on Martha's Vineyard, Massachusetts, was led by Aykroyd on a motorcycle. In May 1983, because fans were desecrating the grave and Judy feared the body would be dug up, she had it reinterred at an unmarked location eleven feet to the north. During the secret operation the original wooden coffin collapsed and a new copper casket was employed. As a further deception, the original gravestone, a large boulder bearing the name BELUSHI, was moved well away, to a spot near the cemetery gate.

Cathy Evelyn Smith was questioned by police and released; hardly able to believe her good luck, she fled to her native Ontario. There, in return for $15,000, she gave an interview to the *National Enquirer*, admitting, "I killed John Belushi." A full investigation followed. After fighting extradition she returned to Los Angeles in 1985. She pleaded "no contest" to involuntary manslaughter and in September 1986 was sentenced to three years in prison. *See* Bob Woodward, *Wired* (1984).

Berg, Alban (1885-1935)

The Austrian composer, who developed Arnold Schoenberg's twelve-tone technique, was singularly prone to abscesses, as well as to asthma, jaundice, muscular pains, and splitting headaches. The unfortunate man also seemed to attract the attention of insects. He was set upon by a swarm of wasps in 1932, and it was to an insect bite or sting in August 1935 that he attributed his fatal carbuncle of the lower back. However, the presence of another carbuncle on the left foot suggests a recurrence of the general staphylococcal infection he had experienced more than once before.

Berg's final year was taken up largely with his *Violin Concerto* and the opera *Lulu* (in which a prostitute is murdered by Jack the Ripper), left unfinished at his death. He was able to attend symphonic excerpts from the opera—the so-called *Lulu Symphony*—in Vienna on 11 December 1935. On the sixteenth his pain abruptly ceased: the lumbar abscess had evidently burst internally. As he was taken to Rudolf Hospital, Vienna, he quipped that he was halfway to the cemetery already. In two operations surgeons failed to discover the septic focus. A blood transfusion produced only temporary improvement. Berg, on being introduced to the donor, a local youth, joked that maybe he would now write light Viennese operettas. By the twenty-second his heart was affected. The number 23 had always been a fateful one for him. Next morning, therefore, he announced that this would be a decisive day. In his last hours his thoughts were of *Lulu,* and he made conducting gestures, calling more than once for "an up-beat." He died at 1:15 A.M., 24 December 1935, succumbing, like Gustav Mahler (q.v.) to septicemia. It was Mahler's daughter Anna ("Gucki") who prepared Berg's death mask. He was buried in Hietzing Cemetery, Vienna.

Bergman, Ingrid (1915-1982)

The Swedish actress won an Academy Award for *Gaslight* (1944). For many years she was shunned by Hollywood after she deserted her husband Dr. Petter Lindstrom and their daughter Pia and settled in Rome with the Italian director Roberto Rossellini. The birth of their son in February 1950 produced worldwide headlines. Bergman later married Rossellini and had twin girls; she and the director were divorced in 1958 and Ingrid married Lars Schmidt, a Swedish theatrical producer. Bergman's second Oscar—for *Anastasia* (1956)—marked her return to the United States; her third was a supporting actress award for her cameo role in *Murder on the Orient Express* (1974).

In November 1973 she was acting in a London West End revival of Somerset Maugham's *The Constant Wife*. After a performance later that month she was lying in bed in her Mount Street apartment, leafing through a magazine, when she came upon an article about breast cancer. While conducting a self-examination with her fingers, she discovered a small lump under her left breast. She was persuaded to see a doctor, but despite his urging she put off essential surgery for more than six months, until the play's run and her work on *Orient Express* were over and she had made inessential trips to New York and Europe. At last, on 11 June 1974 she entered the London Clinic; the tumor was malignant and the breast was removed.

Ingrid Bergman's final theatrical film was Ingmar Bergman's *Autumn Sonata* (1978), in which she plays Liv Ullmann's anguished mother. The Ingrid-Ingmar relationship during the forty days of filming in Norway was tense and demanding on both sides. "The first days were terrible," recalled the director. "She went to a limit and objected to go beyond the limit. I had to take her with me by the hand and by violence. We were fighting all the time . . . " The original shooting schedule was cut by three weeks to allow Ingrid to return to London for further surgery; swollen lymph glands had produced an egg-sized lump under her arm that needed to be excised. By now, Schmidt was an absentee husband, engaged in a separate relationship, and Ingrid had turned for support to a new friend, Griffith James, a Britisher. While acting in a revival of N. C. Hunter's *Waters of the Moon* at the Haymarket Theatre she had daily radiation treatment at the Middlesex Hospital. At the end of the play's run in July 1978 she felt a pain in her remaining breast; it too harbored a cancerous tumor, and it was removed at the Harley Street Clinic. She spent much of her time now in the town house she had bought at No. 9 Cheyne Walk in the arty, upscale district of Chelsea, near the Thames in southwest London. But she toured the United States and Europe in 1980 to promote her autobiography, *My Story,* and late in the year was with difficulty persuaded to tackle the role of the late Israeli leader Golda Meir in a television movie. During the filming in Israel a year later Ingrid was quickly fatigued by the unusually warm October weather; besides, removal of lymph glands during the second mastectomy had led to a chronically swollen right arm. For a crucial close-up of her hands she spent the previous night with the arm strapped above her head and had the scene shot first thing next morning.

Back in London, the British cook-masseuse Margaret Johnstone, who had accompanied the actress to Tel Aviv, stayed with her as a resident helper. Bergman spent five separate weeks in St. Thomas's Hospital undergoing chemotherapy. In June 1982 she was able to fly on the Concorde to New York for the thirtieth birthday of her twins, Isabella and Isotta, and to visit Pia. By now a painful back was added to her other problems, but, lonely after her return to London, she longed to see again Lars Schmidt's tiny island of Danholmen, off the village of Fjällbacka, eighty miles north of Göteborg on Sweden's Atlantic coast. Though they were now divorced they were still friends, and Schmidt kept a bedroom at his island home full of her things. She enjoyed her stay there and was able to say good-bye to friends in her native Stockholm before flying back to England on 23 August. "I'm not afraid to die," she told them. "I've had a rich life; I am content."

On Sunday, 29 August 1982, Ingrid Bergman's sixty-seventh birthday, her cousin Britt Bergman, Lars Schmidt, Griff James, and Margaret Johnstone gathered at her bedside to toast her in champagne and brushed her lips with a glass of it. Then they left quickly. The previous morning, as she stepped out of the bathtub, she felt a terrible pain in her spine; the cancer had collapsed her twelfth thoracic [or dorsal] vertebra. Now, under the merciful influence of diamorphine, she was only half-conscious. One lung was out of action and the other barely functioning.

At 3:30 A.M. on the thirtieth, Britt in the next room could no longer hear her cousin's breathing. She went in and peered anxiously at Ingrid's face; there were tiny beads of blood on her dead lips.

Twelve hundred attended her memorial service in Trafalgar Square at the Church of St.-Martin-in-the-Fields. A violin evoked Bergman's role in the movie *Casablanca* (1943) by playing "As Time Goes By." In June 1983, Isotta Rossellini and Lars Schmidt rowed out from Danholmen and scattered Ingrid's ashes into the waters of the Skagerrak. *See* Laurence Leamer (1986).

Berlin, Irving (1888-1989)

The Russian-born U.S. songwriter produced both the lyrics and the music for some fifteen hundred songs, of which twenty-five reached the very top of the charts. One of them, "God Bless America" (donated to the Boy Scouts of America), has become the unofficial national anthem; another, "White Christmas," is the most popular song of all time, having even by the mid-1960s sold 40 million recordings and 5.5 million copies of the printed version. Yet the songwriter never learned to read music and, of course, could not write down his own compositions; instead, he dictated them to his musical secretary, Helmy Kresa.

Berlin's last visit to the theater was with his second wife Ellin in 1970 to see the hit play *Sleuth*. In his eighties his insecurities grew. Always jealous of his reputation, by now he would make abusive phone calls to anyone he feared might jeopardize it. There was a call, for example, to the sixty-four-year-old musicologist James T. Maher, coauthor of *American Popular Song,* due for publication by Oxford University Press. Berlin had been sent the eighty-page section dealing with himself, which was, in fact, a very laudatory account of his work. Yet the octogenarian, beginning loudly with "Who the hell do you bastards think you are?" worked himself into a hysterical rage with a nonstop stream of profanity that left Maher white and shaking.

Apart from his ceaseless use of the telephone to call enemies and friends, especially fellow songwriter Harold Arlen—like himself a Sunday painter and the son of a cantor—he did little in his final years except for his daily walk and much television watching. He kept a sharp eye on his copyrights, refusing to sell any of them outright and placing strict limits on their use. He avoided agents and made all deals himself.

Gradually he withdrew from the public gaze; he was never seen, except occasionally while taking a walk, escorted by a bodyguard near his town house in New York's Beekman Place. Most of his neighbors were unaware of his identity; the few who recognized him were ignored. He would chase away any children who came near him. One woman was known to cross the street whenever the diminutive, forbidding figure approached.

On Christmas Eve 1983, a very cold night in Manhattan, a nodding acquaintance and admirer of Berlin's, John Wallowich, collected some friends to sing "White Christmas" and "Always" outside his Beekman Place home; they were astonished when invited in afterward to be thanked and hugged. It was Berlin's last appearance before the public.

Though Berlin was known to boast on the phone that "my health is perfect—from the neck up," his eyesight was failing. The deaths of Arlen in 1986 and of his favorite performer Fred Astaire a few months later greatly depressed him. By now his household routine was invariable. He dined with Ellin at 5:00; she would dress appropriately and "fix the left side of my hair because Irving sits to the left of me at dinner, and it is the only side he will see." His cardiologist called every week, his barber every month.

The songwriter reluctantly agreed to a televised celebration of his centenary in May 1988 at Carnegie Hall, but refused to cooperate, refused to appear, refused to comment on it, refused even to watch it at home.

Three months later, Ellin Mackay Berlin died, after a series of strokes, aged eighty-five; her desolated husband, unprepared to attract publicity, stayed away from her funeral service in St. Patrick's Cathedral, where the blessing and a short tribute were given by John Cardinal O'Connor.

At last even the telephone was silent as Berlin, without the essential support of his wife, went rapidly downhill. By mid-1989 he needed around-the-clock nursing care. When he died at last, quietly on the afternoon of 22 September 1989, he was 101 years and four months old. "He just fell asleep," said his son-in-law, Alton Peters.

The funeral was very private. The family attended a short service at the Frank E. Campbell Chapel in Manhattan. Only his three daughters and a few employees of his publishing corporation were present at Woodlawn Cemetery in the Bronx, New York, for the burial service, conducted by a Reform rabbi, Daniel Wolk, as Irving Berlin was interred beside his first wife Dorothy, who had died way back in 1913 after only five months of marriage. *See* Laurence Bergreen (1990).

Bernstein, Leonard (1918–1990)

The U.S. musician's gifts were protean, encompassing, as a composer, three symphonies, Broadway musicals (including *West Side Story*), ballet, and opera; he was also a world-renowned conductor, music publicist, and author. He sprang into the limelight when he took over the New York Philharmonic at short notice after Bruno Walter fell ill. "Typical Lenny luck," said some envious colleagues; but he had given luck a helping hand: when he heard Walter was ailing, he paid extra attention to the scores for the concert. (He was to become music director of the orchestra, 1959–69.)

Bernstein's early career was jeopardized by rumors of homosexuality (only publicly disclosed in Joan Peyser's 1987 biography) and by his sympathy for radical causes (he once threw a party for the Black Panthers). His marriage to Chilean-born Felicia Montealegre Cohn in 1951 stabilized his life and enhanced his reputation; they separated in 1976 and she died in 1978.

Bernstein's health was threatened by heavy cigarette smoking. At a memorial service for the lyricist Alan Jay Lerner in 1986, Bernstein admirers confronted him with signs: "We love you—stop smoking." An orchestral official commented, during the maestro's final, painful months, "Lenny is the only conductor I have ever seen who simultaneously gasps into a respirator and lights up a cigarette the minute he comes off the stage."

During the first months of 1990, he was forced to cancel several engagements in the United States and Japan. He conducted for the last time on 19 August at Tanglewood, Massachusetts, when he led the Boston Symphony Orchestra in Britten's *Four Sea Interludes* and Beethoven's *Seventh Symphony*. In the third movement of the symphony he began coughing into a handkerchief, and at the end left the stage obviously exhausted, with a look of agony in his eyes. A European tour was immediately canceled.

Bernstein withdrew to his spacious apartment in The Dakota on Manhattan's Upper West Side (where John Lennon had lived) and was said to have turned his attention to the composition of new works. But longstanding emphysema and bronchial problems worsened. His permanent retirement was announced just five days before his death; a pleural tumor had added to the strain on his heart.

Adamant in his refusal to go to a hospital, he was cared for at home by Dr. Kenneth M. Cahill and his three assistants. Though hooked to an oxygen supply and breathing with great effort, his hopes ran high to the end, with ideas about a chamber composition, a musical and the writing of his memoirs. Just two hours before his death on 14 October 1990 he was watching a concert on television and humming along with a Rachmaninoff concerto. A visitor said of him, "He looked himself. . . . He was lucid, even witty. I was happy for him at that moment." His secretary had warned the visitor, the thirty-four-year-old Chinese composer Bright Sheng, not to be shocked by the invalid's appearance, but "I thought he looked very well." Only once did Bernstein refer to his illness, when he told Sheng, "All of a sudden the body is giving up." It gave up, finally, at 6:15 P.M. with a severe heart attack.

A memorial concert was staged at Carnegie Hall on 14 November 1990. Most of his multimillion-dollar estate was left in equal shares to his three children.

Bettelheim, Bruno (1903-1990)

The U.S. psychoanalyst during his lifetime was viewed as a pioneer in the treatment of autistic and other "problem" children. Born in Vienna, he spent over a year in Nazi concentration camps at Buchenwald and Dachau and gained insight into the behavior of human beings under extreme stress. His views could arouse bitter criticism, as when he referred, especially after his retirement, to the "ghetto mentality" which, he charged, led many of his fellow Jews to placate their oppressors instead of fighting back.

For thirty years he headed the Sonia Shankman Orthogenic School for disturbed children at the University of Chicago. In several books he preached the need for a stable, loving environment in which youngsters could be treated with respect. All the more startling was it that, after his death, former students at the school came forward with tales of gross cruelty and humiliation perpetrated by Bettelheim over many years, not sporadically but as a deliberate policy (A news magazine carried the headline: BENO BRUTALHEIM?) One of his most admired books, *The Uses of Enchantment: The Meaning and Importance of Fairy Tales* (1976), was attacked by the folklorist Alan Dundes in 1991 for its errors and plagiarism.

Bettelheim's wife Gertrud died in 1984, and three years later a stroke put an end to further writing. Until six weeks before his death he lived near his elder daughter Ruth, a clinical psychologist, in a well-appointed apartment overlooking the ocean in Santa Monica, California. Often in pain and feeling useless, he would ask visiting friends why he shouldn't emulate Socrates and drink hemlock.

After becoming estranged from Ruth he moved to a retirement home, Charter House, in Silver Springs, Maryland, to be near his other daughter, Naomi, but he was disappointed by the change and felt restricted there. The current director of the Orthogenic School, Jacquelyn Sanders, was the last colleague to talk to him. On the eve of his suicide she called to ask whether she could see him in Washington the following week. His reply: "It depends on what shape I'm in."

Next day, 13 March 1990, Bettelheim scribbled a note, the contents of which were not disclosed, and swallowed an overdose of barbiturates; then he pulled a plastic bag over his head and shortly expired.

Biko, Steven (1947-1977)

The South African leader, who preached the nonviolent gospel of black consciousness, was arrested near Grahamstown in the Eastern Cape Province for being outside the small area to which he was confined. He died 12 September 1977 while in police custody, the twentieth black in eighteen months to do so. During his final twenty-two hours of questioning at Port Elizabeth, naked and in chains, he sustained extensive brain injuries. He was taken, unconscious, not to the hospital but, scantily clad, 750 miles north by station wagon to the Central Prison in Pretoria, where he died alone in a cell a few hours later. He was buried near his home in King William's Town.

After an inquest, magistrate Marthinus Prins ruled that Biko died in a scuffle with security police and that "the death cannot be attributed to any act or omission amounting to a criminal offense on the part of any person." He added no word of censure. In 1985 two prison doctors who authorized Biko's transfer from Port Elizabeth were reprimanded but the torture and beating of prisoners there continued unchecked.

Billy the Kid (1859-1881)

Henry McCarty, alias William H. Bonney, alias Billy the Kid, infamous young outlaw of New Mexico's Lincoln County cattle war, was captured and tried in March 1881 for the murder of one Andrew L. "Buckshot" Roberts. He was acquitted on this charge but was found guilty of killing Sheriff William Brady of Lincoln County. Sentenced to hang in Lincoln on 13 May, he was escorted there from the trial venue at Mesilla and held under guard by Sheriff Pat F. Garrett in the newly acquired county headquarters building.

Garrett was out of town on 28 April and the less dangerous prisoners were across the street at the Wortley Hotel under guard having supper when the Kid escaped. According to Garrett's account, Billy asked the remaining guard, James W. Bell, to be taken down to the privy in the rear of the building. Running rapidly ahead as they returned to the second floor, the prisoner forced the door of the armory, grabbed a six-shooter and fired at the fleeing Bell, killing him with a ricocheting bullet before he could reach the back gate. The other guard, Deputy Marshal Robert Olinger, heard the shots and raced across the street, only to be gunned down by his own breechloader, containing thirty-six buckshot in the two barrels, which the outlaw found in Garrett's office.

Billy escaped on horseback and was at large for over two months. Garrett heard scattered reports of his being seen in and around Fort Sumner, a hundred miles to the northeast, and early in July he left Lincoln surreptitiously with two deputies. They spotted the fugitive after dark on the fourteenth without recognizing him. He was in a group talking Spanish near a cluster of converted military housing on the northern edge of Fort Sumner, and seems to have been hiding out with a Mexican family. That Garrett knew more than he admitted in his account about the wanted man's whereabouts is clear, otherwise it is difficult to explain how he came to be in Pedro "Pete" Maxwell's bedroom when the final scene took place.

Maxwell lived in one of the converted buildings, and it was close to midnight when Garrett crept into the darkened room and sat near the head of the bed where Pete was lying in the dark. "Where is the Kid?" he asked. "He's been around," said Maxwell. Just then a barefooted man sprang quietly into the room and called out in Spanish, "Who comes there?" The sheriff was silent, knowing full well that "the sound of my voice (which he knew perfectly well), would have been his signal to make a target of my physical personality, with his self-cocker."

"Who is it, Pete?" whispered Garrett. The newcomer crept forward, leaned on the bed, "his right hand almost touching my knees" as Garrett wrote later, and—referring to the sheriff's deputies, whom he'd seen near the house—"Who are they, Pete?" At the same moment Maxwell whispered to Garrett, "That's him!" Sensing the presence of a stranger beside Maxwell, the intruder raised his pistol and retreated rapidly. The sheriff drew his revolver and fired twice. Billy the Kid dropped dead with a strangled sound; the second bullet had missed, but the first hit him just above the heart.

The outlaw, just twenty-one years old, was laid to rest next day in the military cemetery beside the Rio Pecos, seven miles southeast of Fort Sumner. *See* Pat F. Garrett (1882, 1954)

Blitzstein, Marc (1905-1964)

The U.S. composer, a pioneer in the creation of indigenous American opera, made the headlines in 1937 with his antifascist, prolabor musical *The Cradle Will Rock* when it was produced, in the face of stiff opposition from unions and the government, by Orson Welles and John Houseman. He is also remembered for *Regina* (1949), his operatic version of Lillian Hellman's play *The Little Foxes,* and for his masterful American adaptation (1952) of Kurt Weill and Bertolt Brecht's *The Threepenny Opera.*

During the last year of his life, Blitzstein worked on *Sacco and Vanzetti,* based on the cause célèbre of the 1920s and funded by both New York's Metropolitan Opera and the Ford Foundation. In November 1963, unknown to anyone, he left the score behind in the trunk of his Peugeot at a friend's house in New Rochelle, New York, before flying to Martinique for the winter. There, on the West Indies island, he worked on two one-act operas based on stories by Bernard Malamud. He rented a three-bedroom house near Frégate-François, across the island from the capital, Fort-de-France, and soon made friends with an American couple living nearby. Applying himself mainly to one of the short operas, *The Magic Barrel,* he was able to describe himself, in a letter to his sister Josephine, as "healthy-looking enough, if skinny." A 1947 Veterans Administration report had characterized him as a "rather detached withdrawn individual with marked depressive features" and suffering "marked inhibitions in his inner personal contacts with some suicidal preoccupation"; physically, he had needed repeated surgery for a hernia and suffered from a weakened liver, exacerbated, his biographer Eric A. Gordon believes, by excessive drinking.

The mystery that for many years surrounded the composer's death was resolved by Gordon's *Mark the Music* (1989). As he chronicles the events, the composer had dinner with his friends on 21 January 1964 and then drove alone to Fort-de-France, where he visited the waterfront taverns. "He fell in with two Portuguese [from Madeira] and a native Martiniquan," writes Gordon, "and together they toured several of the low-class dives around the Place de Stalingrad."

As they drank, Blitzstein fished for bills from his wallet, revealing the tidy sum he was carrying. After two or three hours, en route to the next bar, Blitzstein and one of his companions slipped into a nearby alleyway, the lure of sex in the air. The other two followed. Then suddenly, all three set upon him. They beat him severely, robbed him of his valuables, and left him there in the alley stripped of every piece of clothing but his shirt and socks. Hearing his cries and moans, policemen found him between three and four in the morning and took him to Clarac Hospital.

Later that morning, Blitzstein told a consular official his injuries were due to an auto accident, and his sister in Philadelphia was so informed by cable. That afternoon, looking gravely jaundiced and deeply embarrassed while retailing to his new friends the circumstances of the attack, he begged them to say nothing to the press. It was this, not the prospects for his recovery, that concerned him most. His condition worsened rapidly and around 8:00 P.M. that night, 22 January 1964, he died, "brought down," writes Gordon, "by the very type of men he had held so high."

The conductor Leonard Bernstein broke the news the following evening at a New York Philharmonic concert and dedicated a performance of Beethoven's *Eroica Symphony* to the dead man's memory. Blitzstein's ashes were buried without ceremony in a Germantown cemetery in suburban Philadelphia.

At a memorial concert in New York three months later, arias from the unfinished Malamud operas and from *Sacco and Vanzetti* were performed, and Bernstein announced that the manuscripts for the latter opera were missing. By that date the Peugeot had been taken to a used-car lot in Long Island City; the manager, who happened to read the announcement in a newspaper, found the score and turned it over to Bernstein, who was pressed on all sides to complete it, but declined. (It is still unfinished.) Of the two Malamud derived one-act operas, *Idiots First* was "almost complete," according to Bernstein. He announced to the press his intention to complete and orchestrate it; later he backed out and it was completed by Leonard J. Lehrman. It has been staged in two-piano versions and given an orchestrated concert reading, but no full production so far.

In March 1965, Armando Fernandez, 27, and Alfredo Rodriguez, 35, received three-year and fourteen-month prison sentences, respectively; the Martiniquan youth, Daniel Yves Charles Nicholas, 18, was given a suspended sentence and put on probation.

Borden, Lizzie (1860-1927)

Lizzie Andrew Borden was accused of murdering her hated stepmother Abby with twenty blows of an axe in the midmorning heat of 4 August 1892 and of dispatching her father Andrew with ten blows when he returned home to 92 Second Street, Fall River, Massachusetts, a little later. She was acquitted by a New Bedford jury who were never told, among other things, that she had tried to purchase cyanide in the days before the crime.

With her substantial inheritance she was able to buy a house, Maple-croft, on French Street in a better part of Fall River, and employ four servants. Once or twice a year, Lizbeth A. Borden, as she now called herself, would travel to Boston, New York, or Washington to enjoy a pleasant anonymity.

She failed to regain her health after surgery of an undisclosed nature in 1926 and died at Maplecroft 1 June 1927. Her few friends, invited to the house for the funeral, were astonished to learn that Lizzie had been interred the previous night after an unattended ceremony at the undertaker's. The black-draped coffin was surreptitiously taken to Oak Grove Cemetery, where men in dark clothing, unbetrayed by a single pale gleam, buried it in the family plot. The grave bears the single name LIZBETH; the family monument adds another subtle change: it reads LIZBETH ANDREWS BORDEN. *See* Victoria Lincoln (1967).

Bormann, Martin (1900-1945)

Adolf Hitler's right-hand man was last seen alive while trying to escape on foot across Berlin from encircling Soviet forces. Near the Lehrter railroad station on 2 May 1945, trapped by crossfire, the stocky Bormann and the tall Ludwig Stumpfegger, one of the Führer's physicians, crushed cyanide ampoules between their teeth and died on the spot. Under Russian direction, post office workers buried the decomposing, unidentified corpses in a plot of ground nearby.

In December 1972 a construction crew unearthed two skeletons, one short and one tall. Dr. Reidar F. Sognnaes, a forensic dental specialist at UCLA, who had just announced a conclusive identification of Hitler's remains, undertook a detailed comparison of the skulls with diagrams prepared by Hugo Blaschke, dentist to several top Nazis. The skull belonging to the shorter skeleton showed many points of agreement and no discrepancies; also, a healed collarbone fracture corresponded to a known riding accident of Bormann's. Sognnaes's findings on Hitler, Bormann, and Eva Braun were published in *Legal Medicine Annual, 1976*.

Bow, Clara (1905-1965)

During Hollywood's final silent decade, Clara Bow's saucer eyes and Cupid's-bow lips, her vivacious manner and sidelong "come-on" looks sent her to the top of the charts. Her role in *It* (1927) led to her nickname, the "It" girl, and in 1929 she was voted the most popular cinema actress. Despite an atrocious Brooklyn twang, she made an effortless transition to the "talkies," but in the early 1930s her star plummeted. Her reputation had survived numerous affairs with the biggest names in the business, Roland Gilbert, Gary Cooper, and Victor Fleming among them; but when she sued her former secretary Daisy De Voe for embezzlement and blackmail, court revelations of drink, gigolos, and drugs were too much and her public turned away.

She could have fought her way back, for she had an indomitable spirit, but her pitiable heredity doomed her to early invalidism. Before she escaped into films, her schizophrenic-epileptic mother chased her with a kitchen knife, called her a whore, and tried to slit her throat; her would-be killer, like her own mother before her, ended life in an asylum.

Sexual abuse by her father probably twisted all her future relations with men. Her marriage to cowboy-actor (and future Nevada lieutenant-governor) Rex Bell began hopefully, but her chronic insomnia and barbiturate dependency gradually undermined it. The two separated but remained fairly friendly until his death in 1962. After her diagnosis as a schizophrenic in 1949 she lived quietly at 12214 Aneta Street, Los Angeles, with a resident nurse. She finally won her battle with barbiturates but never with insomnia. She seldom left home, but she became a speed typist with a worldwide correspondence, read widely, and welcomed visits from her two sons, Tony and George.

On Sunday night, 26 September 1965, Clara Bow sat with a substitute nurse watching *The Virginian* (1929), starring Cooper and directed by Fleming. Suddenly her head fell to the side; it was 12:06 A.M. on Monday morning. The autopsy showed severe heart disease; the attack that killed her was not her first. After an Episcopal service she was buried beside Rex at Forest Lawn, Los Angeles. She had long before planned her funeral to the last detail, including makeup and casket lining: "either satin or silk . . . preferably in apricot or egg-shell." *See* David Stenn (1988).

Boyer, Charles (1899-1978)

The screen's great lover was still able to project a remarkable presence in his mid-seventies in the French-made movie *Stavisky* (1974). In 1977, he and his Yorkshire-born actress-wife Pat Paterson flew from their Geneva home to New York for medical check-ups. Boyer kept from Pat the knowledge that she was suffering from liver and colon cancer and had only a year or so to live, but, under a pretext, he retired with her to Arizona with the hope of improving the time she had left. In February 1978 they celebrated their forty-fourth wedding anniversary.

Charles nursed his wife devotedly in their Scottsdale home as her condition worsened, reading to her from newspapers, plays (in which he took all the parts), and Dickens's *Martin Chuzzlewit*. On 23 August she felt better, but stayed in bed. They played gin rummy, and then she fell asleep for the last time; she died peacefully at 3:00 A.M. on the twenty-fourth.

During her funeral service in California next day, Boyer stayed in Arizona and put their papers in order. On the twenty-sixth he swallowed an overdose of barbiturate; it was two days before his seventy-ninth birthday. They lie side-by-side in Holy Cross Cemetery, Los Angeles. *See* Larry Swindell: *Charles Boyer, The Reluctant Lover* (1983).

Braun, Eva (1910-1945)

Adolf Hitler's mistress married him on 29 April 1945 in the bunker under the Berlin chancellery as the Soviet army overran the city in the last days of World War II. On the thirtieth they committed suicide, Eva by swallowing cyanide. The bodies were carried up to the courtyard and partly cremated with the aid of limited stocks of gasoline.

In the *Legal Medicine Annual, 1976*, Dr. Reidar F. Sognnaes, a dental professor at the University of California, Los Angeles, reported that, whereas Hitler's remains could be conclusively identified by a comparison of dental X rays with Soviet postmortem data released in 1968, this was not the case for Eva Braun. The autopsy performed in a Berlin suburb on 8 May 1945 by a Soviet pathology team on "the partially burned corpse of an unknown woman (presumably the wife of Hitler)" revealed that much of the skull had been destroyed by fire and most of the teeth were missing or dislodged.

Moreover, a gold bridge found under the tongue "replacing the right mandibular first and second molars" does not correspond with the records of Hitler's (and Braun's) dentist, Dr. Hugo Blaschke, which indicate that these teeth, though missing, had not been replaced by a bridge up to the last time he saw her, shortly before her death. Though Eva Braun undoubtedly killed herself, no positive identification of her body has ever been made.

Britten, Benjamin (1913-1976)

The British composer added several operas to the international repertoire, including *Peter Grimes* (1945) and *Billy Budd* (1951); he also wrote the *War Requiem* (1962) for the dedication of the rebuilt Coventry Cathedral. Many of his compositions were tailored to the voice of his lifelong companion, the tenor Peter Pears, with whom he established the Aldeburgh Festival near their Suffolk home in 1948. The most personal of his operas, *Death in Venice*, which was based on Thomas Mann's novella, supplied in the main role (Aschenbach) an ideal role for Pears; it received its premiere at Aldeburgh in June 1973.

The previous month, Britten had undergone surgery at the National Heart Hospital in London for replacement of a faulty cardiac valve. During the operation he suffered a slight stroke that disabled his right arm and brought his career as accompanist and conductor to an end. But he could still write, and though confined much of the time to a wheelchair, he continued to travel—to performances at Covent Garden and even, for the last time, to Venice. In his last months he continued to produce new works and was able to attend some of the Aldeburgh Festival performances in June 1976. In that month, too, he was honored by the queen with a life peerage, becoming Baron Britten of Aldeburgh. His old friend, the writer Christopher Isherwood, visited him and said later, "I knew Ben was ill, but I didn't know how ill he was . . . the others left us, and Ben and I sat in a room together, not speaking, just holding hands."

After a vacation with Pears in Norway, Britten was able to hear his final major work, the *Third Quartet,* rehearsed by the Amadeus Quartet in September. Mstislav Rostropovich, for whom the composer had written his *Cello Sonata* in 1961, visited him and was shocked by his appearance and trembling hands.

The dying man's nurse, Scottish-born Rita Thomson, recalled his thoughts as he neared the end: "He used to say, what will it be like? And I said, well, we'll be with you and we'll just make it as gentle as possible. And he said well, is it going to be painful? And I said no, we wouldn't want it to be painful—and of course it wasn't. I said I would be with him and probably Peter; *obviously* Peter would be with him when the time came that he was going to die!"

Benjamin Britten died of heart failure at 4:15 A.M. on 4 December 1976 in the rambling home, the Red House outside Aldeburgh, that he and Peter Pears had shared for three decades. He had no terror of dying, said Pears. "He died—in my arms, in fact—peacefully [with] no struggle to keep alive, except a purely physical one . . . to breathe . . . He'd always said earlier, to me, I must die first, before you, because I don't know what I'd do without you."

Britten, though not a regular churchgoer, was a devout Christian pacifist. At his funeral in Aldeburgh Parish Church, the Bishop of Ipswich delivered a short address. The composer was buried in the churchyard; the gravestone has a simple inscription: BENJAMIN BRITTEN 1913–1976. In his will, Britten left £50,000 to Pears and double that amount to a charitable trust. The total net estate amounted to £1.5 million, all but a small fraction representing the estimated value of the composer's manuscripts.

Little or nothing was said publicly about Britten's homosexuality during his lifetime, but after his death Pears was happy to discuss what both had regarded as a long and happy marriage. In a radio interview he summed it up quite simply: "He loved my voice—and he loved me."

The tenor lived on in the Red House and continued his singing career until he suffered a stroke in his seventies. After that he busied himself in Aldeburgh with the annual festival and the Britten/Pears Library and School. He was knighted in 1978 and was present in November of that year when a memorial stone for his friend was unveiled in Westminster Abbey. Sir Peter Pears died suddenly at the Red House, apparently of a heart attack, on 3 April 1986 at the age of seventy-five. *See* Christopher Headington (1981).

Brown, Christy (1932-1981)

The Irish novelist and poet, the tenth of twenty-two children, was born with crippling cerebral palsy. His mother and a Dublin pediatrician, Robert Collis, encouraged him to paint and type with his sole controllable member. His first book, *My Left Foot* (1954), was an autobiography filmed under the same title in 1989. (Daniel Day-Lewis's portrayal of the adult Brown won him an Academy Award; Hugh O'Conor as the young Brown was also brilliant.) The movie ended with the 1972 marriage of Christy with Mary Carr, a dental technician.

He died in his English home in the Somerset village of Parbrook, near Glastonbury, on Sunday evening, 6 September 1981. At the inquest, a tearful Mary Brown explained that her husband drank "quite a bit of vodka" on Saturday night, and next day had a bottle of red wine and some brandy. That evening she gave him two sleeping pills. "Isn't that dangerous?" asked the coroner. "Didn't you know drink and pills can be a dangerous combination, resulting in vomiting and asphyxiation?" "Yes," she replied, but "I thought by giving him sleeping pills it would let him sleep for a few hours and not have more alcohol, which was the demon of the case, if you like." Of course, Christy always had to be hand-fed; that evening she fed him roast lamb and then left him for a few minutes. When she returned he was choking and she called the ambulance. The coroner offered his sympathy to the grieving widow; she had obviously looked after her husband very well. A death by misadventure, caused by shock and asphyxiation, was recorded.

Brown, John (1800-1859)

The fanatical U.S. abolitionist's sanity has been fiercely debated, but his raid on Harpers Ferry, Virginia, though impractical, had noble aims. On Sunday, 16 October 1859, he led his force of sixteen white and five black recruits across the Potomac from Maryland with the aim of barricading two bridges, occupying the federal armory and the rifle manufactory nearby and awaiting the rebellion of slaves in Virginia.

In less than thirty-six hours, marines under Colonel Robert E. Lee had broken into the armory and taken Brown captive; he had lost ten men, including two of his sons, five escaped, and six were all executed later. At his trial at Charlestown, Virginia, now Charles Town, West Virginia, the wounded Brown lay on a cot, refusing to permit an insanity plea to be entered; he was condemned to hang 2 December. Lincoln applauded his motives but abhorred his violence and treason. Thoreau prayed he would die a martyr to the cause and Brown agreed, rejecting a jail-break plot.

His wife Mary visited him on 1 December; next day he rose early and composed inscriptions for his own and his dead sons' tombstones. His farewell message read, in part: "I John Brown am now quite certain that the crimes of this guilty land will never be purged away but with blood."

On the outskirts of Charlestown, Brown stood quite patiently on the gallows for ten minutes, hooded and with arms and legs tied. With the surrounding troops at last in their allotted positions a hush descended on the crowd. Then, as Stephen B. Oates records in his 1970 biography:

> Below, the sheriff raised the hatchet and severed the rope with a single blow; there was a crash as the platform fell and Brown plummeted through space . . . the rope caught, his arms below the elbow flew up and his body struggled convulsively . . . then at last John Brown "was hanging between heaven and earth," while the crowd looked on in silence. In a moment the voice of Colonel J. T. L. Preston of the Virginia Institute rang out on the wind: "So perish all such enemies of Virginia! All such enemies of the Union! All such foes of the human race!"

Mary received her husband's coffin at Harpers Ferry and sent it by sea from Philadelphia to New York where a friend transferred the body to a casket of Northern manufacture. John Brown was buried in his beloved Adirondacks on his North Elba, New York, farm beside a large boulder. The Civil War and the Thirteenth Amendment of 1865 (abolishing slavery) were hastened by the emotions stirred up by the angry old man.

Brutus, Marcus Junius (85?-42 B.C.)

Most historians are agreed that Shakespeare's portrait of Julius Caesar's chief assassin is better than he deserved. Brutus had returned to Rome after being governor of Cisalpine Gaul and held the rank of city praetor (magistrate) when his colleague Gaius Cassius Longinus persuaded him to head the Republican plot to murder Caesar in March 44. After the deed the Liberators, even with the powerful oratorical assistance of Cicero, were unable to bring back the Republic. The young Octavian (Caesar's heir and the future Emperor Augustus) in October joined in a triumvirate with Mark Antony (Caesar's self-appointed representative) and the army commander M. Aemilius Lepidus. A bill was rushed through the senate outlawing the assassins; Cicero (q.v.), though not a conspirator, became the most notable victim of the cruel proscription that followed.

In the fall of 42 Brutus and Cassius selected with care the site in Macedonia where they were to fight to the death against Antony and Octavian. Their separate, locally mustered armies occupied camps on two hilltops to the west of Philippi, which lay about fifteen miles northwest of the present-day northern Greek city of Kavalla. In the initial engagement Cassius suffered a setback and, not realizing that Brutus had been victorious, killed himself with the aid of his freedman Pindar. Nevertheless, the Liberators were still in a superior position. The Caesarians were far from home and, with diminishing supplies, faced steadily worsening weather. All Brutus had to do was wait. But his troops became impatient and three weeks after the first battle their leader gave way. On 23 October 42 B.C., his men stormed Antony's position. In forcing the enemy back they overextended their line, which was broken by Antony's counterattack and overwhelmed when Octavian entered the fray. Brutus withdrew northward toward the mountains with about fourteen thousand men as darkness fell. By morning most of his men had drifted away. After his slave and his attendant declined to do what Pindar had done for Cassius, Brutus prevailed on a Greek rhetor, one Strato, to point his sword at his commander's heart so that he might run upon it.

Octavian ordered the head sent to Rome to be placed before Caesar's altar, but it was reportedly lost at sea. The corpse was ceremonially burned, and the ashes were despatched to the dead man's mother Servilia, who had never ceased to idolize him. *See* Max Radin (1939).

Brynner, Yul (1915?-1985)

The Russian-born actor's date and place of birth remain uncertain, thanks to the varied accounts he gave interviewers. He was a well-paid CBS television director when he was reluctantly persuaded by Mary Martin (with whom he had worked in the 1946 play *Lute Song*) to audition for the leading male role, opposite Gertrude Lawrence, in the 1951 Rogers and Hammerstein musical *The King and I*. Brynner made many movies of variable quality, but they include the 1956 film version of *The King and I* with Deborah Kerr, for which he won an Oscar, and it is his decades-long appearances as King Mongkut in repeated revivals of the musical onstage for which he is best remembered.

Late in September 1983, during a nationwide tour of *The King and I* and shortly after his fourth marriage, to the diminutive Malaysian-born dancer Kathy Lee, Brynner went with his wife, who had a cold, to see her

Los Angeles doctor Paul Rudnick. While there the actor asked Rudnick to check a lump in his neck that he'd noticed while making up during the past two weeks. An aspiration, followed by a complete biopsy, revealed that Brynner, at one time a five-packs-a-day cigarette smoker, had cancerous tumors (poorly differentiated adenocarcinoma) of both lungs, and the disease was now invading his lymphatic system. It was too late for surgery. Only one of the half-dozen oncologists the actor thereafter consulted, Steven Greenberg at Cedars-Sinai Medical Center, gave him any hope of living much beyond two months. Brynner determined to keep his condition secret and fight the scourge. Six times a week for eight weeks Brynner underwent radiation therapy before his Los Angeles performances and, though often ill and nauseated, missed not a single performance. He told only the show's producer, his agent, and his two oldest children.

Yul and Kathy went to Germany in 1984 for treatment by a Hanover immunologist, Hans Nieper, who professed to cure cancer patients with special diets and herbal injections. Back in New York, feeling better and with all tests negative, Brynner was told he was in remission. "Those doctors are being too conservative," he said happily. "I'm in *permanent* remission. I've licked the Big C."

The national tour continued and was due to end on Broadway in May 1985. Audiences, paying record prices, began to notice that the star was losing some of his sparkle. Mary Beth Peil, his leading lady in six hundred performances, later revealed that Brynner was barely able to walk from his dressing room during the final weeks; yet on reaching the stage he would glide "into the light, erect, with the body of a sleek jungle cat." To those who sensed that something was seriously wrong, the actor would admit to suffering the effects of a back injury dating from his circus days in Paris, and the management would sometimes announce that "Mr. Brynner has a serious throat and ear infection." The run was extended to 30 June, but Yul missed only seven of these extra performances. When he did appear, the "Shall We Dance?" number, in which he was whirled around the stage by Peil, was slowed down and "A Puzzlement," his solo number, was omitted. But still, thirty-four years after creating the role, the short-statured Brynner dominated the show to the end by sheer force of character. When the final curtain came down the audience rose to sing "Auld Lang Syne." Brynner took his bows for the 4,625th time, grasped the hand of his wife Kathy, who played the principal royal dancer, and at the top of the rear stairway waved a final good-bye. An estimated 3.6 million theatergoers had seen him in the role on Broadway since 1951 and a further 4.5 million Americans during his numerous tours.

The couple spent a month at their home in northern France, then returned to New York. On 4 September Yul was admitted to New York Hospital under the name Robby Lee and the staff were sworn to secrecy. He lapsed into a coma two weeks later and died on 10 October 1985. His press agent said, "He faced death with a dignity and strength that astonished his doctors." At the actor's bedside were Kathy and his four children, two of them adopted. A private funeral service took place the same day.

After Yul Brynner's death his half-minute antismoking message, filmed not long before for the National Cancer Institute, was repeatedly shown on television. At a memorial service in Manhattan's Shubert Theater in January 1986 the TV interviewer Mike Wallace said Brynner "was born with an extra quart of champagne in his blood—and knew how to pass it around."

Buck, Pearl S. (1892-1973)

The only woman to win both of the top literature prizes, the Pulitzer Prize in 1933 (for her novel *The Good Earth*) and the Nobel in 1938, set up her foundation for Asian-American children in 1964. Four years later it was beset by scandal when she fell under the influence of an ex-dance instructor, Thomas F. Harris, who was forty years her junior and who was accused of major financial irregularities in his running of the organization.

After Harris's resignation, she financed for him an antique business in Danby, a small Vermont village where she took up residence late in 1968. Approaching eighty, she wrote in an article about death: "I did not ask to be, but I have been and I am. My reason tells me I shall continue to be. I am on my way somewhere, just as I was on the day of my birth."

Ambitious plans to revisit China in 1972 after Richard Nixon's trip there collapsed when the Beijing government denied her a visa. She returned to her former home, Green Hills Farm in Perkasie, Pennsylvania, for an eightieth birthday reception on 26 June 1972, at which hundreds of guests passed by the stately seated figure. Immediately after it was over she collapsed and was taken to the hospital at Rutland, Vermont, and was put on a diet to shed twenty pounds.

In September she underwent gallbladder surgery in Burlington, where part of the medical center had to be taken over to handle her worldwide correspondence and the numerous assistants commuting from Danby. More surgery was needed the following month. Back home in Danby House for Christmas, she spent the first weeks of 1973 confined to her bed, surrounded by the Dickens volumes she had first enjoyed during her childhood in Chinkiang (Xinjiang).

Pearl Buck died quietly early on 6 March 1973. Shortly before, Harris had summoned her sister Grace, and she and several of her adopted children went upstairs for a final good-bye. There they were astonished to find the dying woman sitting erect in an armchair, wearing a long red and black Chinese robe, red earrings and necklace and a ruby bracelet, which had been brought to her by Harris moments before from the adjoining antique shop.

She was buried after a private service under an ash tree on the lawn at Green Hills Farm. All nine of her adopted children were present; only her natural daughter, the retarded Carol Buck, was absent. Her will, leaving most of her estate to Harris, was challenged by the family and later by the Pearl S. Buck Foundation, which had been left without income. A secret out-of-court settlement was reached.

Burton, Richard (1925-1984)

During a U.S. tour of *Camelot* in 1981, the golden-voiced Welsh actor was felled by partial paralysis brought on by a pinched spinal nerve. When he married Sally Hay, a production assistant, in 1983 during a run of *Private Lives* with Elizabeth Taylor, his health was poor. He had been mildly epileptic most of his life; now his back pains were recurring, his arthritis was worsening, and always he lived under the threat of cirrhosis of the liver if he failed to moderate his frequent alcoholic binges. In July 1984 he appeared with his daughter Kate in a TV drama, *Ellis Island*. The last of his fifty-five movies, released after his death, was George Orwell's *1984*.

Back home with Sally in the Swiss village of Céligny, on the lake north of Geneva, he studied scripts for future work on *Wild Geese II* and *The Quiet American* and took calls from Elizabeth Taylor, his partner in two tempestuous marriages (1964–74 and 1975–76), who wanted to work with him again and who was not far away in Gstaad. ("I am obsessed with that woman," he never ceased to admit to interviewers.) On the evening of Friday, 3 August 1984, he got drunk at the local Café de la Gare and next day complained of a headache. Retiring early to read and make notes, he was asleep when Sally joined him. Early on Sunday, the fifth, he was breathing heavily and she could not rouse him. He was rushed north to the little hospital at Nyon, then south to Geneva. He had suffered a cerebral hemorrhage and died the same afternoon. "I remember thinking 'Well done,' " said Sally. " 'You've thrown off that old body. You're on your next adventure. Well done!' "

The funeral was marked by Sally's bitter determination to keep Elizabeth Taylor away. After the Presbyterian service in Céligny, complete with hymn singing in Welsh by his visiting family, he was buried in the tiny Protestant cemetery nearby. Elizabeth, in a dawn visit, prayed at the grave a few days later; she was accompanied by Maria, her and Burton's German-born adopted daughter, and a four-man escort to keep the press at bay. She went on to visit his birthplace, Pontrhydifen near Port Talbot, and attended a memorial service in London. His last words, in red ink on his bedside notepad, were: "Our revels now are ended." See Melvyn Bragg (1988).

Burton, Sir Richard Francis (1821-1890)

The flamboyant British Arabist, world traveler, explorer, anthropologist, and linguist first achieved fame with his earthy chronicle of a pilgrimage to Mecca he made in disguise in 1853. The most monumental of his fifty-odd published books is the sixteen-volume translation of The Thousand Nights and a Day (1885–88), often called The Arabian Nights. He entered the diplomatic service in 1861 and at the time of his death had been for nine years British consul in Trieste.

In his final month, Burton worked for hours each day on his translation of The Perfumed Garden, an erotic work in Arabic that had engaged him on and off for fourteen years and was said to be within twenty-four hours of completion when he died. He wandered aimlessly in his garden most of Sunday, 19 October 1890, at one point rescuing a baby robin that had fallen into a water butt and dwelling mournfully in remarks to his wife Isobel on the imminent migration of the swallows that were to be seen flocking around the house. He assured Isobel that when he retired the following March at the age of seventy they would indeed settle down back in England in a little place of their own; and he would never again write a book on "this subject," but would turn to autobiography. "What happiness that will be," responded Mrs. Burton, a devout Catholic.

At 9:30 Burton retired, but at midnight complained his gout was troubling him. His resident physician F. Grenfell Baker came by with routine medicines at 4:00 A.M. but had to be summoned again a little later when Burton cried out, feeling suffocated. It was evident his heart was failing.

Isobel held him as he called out, "Oh, Puss, chloroform—ether—or I'm a dead man." But neither was appropriate, or at hand. "My God," he shouted again, "I am a dead man," and died. The time was around 5:00 A.M. on 20 October 1890.

Frantic, Isobel Burton sent off for a priest. Refusing to believe her husband had died unabsolved, she urged Baker to apply the terminals of a battery to his heart while she alternately sought for a priest and fervently prayed. At 7:00 A.M. Father Pietro Martelani called at the house but refused to give the last sacraments to one he had heard was a notorious unbeliever. "No, no," protested Isobel, "he is a Catholic. You *must* give him Extreme Unction." After this was done she cried, "Let the world rain fire and brimstone on me now."

There were a hundred thousand at the grand military funeral conducted with Catholic rites by the Bishop of Trieste. Mrs. Burton claimed that her husband's spirit appeared to her in a dream, commanding her to burn his writings. (As Vincent Starrett once wrote, "If you believe this, you'll believe anything.") The task of sorting through a twenty-seven-year accumulation of manuscripts, journals, and letters and the burning of most of them required sixteen days. The family's reaction to their dead relative's posthumous conversion was as nothing to the public outcry at this act of literary vandalism. As many as forty-one books in various stages of completion were destroyed; seven were quite or almost finished, including *The Perfumed Garden,* described even by Isobel as her husband's magnum opus.

For Burton's resting place in the Catholic cemetery at Mortlake in southwest London, his wife raised £688 from friends and commissioned a memorial in the form of an Arab tent; eighteen feet high, built of dark stone and Carrara marble. Only one relative of Burton's was among the eight hundred who turned up for the second funeral in June 1891. Mrs. Burton, who was to die of cancer in 1896, took a cottage nearby and spent many hours in prayer at the grave; she also completed in 1893 a rambling and inaccurate biography of Sir Richard.

The burial ground is unkempt and abandoned now behind its high wall. The Burton memorial stands neglected in its weedy plot, the stained glass window in the rear smashed. After Isobel Burton's death, meetings were held there by a cult headed by a certain Goodrich Freer, who called herself "Miss X," but three years later she was no longer heard of. *See* Byron Farwell (1963).

Callas, Maria (1923-1977)

Born in New York of Greek parents, the famous diva early in 1970 attempted to resume her notorious love affair with Aristotle Onassis when his 1968 marriage to Jacqueline Kennedy began to show signs of failure. The rapprochement did not last and in May, Callas was briefly admitted to the American Hospital in Paris suffering from an overdose of barbiturates and tranquilizers. In October 1971 she began a notable series of master classes at the Juilliard School in New York, but the select audiences could hear that her voice was by then undependable. In her last years her loneliness was assuaged by the tenor Giuseppe di Stefano, and with him she embarked on a world concert tour late in 1973. Her voice was last heard on stage at the end of their tour in Sapporo, Japan, on 11 November 1974.

Thereafter she retired to her Parisian apartment at 36 Avenue Georges Mandel, practicing from time to time but soon sinking lethargically into television viewing. On 16 September 1977 she awoke late and breakfasted in bed. According to varied reports she collapsed, apparently from a heart attack, on the way to or from her morning bath. Her maid Bruna and her butler lifted her onto her bed and called around for medical help, but before a physician could reach her she was dead.

The funeral service was at the Greek Orthodox Church on the Rue Georges Bizet. Her ashes were laid to rest in the Père Lachaise Cemetery; three months later they were stolen, but were retrieved a few hours later in a remote corner of the cemetery. In 1979 they were scattered over the Aegean Sea. Callas's ex-husband G. B. Meneghini (1895–1981), suspicious that neither an inquest nor an autopsy took place, that no recent will was found, and that the cremation was unduly hastened, believed that she may have died by her own hand. *See* biographies by A. Stassinopoulos (1981) and G. B. Meneghini (1981).

Capone, Al (1899-1947)

The Brooklyn-born Chicago mafioso Alphonse "Scarface" Capone was never convicted of a capital offense; he was put away in October 1931 to serve ten years for federal income-tax evasion. While on library duty at Alcatraz prison in February 1938 he first showed the symptoms of neurosyphilis. He was treated before and after his release with arsphenamine (an arsenic compound), which slowed but did not arrest the disease, and he continued to have confused episodes.

During his last years, spent with his wife Mae and his son at their Florida home, 93 Palm Avenue on Palm Island in Biscayne Bay, Capone's pudgy figure became ever more gross. Penicillin, when it became available after 1942, stabilized his condition, but nothing could reverse the extensive brain damage. Early on 19 January 1947 he suffered a cerebral hemorrhage and last rites were said. He rallied, only to succumb to bronchial pneumonia on the evening of 25 January; no autopsy was performed.

The Roman Catholic Church forbade elaborate ceremonies. On the family tombstone in Mount Olivet Cemetery, Chicago, he is named simply as AL CAPONE / 1899–1947. The family, annoyed by sightseers, within a few years secretly removed Capone's remains to Mount Carmel Cemetery at the other end of the city. The genuine grave is marked by a small black marble stone bearing only the words: MY JESUS MERCY. *See* John Kobler (1971).

Capote, Truman (1924–1984)

The elfin writer from New Orleans, author of the insouciant *Breakfast at Tiffany's* and the chilling "nonfiction novel" *In Cold Blood,* had been neglected by his mother and raised by elderly female relatives. As his powers failed he turned in his last years to retailing malicious gossip about his friends in New York's jet set on TV talk shows and in his never-to-be-completed novel, *Answered Prayers.*

An alcoholic hooked on tranquilizers and other drugs, he turned for comfort to the few friends who never abandoned him. Joanne Copeland, divorced from NBC's *Tonight Show* host Johnny Carson in 1972, supplied the mother's love he had never known. She set up a guest room just for him at her Bel Air, Los Angeles, home, and it was there that she found him, struggling to put on his swimming trunks, at 8:00 A.M. on 25 August 1984.

"I'm a little tired and very weak," he murmured, and said he felt cold. As Joanne turned to fetch him hot tea he grasped her and begged her to sit with him; as they held one another in a tearful embrace he moaned, "Mama, Mama." At last he fell back, hands on his chest, and she left him to rest, looking in every half hour. It was close to noon when she saw his color had worsened and his forehead was cold to the touch. "I tried to revive him," she said, "but I knew he was gone." His system, undermined by drug use, had succumbed to liver disease complicated by phlebitis.

Capote's ashes were sent to his lover of thirty-six years, Jack Dunphy in New York, but Mrs. Carson kept some of them back as a keepsake. She placed the small package in the room where he died, between photographs of his two mothers, the real and the substitute. For four years it was her "sanity," she said. Then, after a Halloween costume party, she found it gone along with some jewelry and memorabilia. The ashes, but nothing else, were returned to her back steps mysteriously six nights later. Regretfully, on 11 November 1988 she placed them for safety, along with mementos and a good-bye note to Capote, in a crypt, near those of Marilyn Monroe and Natalie Wood at Westwood Memorial Park, Los Angeles. The note, recalling Capote's story "A Christmas Memory," said in part, "Wait for me, I'll be joining you in time and we'll sail kites against the clear blue sky . . ."

Cassidy, Butch (1866-1937)

In the 1969 movie *Butch Cassidy and the Sundance Kid* the two outlaws were killed in a spectacular shoot-out at San Vicente, Bolivia, after a payroll robbery. This story, long believed to be true, was based on a 1930 magazine account by Arthur Chapman. In 1975 Cassidy's sister revealed much of the truth, and Larry Pointer in his 1977 book *In Search of Butch Cassidy* tied up the loose ends.

Butch (real name: Robert Leroy Parker) returned to the United States in 1908 and surfaced in Adrian, Michigan, as William Thadeus Phillips. He married a local woman and moved on to Spokane, Washington, where he founded the Phillips Manufacturing Company. Ruined by the Depression, he died of rectal cancer at Broadacres, the county poor farm at Spangle, south of Spokane, on 20 July 1937. His widow, Gertrude Livesay Phillips, scattered his ashes over the Little Spokane River. The fates of the Sundance Kid (Harry Longabaugh) and his sweetheart Etta Place, and indeed Etta's true identity, remain unknown.

Cézanne, Paul (1839-1906)

The French artist's paintings were not only anathema to the Academy through most of his life but incomprehensible to the critics. A surly, puritanical man who generally painted nudes only from photographs, he subordinated all other matters to his art and swore he would die painting.

Success came slowly, beginning with a one-man show in 1895; by 1904 he was being sought out by collectors and dealers, but his growing fame had little influence on his life. He had long since abandoned Paris for his native Aix-en-Provence, leaving his wife and son in the capital. The heat of the Provençal summer in 1906 weakened the artist, who suffered from diabetes, swollen eyes, and a festering sore on the right foot. For ten years he had hired the same dilapidated carriage to take him from his rooms at 23 rue Boulegon in Aix to his chosen work site, but as the cooler weather brought some relief in October, the cost of the carriage was abruptly increased and the outraged artist sent the driver packing. No longer able to handle the oil-painting equipment, he turned to watercolors and executed some of the finest ever seen. Still, carrying his gear on his back was almost beyond his strength, and he tottered home every night completely exhausted.

On 15 October Cézanne was drenched to the skin during a violent storm while working outside the village of Le Thelonet, near Mont Sainte-Victoire. Chilled to the bone, he staggered homeward; the driver of a laundry cart found him collapsed beside the road and took him to the rue Boulegon, where the housekeeper, Mme. Brémond, sent for Dr. Guillaumont. Next day, ignoring the doctor's orders, the truculent artist set out into the chill dawn and tried to finish a portrait of his gardener Vallier in the shadow of lime trees on a hill. Toward evening his legs trembled and he felt feverish and light-headed. Despite his lifelong dread of being touched, he begged Vallier to help him down the hill.

Beset by pneumonia complicated by diabetes, he lay, coughing and restive, in his bare, cheerless room, watched over by his sister Marie. Mme. Brémond wired to Paris for his wife Hortense and son Paul but, busy with fittings at the dressmaker's, she hid the telegram from her son and did nothing. By now delirious, Cézanne could be heard murmuring the name of his dead friend, Émile Zola, and calling repeatedly for Paul. A priest, Canon Joseph Lauie, administered the last rites. While Marie was at confession on 22 October 1906 Mme. Brémond found the artist dead, his face turned to the wall. The death announcement was delayed until next day so that the funeral could be legally postponed until the twenty-fourth. Hortense and Paul were therefore able to be present when Paul Cézanne was interred in the cemetery of St. Pierre in Aix-en-Provence.

Chandler, Raymond (1888-1959)

The Chicago-born, English-educated creator of Philip Marlowe, the tough but humane private eye, moved to La Jolla, California, in 1946. When his wife Cissy, eighteen years his senior, died in 1954 he fell apart. "She was the beat of my heart for thirty years," he wrote later. First he tried to shoot himself while in the shower and spent a short time under psychiatric care; then, seeking companionship, he traveled repeatedly in England, where his books are highly regarded.

Returning to La Jolla, he completed his final novel, *Playback,* and tried quixotically to help his secretary with her hopelessly tangled affairs. His London agent Helga Greene flew over to help him, even at last agreeing to marry him; however, feeling rebuffed at a New York meeting with her father, he returned alone to his rented cottage at 824 Prospect Street, La Jolla, and began drinking again. He died of pneumonia at Scripps Clinic 26 March 1959 and was buried in Mount Hope Cemetery, San Diego. *See* Frank MacShane (1976).

Chaplin, Sir Charles (1889-1977)

The British movie comedian and producer settled at Corsier-sur-Vevey, Switzerland, near the eastern tip of Lake Geneva, after being denied a re-entry visa by the United States during the McCarthy era. (He was constantly accused of Communist sympathies, and many resented his failure to become an American citizen.) He and his young wife Oona O'Neill raised their eight children on a thirty-two-acre estate. In his last months, Chaplin—knighted in 1975—was confined to a wheelchair with sight, hearing, and speech impaired. He died peacefully at home aged eighty-eight, at 4:00 A.M. Christmas Day 1977, and his body was laid in a simple grave overlooking the lake.

On the night of 1–2 March 1978 the three-hundred-pound coffin was stolen. (The grave robbers had tried to hide it below the original grave but had found the digging too laborious.) It was found buried in a cornfield on 17 May; the public then learned that twenty-seven phone calls had been made by the criminals, Roman Wardas and Gantscho Ganev, demanding a ransom from the family. Wardas was apprehended making the final call from a Lausanne phone booth; he was sentenced to four and a half years in prison and Ganev was given an eighteen-month suspended sentence. The coffin was reinterred in a specially constructed concrete vault in the same cemetery.

Charles II (1630-1685)

Eleven years after his father Charles I had been beheaded, Charles II entered London on his thirtieth birthday amid great rejoicing to be proclaimed King of Great Britain and Ireland. The people who had suffered through the Civil War and Oliver Cromwell's regime were ready for what were to be the twenty-five years of "Good King Charles's Golden Days."

Apart from several convulsive attacks in 1678 and the following year, the king's health was good until, early in 1685, gout prevented him from taking his daily exercise in the park. His final Sunday evening, as recorded by the diarist John Evelyn, was one of "inexpressible luxury and profaneness, gaming and all dissoluteness." The king was "toying with his concubines," the Duchess of Portsmouth (Louise de Kéroualle, detested by her rival Nell Gwyn), Lady Castlemaine, and the Duchess of Mazarin. A French boy was singing love songs in the gallery and a large number of people were playing basset, a card game, with a bank of at least £2,000 in gold.

That night, 1 February 1685, Charles was restless; next morning his speech was thick and indistinct and he seemed absentminded. He made an effort to converse with his attendants in his usual lively manner but suddenly, with a loud cry, fell into the arms of one of his gentlemen-in-waiting. Dr. Edmund King, in charge of the sovereign's private laboratory at Whitehall, happened to be present; he opened a vein in Charles's right arm with a penknife and the unconscious man was carried to bed while his other physicians were sent for.

The first two advocated absolute rest and quiet until the king regained consciousness. But as other doctors gathered around the sickbed a program of cupping, blistering, bleeding, purging, and emetics was agreed upon. Spirits of ammonia were held to his nostrils to stimulate the brain and make him sneeze. Next day he appeared weaker, yet ten ounces of blood were drawn from the jugular vein and purgatives were again given. On the fourth a milder laxative was administered. Physicians keeping watch during the night noticed he was suffering from paroxysms of pain. Peruvian bark in syrup of cloves was given throughout the following day. On the evening of the fifth the king was completely exhausted. Records reveal that fourteen physicians were in attendance and fifty-eight different drugs and treatments were given. Charles bore these ministrations with good humor, even apologizing for being so long a-dying.

Anglican churchmen urged him to think of his immortal soul and receive the last sacraments, but he waved them away. When James, Duke of York, received word from Louise de Kéroualle that his brother the king had secretly embraced the Roman Catholic faith, he whispered to the dying man that he, James, should find a priest. "For God's sake, brother, do, and please lose no time," murmured Charles. The room was cleared except for two trustworthy attendants, and Father John Hudleston, who had saved his life after the battle of Worcester in 1651, was spirited in. Charles welcomed him: "You that have saved my body, is now come to save my soul." The king's confession was heard and absolution given. The queen, Catherine of Braganza, sent a plea for forgiveness for any wrongs she had done him. "Alas, poor woman," he replied, "she beg my pardon? I beg hers with all my heart: take back to her that answer."

His illegitimate sons (he had no other) knelt for his blessing. He entreated James to look after Louise and all his children, adding, "And let not poor Nelly starve." At 6:00 A.M. on 6 February 1685 he asked that the curtains be drawn back so that he could watch the dawn for the last time. A few hours later he lapsed into a coma, breathing loudly and with difficulty; he died about midday.

Rumors that the king had been poisoned were so prevalent that a postmortem was performed. The report, still extant, makes it clear that Charles II died a natural death. Modern authorities conclude that the convulsive fits and final illness were due to chronic nephritis (Bright's disease) ending in a uremic coma.

For several days his body lay in state in the Painted Chamber at Whitehall dominated by an upright wax effigy dressed in crimson robes. At dead of night on the fourteenth the body, enclosed in a lead coffin, was taken to Westminster Abbey and lowered into an unmarked tomb in the chapel of Henry VII. In 1867, when heating ducts were being installed, the coffin was seen to have collapsed and the king's remains were visible. They were seen again when the vault was opened in 1977.

Cheever, John (1912-1982)

The U.S. short-story writer and novelist was the unwanted child of alienated parents. His first novel, *The Wapshot Chronicle* (1957), was a great success, but was not immediately followed by other triumphs. He suffered the first of three heart attacks in 1973; in 1980, at the Yaddo writer's colony in Saratoga Springs, New York, of which he was vice president, he was felled by the first of two grand mal seizures; and in his last months he was afflicted by strange incidents of "otherness," when his mind would slip from the present into a timeless dimension.

Cheever's daughter Susan, in her painfully honest biography, *Home Before Dark* (1984), chronicles her father's alcoholism and his numerous affairs, which undermined but did not quite shatter her parents' marriage. Alcohol, combined with Valium, Librium, and Seconal, reduced Cheever by the spring of 1975 to his lowest point. A writing course he was teaching at Boston University was canceled, and he was admitted to a New York drying-out clinic. In a dramatic turnaround, he never drank again; he gave up the tranquilizers and in 1978 gave up smoking. In just three years the effects of the previous fifteen years of degradation were reversed. "It was like having my old father back," writes Susan. "[He] went from being an alcoholic with a drug problem who smoked two packs of Marlboros a day to being a man so abstemious that his principal drugs were the sugar in his desserts . . . and the caffeine in the dark, room-temperature 'iced' tea that he drank instead of whiskey."

But he craved affection, and at last yielded to a homosexual proclivity that his New England upbringing had long suppressed. His lover "Rip" often lived with the Cheevers at their Ossining, New York, home, near Sing Sing prison.

The writer's most successful novel *Falconer* (1977) is set in a prison. He completed it within a year after his discharge from the New York clinic, by which time he was regularly attending four local Alcoholics Anonymous chapters. His collection, *The Stories of John Cheever,* won the 1979 Pulitzer Prize. Late in 1981 he was found to have renal cancer which had spread to his lungs. He died at his Ossining home on 18 June 1982, three days after breaking his leg as he got out of bed. Late in the afternoon the minister from the village's Trinity Church said the last rites in the dark overheated room as the dying man's head tossed on the pillow. "Under the bedcovers my father kicked his legs and flailed his arm . . ." writes Susan. "It was harder and harder for him to breathe . . . I heard a little coughing noise, and . . . my father was dead."

After a simple service at Norwell, Massachusetts, John Cheever was buried next to his parents and brother in the village cemetery, in a grassy spot under a big maple on a hillside only a few miles from his birthplace in Quincy.

Churchill, Lord Randolph (1849-1895)

Like his son Winston, Lord Randolph was a parliamentary spellbinder, rallying his fellow Conservatives against the Liberals of the Gladstone administration and pushing for his idea of Tory democracy against his personal adversary, the Marquess of Salisbury. Though he was a member of the House of Commons for twenty years, his effective career was shortened by illness to barely a third of that period. He was probably infected with syphilis long before his whirlwind courtship and marriage, at the age of twenty-four, to the nineteen-year-old New York beauty Jennie Jerome. (He once told a woman relative that he liked only "rough women who dance and sing and drink—the rougher the better—great ladies bore me.")

Syphilis is protean in its effects; it kills very slowly, but undermines the body and brain in unpredictable ways. Churchill was a self-willed, impulsive man of great energy, but his ill health and accompanying depression caused him to withdraw from the public scene for long periods, beginning with an unexplained hiatus of seven months in 1882. By 1886 he was partly deaf. He took doses of mercury, the only available remedy for syphilis at that period, but it is a cumulative poison that can itself cause progressive disability and tremors. He was also treated with increasing amounts of digitalis for cardiac weakness. Still, though friends observed the telltale symptoms, and even surviving photographs display the drooping eyelids that are evidence of partial paralysis of their muscles, Lady Randolph worked hard to keep the secret. "[I]t would be hard if it got out," she wrote to her sister after her husband's death. "It would do incalculable harm to his political reputation and his memory and be a dreadful thing for all of us."

Nine years before his death, when only thirty-seven, he looked old, "like a man who has had a stroke." His 1981 biographer R. F. Foster writes that by 1892 "signs of slurring in speech, vertigo, and palpitations were becoming marked. What would follow, in the inevitable pattern of General

Paralysis, were the euphoric delusions which would lead to such embarrassments in the terrible last two years of his life." In his 1905 biography, Lord Randolph's son Winston looks on the brighter side: "But now nature began mercifully to apply increasing doses of her own anaesthetics, and for the space there was yet to travel he suffered less than those who watched him. Indeed, in an odd way he was positively happy in these last few months . . ." Mercifully indeed! By then, according to a 1984 medical study by R. B. Greenblatt, "Walking [had become] stumbling and his feet moved sideways, hitting the ground with a stamp. His legs, feet, and joints were swollen; his body was covered with festering gummatous sores; and he was soon incontinent." His last speeches in the Commons were described as "terrible" and "tragical."

In June 1894 he began a journey around the world which was cut short in Burma when his strength at last failed him. When he arrived back in London in December he was in a coma. He died in his mother's home on 24 January 1895. Large crowds turned out for his funeral procession through the London streets. He was buried at Bladon, a mile from his boyhood home, Blenheim Castle, where his son and first biographer would join him after even greater public tributes seventy years later.

Cicero, Marcus Tullius (106–43 B.C.)

The influence of the Roman statesman, lawyer, scholar, writer, and orator, who was called "the most eloquent of the sons of Romulus," has continued to the present day. At the height of his power he exposed Lucius Sergius Catilina's revolutionary intentions in the senate chamber with a famous oration. The rebel leader fled, but his fellow conspirators were put to death. Soon afterward, Cicero was accused of executing the men without a proper trial and in 58 B.C. he was exiled in Thessalonica.

He returned to Italy in October 48 after Julius Caesar had forgiven him for his half-hearted support of Pompey, the emperor's opponent for control of the Roman world. After Caesar's assassination in 44, Cicero fell afoul of Caesar's adopted son Octavian, who was not amused by Cicero's comment, "*laudandum adulescentem, ornandum, tollendum*" (i.e. that Octavian should be "praised, honored, and promoted"); as the final word can also mean "disposed of" the remark is ambiguous. When the triumvirate of Octavian, Antony, and Lepidus was formed at the end of October 43, Cicero's name appeared on the list of those condemned to death.

Aware of his likely fate, Cicero refused to commit suicide. He left Rome with his brother Quintus Tullius Cicero and returned to his villa at Tusculum, southeast of the city. When they received news of their proscription they fled south. Quintus turned back for some money, but his slaves betrayed him and he was killed. Cicero continued on to his house at Astura, on the Tyrrhenian shore, then put out to sea, perhaps to flee to Greece; with characteristic indecision he returned to the mainland. On 7 December 43 B.C. the assassins from Rome arrived at his villa at Formiae on the Campanian coast. A centurion, Herennius, and a military tribune, Popilius, found the old man in the garden. Realizing he was doomed, he looked steadfastly at the assassins as they approached and beheaded him. His head and severed hands were taken to Antony, who gloated over them and passed them to his wife. She mutilated the head before it was displayed on the *rostra* at Rome. *See* W. K. Lacey (1978).

Cocteau, Jean (1889-1963)

The prolific French poet, dramatist, and film director was a slender man with dark eyes and a brush of wiry hair. His companion before World War II was the blond, blue-eyed actor Jean Marais, but in 1948 Cocteau transferred his affections to his chauffeur, the strapping young Édouard Dermit, and it was Dermit who became his heir.

Cocteau's addiction to opium probably undermined his health. Attacks of angina pectoris began in 1947; among other ailments were a near-fatal uremia in 1953, myocarditis the following year and a massive internal hemorrhage in 1958. His convalescence from a coronary in April 1963 was slow. In July, Marais took him by ambulance from the writer's Paris apartment to the actor's home near Versailles, but Cocteau insisted in September that he move to their old house at Milly-la-Forêt, thirty-five miles south of the capital. To an old friend he complained, "I am surrounded by doctors who have torn me from death without bringing me back to life." Propped up in bed he worked on a book of memoirs, *Le Passé Défini*.

"The ship is sinking," murmured Cocteau when, at 9:00 A.M. on Friday, 11 October 1963 the radio announced the death of Edith Piaf. At noon the dying man was overheard praising the singer: "She died as if consumed by the fire of her fame." Just at that moment Louis Aragon was telephoning to ask Cocteau to write an article about Piaf for the literary weekly, *Les Lettres Françaises*. As Dermit was explaining that his friend was too ill to speak,

Cocteau reached over to take the phone. Sharp pains jabbed through his chest, the blood-tinged froth of pulmonary edema bubbled from his nose and mouth and he began to choke. By the time the doctor and the curé arrived Jean Cocteau was dead.

On Monday, 14 October, his friends came to pay their respects. The dead man, dressed in black, Academic sword beside him, was wearing the red cravat of the Légion d'Honneur. His two-cornered hat lay at his feet and his once-expressive, long-fingered hands were folded across his breast. The last letters addressed to him lay unopened on a side table and the calendar had been left at the date of his death. The room was filled with roses and gladioli. A huge bouquet from the actor and singer Maurice Chevalier was inscribed "To the One and Only."

Cocteau had wished to be buried in his garden, but this was not permitted. On 15 October he lay in state at the *mairie* (town hall) at Milly, and next day villagers, relatives, friends, and representatives of the Government, the French and Belgian academies, and the Comédie Française were present when he was buried in the churchyard of Saint-Blaise-des-Simples at Milly.

In 1958 Cocteau had decorated the tiny twelfth-century chapel with drawings of tall medicinal herbs and scenes of the Resurrection. On 24 April 1964 his body was moved from the churchyard into the quiet chapel and covered by a great stone slab inscribed in his own handwriting, "Je reste avec vous," above the star he always appended to his signature.

Cole, Nat "King" (1919-1965)

The black U.S. balladeer with the husky voice lost much weight in September 1964 while commuting between Hollywood, where he was making *Cat Ballou*, and a nightclub act at Lake Tahoe. Two months later a searing chest pain hit him while onstage at the Sands Hotel in Las Vegas. He was diagnosed as having lung cancer and was taken to St. John's Hospital in Santa Monica, California, in December; his wife Maria and their five children spent Christmas Day with him there. Some days he would be well enough to play the piano in the hospital auditorium, and would scold the audience if he saw them smoking, reminding them he had been a three-pack-a-day man himself. The diseased left lung was removed on 25 January 1965, but it was soon evident that the liver was involved.

On St. Valentine's Day he felt able to enjoy a drive along the coast. He declined a wheelchair on his return and walked back into the hospital. That night he was restless and asked several times for "Skeez." The nurse was puzzled. "Who do you mean, Nat?" "Maria," he said, and never spoke again. He died at 5:30 A.M. on 15 February 1965 and was buried in Forest Lawn Memorial Park, Los Angeles.

Costello, Lou (1906-1959)

The pudgy, innocent partner of Bud Abbott (q.v.) appeared with him in thirty-six movies. He was three times laid up with rheumatic fever between 1943 and 1953. He was taken to Doctors Hospital, Beverly Hills, California, with chest pains at the end of February 1959. On 3 March, feeling much better, he sent a visitor, his manager Eddie Sherman, across the road for an ice-cream soda: "Strawberry, two scoops." Then, discussing future plans, he said, "That was the best ice cream soda I ever tasted." Moments later he fell back dead.

Abbott and his wife were watching a TV rerun of Bud and Lou's famous *Who's on First* when Sherman called them. "Why didn't someone tell me he was sick?" asked Bud tearfully. "I could have brightened him up, made him laugh." Costello was buried in Calvary Cemetery, Los Angeles. *See* Bob Thomas (1977).

Coward, Noël (1899-1973)

The seventieth birthday of Britain's wittiest playwright and entertainer was celebrated by a week-long series of his creations on BBC television. On the great day, 16 December 1969, he lunched with the queen, and a month later she made him a Knight Bachelor. His last public appearance was in January 1973, when he escorted Marlene Dietrich to a New York performance of *Oh! Coward*. Then he hurried away to the warmth of his Jamaica retreat, on the north coast at Firefly Hill near Grant's Town.

By then his health had worsened and he walked with a pronounced stoop. On his final evening, 25 March 1973, he sat on the verandah with his close friend Graham Payn and secretary-companion Cole Lesley, watching the starlings swooping in for a quick dip in the swimming pool and listening to the basso profundo croak of their friendly tree-frog Ezio (named for opera star Ezio Pinza) as lights appeared below in Port Maria. "Goodnight, my darlings," he called after his friends as they walked away down to his big house, Blue Harbor. Later, Coward read E. Nesbit's *The Enchanted Castle* and bade good night to the watchman before closing his door.

Early next morning, Imogene, wife of his servant Miguel, heard him calling for help during a heart attack in the bathroom. Miguel helped him back to bed and held his hand. Should his friends be sent for? "No, it is too early; they will still be asleep." These were his last words, not witty, just considerate, as usual. "I went on holding his hand," said Miguel, "and then he gave a little sigh and died."

His grave is in a spacious underground room dug by his servants on Firefly Hill; it has white walls and is topped by elegant white lattice work.

Crane, Stephen (1871-1900)

The U.S. novelist, short-story writer and journalist is best remembered for *The Red Badge of Courage* (1895) in which, without any firsthand knowledge, he graphically evoked the Civil War. It was around the time of the novel's publication that he conducted his "experiment in misery," living with the downtrodden in New York's Bowery, and soon thereafter his friends observed a hollow cough that shook his slender frame.

He settled in England in 1897 with his common-law wife Cora Taylor Stewart; they were both hopelessly improvident and were soon deeply in debt. The following year he reported on the war in Cuba and returned with malaria added to his tuberculosis. Destitute, Crane wrote frantically for magazines in 1899 to earn a little money. Yet they had rented an enormous manor house, Brede Place in Sussex, and here they threw a magnificent year-end party. After the host fainted on the shoulder of a guest and vomited blood, another guest, the writer H. G. Wells, cycled seven miles to Rye to fetch a doctor.

In April 1900 Crane suffered hemorrhages twice more and, though the twenty-eight-year-old was weakened by a rectal abscess and a recurrence of malaria and eager to die at home, Cora insisted on a journey to Baden-weiler in the Black Forest in a futile search for a cure. It was there, in southeast Germany, that he died quietly after a final severe hemorrhage, in a morphine-induced coma at 3:00 A.M., 5 June 1900. Despite the great expense of the journey, Cora brought her husband's body back to England and then, aboard the liner *Bremen*, to New York. He was buried beside his family in the Evergreen Cemetery at Hillside, New Jersey. Cora, aged forty-six, died in Jackson, Florida, 4 September 1910, after helping push a stranded automobile out of the sand.

Crawford, Joan (1906-1977)

The U.S. movie star was instantly recognizable, possessing—with Garbo, Dietrich, and Swanson—what someone called one of the "four fabulous faces." Though small (four feet four and a half inches), she carried herself imperially. "I never even slump mentally," she said. "She created herself," said columnist Louella Parsons. She won an Oscar for *Mildred Pierce* (1945); the last of her eighty-one films was *Trog* (1970) and she made her final appearance in September 1972 in an episode of NBC television's *The Sixth Sense*. Her fourth and final marriage (1955–59) was to the Pepsi-Cola executive Alfred N. Steele.

She worked tirelessly for Pepsi after Steele's death until her involuntary retirement in 1973. Her relations with the two eldest of her four adopted children were always strained. A year before her death she wrote in her will: "It is my intention to make no provision herein for my son Christopher or my daughter Christina for reasons which are well known to them." (Christina was to write a devastating best-seller, *Mommie Dearest*, about their tempestuous life together.)

Crawford's last years were spent quietly in her Manhattan apartment at 150 East 69th Street; dining regularly at "21" but returning home by 10:00 P.M. She was happy to welcome visits from old friends and spent hours each day writing notes to friends and loyal fans and to television actors whose performances she admired. For years she had been a heavy drinker of 100-proof vodka, but now, after returning to her old faith, Christian Science, she quit drinking and smoking. Her only companions were a housekeeper, her dog Princess and a longtime admirer from Brooklyn who ran errands.

Early in 1977, Joan Crawford's health declined dramatically and a hospital bed was installed in her apartment. Her back ached constantly and her weight fell to eighty-five pounds. Though probably suffering from cancer of the liver and pancreas she angrily rejected medical aid. "I'll be damned if I let myself end up in a cold hospital room with a tube up my nose and another up my ass." On the morning of 10 May 1977 she got up and made breakfast for her two companions, then returned to bed to watch soap operas. Suddenly she died; the medical examiner certified the cause of death as coronary occlusion (blockage of a vital artery by a blood clot). Her ashes were placed next to Steele's at a cemetery in Ferncliff, New York. *See* Bob Thomas (1978).

Crosby, Bing (1903-1977)

America's singing superstar made more than seventy movies and sold half-a-billion recordings of over sixteen hundred songs in his long career. His genial on-stage persona belied his true character; many regarded him as an unhappy, tightfisted man, a near-alcoholic, neglectful as a husband, faithless as a friend. Only once, when he went off on a leisurely trip to Europe in 1952 while his first wife Dixie Lee was widely known to be dying of cancer, did the world glimpse a contradiction of what it thought it knew.

In January 1974 a fast-growing benign tumor of Crosby's left lung was excised. On 3 March 1977, while taping a television program commemorating his fiftieth anniversary in show business, he fell into a twenty-foot-deep orchestra pit at the Ambassador Auditorium in Pasadena, California, and ruptured a disc in his lower spine.

A two-week engagement at the London Palladium ended on 10 October 1977. Just four days later he was playing a round at the La Moralejo Golf Club near Madrid when he collapsed at the seventeenth green. At first his partners believed he had slipped and fallen, but he was victim to a massive heart attack and was pronounced dead at Madrid's Red Cross Hospital. After an autopsy Crosby's body was brought home by his nineteen-year-old son Harry Jr. and his English butler Alan Fisher. A private unannounced Catholic service in Westwood, Los Angeles, was followed by burial five miles away in Holy Cross Cemetery, Culver City, next to Dixie Lee. All the surrounding spaces were occupied, but he left instructions for his grave to be excavated extra deep so that his second wife Kathryn, if she wished, could be laid above him. *See* Donald Shepherd and Robert E. Slatzer (1981).

Davis, Bette (1908-1989)

The U.S. movie actress was nominated a record ten times for Academy Awards and won twice, for *Dangerous* (1935) and *Jezebel* (1938). She earned the reputation of being a fighter with directors and studio bosses; in her last years her frustration and belligerence were turned on her fellow players.

It was in her early seventies that she moved from New England to settle in West Hollywood, near the pink mausoleum in Forest Lawn Memorial Park where her mother Ruth and sister Barbara ("Bobbie") already lay. The move, she said, would relieve anyone of having to make "that long trip across the country with me." All the same, she meant to work until the end: "Work is my morale source . . . and work keeps me from thinking too much."

In 1982 the actress starred in *A Piano for Mrs. Cimino,* a television movie about a spunky old woman who, declared mentally incompetent at her children's behest, successfully fights back. It was typecasting with a vengeance and was thought by many to be Davis's best performance in her last decade. In April 1983, while filming the television series *Hotel,* she was found to be suffering from breast cancer and a circulatory dysfunction. She withdrew from the series, returned to the East and after a mastectomy spent several weeks in New York Hospital. Owing, perhaps, to the effects of a series of three minor strokes, she heaped such abuse and obscenities on the staff that some therapists refused to go near her.

Back home in Los Angeles, Davis fell and fractured her hip. Late in 1984 she was in London for five weeks making *Murder with Mirrors,* an Agatha Christie mystery due to be telecast the following year. The anger she directed against fellow veterans caused even the gentle-natured Helen Hayes to say afterward that Davis "seemed determined to make life difficult for us all." Hayes asked another colleague, John Mills, how he'd gotten along with Bette. "I was never so scared in my life," he replied. "And I was in the war." In 1987 Davis filmed the slow-moving movie *The Whales of August* with Lillian Gish, during which, Hayes reported, Bette made "mincemeat out of poor Lillian, . . . [who] swears she'll never act again."

Davis had extensive dental surgery in 1988, after which her weight fell further, from eighty-eight to seventy-five pounds; she dropped out of the filming of *Wicked Stepmother* (1989) pleading ill health and complaining that director Larry Cohen made her look terrible. Roles began to dry up, but honors kept rolling in—from New York's Film Society of Lincoln Center, the American Cinema Awards in Hollywood, and finally the San Sebastian International Film Festival in September 1989. By then her breast cancer had spread; leaving Spain she stopped over in Paris on 3 October and there suddenly collapsed. Her young secretary-companion Kathryn Sermak rushed her to the American Hospital in suburban Neuilly-sur-Seine and she died there late on 6 October 1989.

In Bette Davis's heyday a director had said her epitaph should read, "She did it the hard way!" But there is no epitaph at all on the pink marble sarcophagus, where she joined her mother and sister after a service conducted by a minister of the First Christian Church in North Hollywood. A memorial service was held later on a Warner Brothers sound stage.

The name of Barbara ("B.D.") Hyman, Davis's only biological child, is omitted from her will; so is that of Margot Merrill, her mentally retarded adopted daughter. The estate, valued at up to $1 million, was divided between Davis's adopted son Michael Merrill and her companion Kathryn Sermak. *See* Lawrence Quirck (1990).

Delius, Frederick (1862-1934)

The British composer is best remembered today for descriptive orchestral pieces, such as *Brigg Fair* (1901) and *On Hearing the First Cuckoo in Spring* (1912), the latter inspired by birdsong in his garden at Grez-sur-Loing, twenty-five miles south of Paris, where he lived the second half of his life.

A vigorous, athletic man until his forties, he began to complain of violent headaches and back pains during an English trip in 1910. In 1921 his worsening health became suddenly alarming: an unsteady gait, uncertain use of his hands, and blurring of vision. By 1924 he was confined to a wheelchair, completely blind. With an undimmed mind imprisoned in a paralyzed body, Delius endured several years of misery. The only bright spots were his music, which in the 1920s was achieving popularity, and musician visitors who called on him at Grez, including Percy Grainger (q.v.), who brought his Swedish bride and the latest musical tidings.

This dismal period ended when in 1928 a twenty-two-year-old fellow-Yorkshireman, Eric Fenby, wrote to the composer out of the blue, offering to take down his music by dictation; for the rest of Delius's life—except for a short period—the young man acted, not without much frustration and discouragement, as an unpaid amanuensis. Delius's wife Jelka Rosen encouraged him: "Stand up to him and I will stand by you." The old man was unaware that he sang in a monotone and could not give a direct indication of melodies. He would shout out the rhythms: "Tar—tar, tar, tar." "Now, on the fifth beat, change the chord; A's to B's and D's to fifths (F sharp, C sharp) and come back to the same position of the D major chord at the next bar . . ."

In a 1980 medical study, S. F. Wainapel surveys the available biographical information. Delius probably contracted syphilis before the turn of the century in Paris, where the disease was rampant. "The visual and neurological symptoms . . . can be explained on the basis of the late manifestation of neurosyphilis, specifically tabes dorsalis . . . Dementia paralytica seems ruled out by the lack of any mental changes . . . ." "He was," writes Wainapel, "a totally dependent quadriplegic man," but Fenby's descriptions of how, when working on a new composition, he was transformed from a slumped figure into an upright one, gesticulating like a pugilist, "demonstrate that he had considerable residual motor functions in his limbs, but lacked fine motor control and coordination."

. In his last days his wife was taken to the hospital suffering from terminal cancer. For many hours every day Fenby read to the dying composer from Mark Twain's novels. Jelka was able to come home and rest in another room as Fenby tended to her husband. He died, heavily sedated with morphine, at 4:00 A.M. on 10 June 1934. After a death mask and cast of Delius's right hand had been made, his coffin was laid in a temporary grave in the village cemetery.

The following May, Frederick Delius was laid permanently to rest in his native England at Limpsfield, near Oxted, Surrey, where the cellist Beatrice Harrison had promised to tend his grave. The interment took place privately at midnight. At the public funeral service on 24 May 1935, Sir Thomas Beecham conducted some of Delius's shorter orchestral pieces. Jelka Rosen Delius lacked the strength to reach Limpsfield; she died two days later in London.

Diaghilev, Sergei Pavlovich (1872-1929)

The dynamic Russian who introduced modern ballet to the world in 1909 was an imposing figure with a large head and an expressive face, but during his final year he had difficulty maintaining his dignified appearance. The ravages of untreated diabetes were evident; he had lost much weight, his face was ashen, his eyes sunken, and running sores covered much of his body. (Insulin was not yet generally available.)

After the Covent Garden season he traveled alone to Venice and took a fifth-floor room at the Hôtel des Baines de Mer on the Lido. When his young secretary Boris Kochno arrived in response to urgent summonses on the sixteenth he found Diaghilev in mercurial mood, first anguished by his physical deterioration, later exhilarated by visits from Coco Chanel and his dearest woman friend Misia Sert. Throughout the night of 17 August Kochno was kept busy opening and closing windows as his master alternately sweated and shivered. At dawn, murmuring "Forgive me," he fell asleep.

By midnight on the eighteenth Diaghilev's temperature had risen to at least 105° and he gasped for breath. Misia hurried over and summoned a Catholic priest. When the labored breathing finally ceased it was 6:00 A.M. on 19 August 1929. As the sun's first rays touched the dying man's face his head fell sideways and a tear rolled down his cheek. Next day, after a Greek Orthodox service at the Church of St. George the Greek, the coffin was placed on a funeral barge and, followed by many gondolas bearing mourners, was taken to the cemetery on the island of San Michele.

Dietrich, Marlene (1901-1992)

The German-born U.S. actress and singer was viewed throughout her long life as a timeless symbol on stage and screen of romantic sophistication.

Approaching sixty, she broke her shoulder when she fell off the stage during a German tour. As she filmed her last important screen role in *Judgment at Nuremberg* (1961) she was suffering from a circulatory ailment, Buerger's disease, brought on by four decades of heavy smoking. Perfection of figure was aided by support garments; surgical needles to which her hair was braided were embedded in her scalp to pull her face taut. Throughout her sixties she maintained her concert schedule. Though cervical cancer was diagnosed in early 1965 and a series of radium implants was necessary, Marlene was well enough to open her own sellout Broadway show in October 1967.

In her last years she gave up smoking, but, "Without her cigarettes she was odious," recalled her secretary-companion Bernard Hall. "She loved being around smokers for the second-hand smoke and encouraged everybody else to puff themselves to death." She fell from the stage again, this time in Washington, D.C., in late 1973; her left thigh was torn open on a protruding nail, but, stitched and bandaged, she soldiered on until complications set in. Bypass surgery on the leg to aid circulation and skin grafts to heal the thigh wound were performed in Houston. She fell in her Paris apartment in August 1974 and broke her right hip; flown to New York, she had a steel pin inserted. The following month, with the aid of her iron will and a wheelchair to bring her to the wings, she was able to walk onstage in London as scheduled, exhibiting only a slight limp.

In September 1975, during an Australian tour, Marlene Dietrich's stage career came to a sudden end. Favoring her right hip as she stepped onstage in Sydney, her "good" left leg, the one that had merely been torn, "bypassed," and skin-grafted, snapped under her. For months, encased in plaster, she proved to be an insufferable patient in New York's Columbia-Presbyterian Medical Center as her compound fracture slowly healed. Shortly after she was released she heard, while recuperating in Paris in June 1976, that her husband of fifty-three years, Rudolf Sieber, had died in California. Though they were rarely together, he was said to be the only one of her many lovers she had really respected. The news was a shattering blow: "I can't go on," she said.

However, she appeared before the cameras one last time, in the West German movie *Just a Gigolo* (1978). Heavily made up, she sang the title song in the inimitable sultry Dietrich style. News emerged late in 1979 from her Avenue Montaigne apartment that she had fallen yet again, breaking her left thigh once more. Sitting at home in a wheelchair, she was interviewed by Maximilian Schell over several days for her last film, *Marlene: A Feature*. It was a retrospective of her movie career that premiered in West Berlin in February 1984 and was a major attraction at the New York Film Festival in September 1986. The stubborn octogenarian refused to appear on camera, but her cranky, shrewd comments delighted theater audiences.

Marlene was now broke. While awaiting money from the movie she was served with an eviction order for nonpayment of rent. The French government, who regarded her by this time almost as a national monument, stepped in, promoted her from Chevalier to Commandeur of the Légion d'Honneur and picked up the tab. When another leg wound in October 1986 threatened her privacy she refused to leave home and had it sewn up on the spot.

Her ninetieth birthday was hailed with great enthusiasm in her newly united native land; across Germany her films and recordings were aired for over a week. She had told Schell that "one should be afraid of life, not death." But, though life had indeed wounded her, she was too proud ever to show it. To the end she maintained the legend she had worked so sedulously to create. As for the future, she told her 1992 biographer Steven Bach that she was, perhaps, "just jealous that I can't believe in an afterlife. . . If it were true, Rudi would be there, and would give me a message." For five years she never left her room. It was rumored that she stopped eating several days before the end.

She died quietly on 6 May 1992 as posters in the fashionable avenue below announced the opening of the Cannes Film Festival the following day, this year to be dedicated to her. Funeral services in central Paris at the Église de la Madeleine, with the French tricolor draped over her coffin, were followed by a flight to Berlin with the Stars and Stripes, the banner of her adopted country, covering her. Finally, with the unified Germany's red, gold, and black flag over the casket, she was lowered into a grave in Friedenau Cemetery in her native Berlin suburb of Schöneberg, beside her mother Josephine, who had died in 1945. The Lutheran minister who conducted the graveside service lamented the widespread misunderstanding many Germans had for the dead woman's long exile and renunciation of German citizenship. The Green party and other liberal groups applauded her anti-Nazi stand, but after opposition from rightist circles a gala tribute at a Berlin theater was canceled.

Dillinger, John (1903-1934?)

According to the Federal Bureau of Investigation, its Public Enemy No. 1 was gunned down by three agents as he left the Biograph Theater on Chicago's Lincoln Avenue on 22 July 1934. The Bureau had been tipped off by a Romanian-born whorehouse madam, Ana Cumpanis, who went by the name Anna Sage and who was fighting deportation. It was to evade this fate and claim the ten-thousand-dollar reward that she turned in her new friend, who was known to her as Jimmy Lawrence. Dillinger, who in less than a year had led his gang in a dozen bank robberies and escaped prison three times, left the movie theater around 10:30 P.M. with Anna and a woman friend after seeing *Manhattan Melodrama*. With half-a-dozen FBI men closing in on him, Dillinger dodged into an alley and reached for his pistol. Three agents fired, hitting the gangster in the neck and face and wounding two women bystanders. He died on the way to a hospital.

His body was put on display at the morgue and thousands filed past. After burial at Crown Hill Cemetery, Mooresville, Indiana, the dead man's father had the soil surrounding the coffin removed and cement, mixed with scrap iron, poured over and around it to discourage souvenir hunters.

Jay Robert Nash, in his *Dillinger Dossier* (1983), advances the claim that a genuine Jimmy Lawrence, who resembled Dillinger, was the victim of the ambush; that no adequate identification of the corpse was conducted (except by Dillinger's sister, who had good reason to aid her brother's escape); that the dead man had brown eyes, not the blue (or gray) recorded in the FBI's dossier; that the Bureau virtually executed their unarmed quarry after he fell in the alley (the Colt automatic he supposedly carried was not put on sale for the first time until five months after the ambush); that the genuine Dillinger was spirited away by a fellow criminal, J. H. "Blackie"

Audett, who in 1979 admitted to driving him as far as an Indian reservation at Hoopa, California; and that he was quite likely still alive forty-five years after his escape.

Nash provides autopsy records as well as several photographs of the living Dillinger and the corpse (and a 1963 snapshot of a man claiming to be Dillinger) by means of which the curious may attempt a judgment.

Dinesen, Isak (1885-1962)

The Danish writer was born Karen Dinesen and by her 1913 marriage became the Baroness Blixen-Finecke; as her pen name she adopted the male pseudonym Isak Dinesen, but her tombstone bears the name Karen Blixen. She was married as she and her husband Bror arrived in Africa, where they had bought land in Kenya for coffee cultivation. Within a year the Baron was notorious for his affairs with the wives of fellow planters and with local Masai women in Nairobi, among whom syphilis was rife. He soon transmitted the disease to Karen, who showed the first symptoms in 1914. During her infrequent visits to Europe she was treated with the new arsenical drug arsphenamine, but she was never cured. In later life she suffered greatly from the tertiary form of syphilis, involving the spinal cord, known as tabes dorsalis or locomotor ataxia, which in her case was localized to the sensory nerves from the digestive organs. Though she was stoical by nature, agonizing cramps often forced her to slip from her chair and writhe on the floor, howling like an animal. She gradually lost her appetite and fell below a body weight of seventy pounds. Surgery in 1946 and 1955 to sever pain tracts in the spine was ineffective and by 1961 she was unable to walk or stand without assistance.

By 1924 she was divorced. The story of her long love affair with the aristocratic Denys Finch Hatton is told in her *Out of Africa* (1937), filmed in 1985 with Robert Redford oddly miscast as her English lover. Hatton, a confirmed bachelor, died when his plane crashed in 1931 around the time she sold the farm and returned to Denmark. Thereafter she gained a reputation, in her *Seven Gothic Tales* (1934) and later works, as a master storyteller.

In the summer of 1962, holding court on her verandah and almost wasted away, she looked, she said, "like the most horrid old witch, a real Memento Mori." Visitors were shown the spot up the hill she had chosen for her burial place. On 6 September she felt very sleepy; she died of emaciation on the evening of 7 September 1962 at her home, Rungstedlund, on the coast of Zeeland, Denmark, fifteen miles north of Copenhagen. *See* Judith Thompson (1982).

Disraeli, Benjamin (1804-1881)

Britain's enigmatic prime minister (1868, 1874–1880) and novelist was of Italian-Jewish origin; only his baptism at the age of twelve permitted his parliamentary career. He outgrew his raffish youth to attain the highest office in the land and the friendship of the queen, who made him the first Earl of Beaconsfield in 1876. Between Victoria and her first minister a close relationship developed during his six-year administration. Though grounded in mutual self-interest, it was nonetheless sincerely felt on both sides. The sovereign was Dizzy's masterpiece, his Faerie Queene, transformed by his sound counsel and evident esteem from an insecure, hypochondriacal widow, helpless without her beloved Albert, into a confident, self-assertive ruler, restored to sound health. So it was that, when the Tory government was unexpectedly overwhelmed by W. E. Gladstone's Liberals in the April 1880 elections, the blow to Victoria was severe. Her favorite's downfall, she assured herself, was entirely due to the Scots rhetorician's vicious slanders, and for some time she could not face the prospect of sending for him to form a government.

Until Disraeli's death a year later, the queen wrote to him in secret, signing herself, "Ever your affectionate and grateful friend V.R.I." From time to time he dined with her at Windsor. In retirement at Hughenden Manor, twelve miles north of Windsor, he completed his novel *Endymion* and began another. His old enemies, gout, asthma, and bronchitis, renewed their attacks on his stooping body. Returning to his London home at 19 Curzon Street on 19 March he caught a chill and took to his bed. Victoria's final letter of 5 April to "Dearest Lord Beaconsfield" accompanied "a few of your favourite spring flowers" from the castle grounds. He maintained an ironic detachment from his physical dissolution. It was suggested he might welcome a personal visit from the queen. "No," he replied, "it is better not. She would only ask me to take a message to Albert." Terrible fits of coughing weakened him; as the kidneys failed, uremic poisoning clouded his mind. His last recorded words were: "I had rather live, but I am not afraid to die."

He remained in a coma throughout Easter Monday, 18 April 1881. Just after 4:15 A.M. on the nineteenth the dying man half-lifted himself from the pillows and leaned forward in the gesture he had adopted so often in addressing Parliament. His lips moved, but no sound came. He sank back and died ten minutes later at 4:30 A.M.

The queen was desolated and could hardly see to write to his devoted secretary, Montagu Corry, "for my fast falling tears." Gladstone suggested burial in Westminster Abbey, but Disraeli, following the wish expressed by his wife Mary Anne, who had died nine years before at the age of eighty, left instructions that he be laid beside her in Hughenden Church. Victoria was prevented by protocol from attending the funeral; she sent three of her sons and two wreaths of primroses. (The protocol was not breached until 1965, when Elizabeth II attended Sir Winston Churchill's funeral service in St. Paul's Cathedral.) Victoria made a pilgrimage to Hughenden four days after the interment and instructed that an enormous marble tablet be erected above his seat in the chancel. Upon it are engraved the words: THIS MEMORIAL IS PLACED BY HIS GRATEFUL SOVEREIGN AND FRIEND, VICTORIA R. I. KINGS LOVE HIM THAT SPEAKETH RIGHT, a quotation from Proverbs. *See* Robert Blake, *Disraeli* (1966).

Donne, John (1572-1631)

The literary reputation of the English poet and cleric, dean of St. Paul's Cathedral, London, has burgeoned in the present century after three centuries of eclipse. He was a witty man of an essentially melancholic turn of mind, much preoccupied with his health and frequently examining his urine and checking his pulse. His most-quoted words (" . . . and therefore never send to know for whom the bell tolls; it tolls for Thee") came from his finest prose piece, *Devotions upon Emergent Occasions* (1624), in which he set down recollections of his recent near-fatal attack of "spotted fever," questioning, well in advance of his time, such procedures as purging. The nature of this illness is mysterious, but W. B. Ober in a 1990 study agrees with an earlier physician, Clara Lander, in diagnosing it as most probably "epidemic louse-borne typhus fever "

In January 1631 Donne complained of a cough, toothache, and deafness, but his death just two months later was possibly caused by cancer of the stomach. As his end approached it is said he posed for his monument by standing on an urn in his shroud while an artist sketched him life-size on a wooden plank, but this report (by Sir Izaak Walton) has been questioned. Those who heard him deliver his final sermon on 12 February 1631 declared him to be obviously dying. In his last hour on 31 March he said, "I were miserable if I might not die," and murmured repeatedly, "Thy kingdom come, Thy will be done," until he breathed no more. He had so disposed his hands and body that they "required not the least alteration by those who came to shroud him."

The monument, of black and white marble, was completed by Nicholas Stone in November 1632; in the great fire of 1666 the cathedral was demolished, only Donne's memorial emerging intact. When Sir Christopher Wren's masterpiece was completed, the monument was erected again as near to the original site as possible.

Eastman, George (1854-1932)

The U.S. inventor of the dry photographic plate introduced the Kodak camera in 1884. By the time Kodacolor arrived in 1928, the multimillionaire had gained a virtual monopoly of the photographic industry in America. His philanthropy was impressive; he gave away $80 million, more than half his fortune, during his life, the University of Rochester and the Massachusetts Institute of Technology being the chief beneficiaries. He lived with his mother until her death in 1907 and never married.

Late in 1930, Eastman at seventy-six noted the first signs of degeneracy of the lower spinal cord, which soon led to a slow shuffling walk. Specialists confirmed what he had suspected: that the disease was progressive. By then it was observed that he had to lean against the wall as he approached the elevators at his office in downtown Rochester, New York. One day he said to his physician, Dr. A. D. Stewart, "Audley, you're always fooling around with that stethoscope. Just where is my heart? Outline it for me." He did so, thumping Eastman's chest professionally with his fingers.

In March 1932 Eastman revised his will, leaving nearly all his remaining assets to the University of Rochester. Sometime during the revision, which required several days, he hid a Luger automatic pistol in a desk drawer in his bedroom, and a spare behind some books nearby. On Saturday the twelfth he left his mansion at what is now 900 East Avenue for a last drive around the University campus and the fifty-five-acre Kodak Park. Two days later several witnesses, all from the Kodak Company, came to his room for the signing of the will. He seemed in the best of humors, joking about his malfunctioning fountain pen. The witnesses left and his secretary, Mrs. Alice Hutchison, was sent to the bank to obtain twenty-dollar gold pieces to reward them. Puzzled, she retraced her steps; her employer's usual fee was ten dollars. As she half-opened the bedroom door, Eastman turned sharply. "What is it?" he snapped, but relaxed when Mrs. Hutchison asked her question. "That's right," he replied; twenty dollars was correct. The moment he was alone again he calmly scribbled a short note with his balky pen:

> To my friends
> My work is done. Why wait?
> G.E.

He then replaced the cap on the pen, put down in an ashtray his cigarette in its black and gold holder, and removed his glasses. Taking the pistol from the drawer, he lay on his bed, placed a wet towel over his chest, probably to prevent powder burns, turned the muzzle of the gun to the spot his doctor had indicated and pulled the trigger.

At the sound of the report, Stewart and the nurses rushed to Eastman's room and found him dead. The note was on his night table; beside it was his mother's sewing basket containing two of her gloves rolled up in little balls.

It was a few minutes after noon on 14 March 1932. During the last hour of trading on Wall Street news of Eastman's death caused Eastman Kodak shares to drop from 78¼ to 73, though the fact it was a suicide was withheld until after the close of business.

The funeral took place without eulogies, as the dead man had wished, at St. Paul's Episcopal Church, Rochester. Loudspeakers carried the service to a crowd of five thousand outside and it was also broadcast. Production was halted at the Kodak factory and classes were suspended at the University and at the Eastman School of Music. The philanthropist's ashes were buried beside the graves of his parents at his native Waterville, near Utica, New York. *See* Roger Butterfield: "The Prodigious Life of George Eastman" in *Life*, 26 April 1954.

Eddy, Mary Baker (1821-1910)

The founder of Christian Science moved to her final home at Chestnut Hill, near Boston, Massachusetts, in January 1908 after discovering her life to be endangered in her native New Hampshire by "malicious animal magnetism." This evil influence, she was convinced, had killed her third husband,

Asa Gilbert Eddy, in 1882. Embarrassed because, although by now a famous healer, she had failed to save him, she had at first ascribed his death to arsenic poisoning by unnamed enemies, but no trace of arsenic was found at autopsy.

During her eighties many adulatory articles about Mrs. Eddy were published, but also growing criticism, including a book by Mark Twain in 1907 and a well-documented series in *McClure's Magazine* the same year. The psychoanalyst Julius Silberger Jr. in his 1980 biography says, "the writers of the *McClure's* series felt that Mrs. Eddy was a talented and impressive mistress of humbuggery." Nevertheless her admirable fortitude, inventiveness, and determination were a model for other women during a period when their options in life were severely limited. Silberger concludes,

> Many religions have been founded by troubled visionaries . . .[who] left to others the task of organizing, giving structure, writing the books, establishing the ceremonies and rules of membership, struggling with the rebels, and preserving the memory of the founder. Mary Baker Eddy did all of it herself, working purposefully into her eighty-ninth year . . .

In her Chestnut Hill mansion Mrs. Eddy ordered the founding of the *Christian Science Monitor*. When, in 1909, a threat to her dominance appeared in the person of Mrs. Augusta E. Stetson, founder and leader of the Church of Christ, Scientist in New York City, she was disciplined by the Mother Church in Boston (for using "absent treatment" on her enemies with intent to harm them) and expelled by her own church.

Mrs. Eddy's great support in her final twenty-eight years was Calvin Frye, twenty-four years her junior, who devoted himself to her interests singlemindedly. He tolerated her frequent temper tantrums and soothed her in the wee hours when nightmares and "malicious mesmeric influences" threatened her with suffocation. As her strength gradually waned she begged Frye to record, if she should die from natural causes, that she had been "mentally murdered" by malicious animal magnetism.

She died at home on 3 December 1910 of pneumonia. The next day, Sunday, the First Reader at the Christian Science service simply announced that she had passed from earthly sight. There was a modest funeral, but burial in Mount Auburn Cemetery had to await the construction of an appropriate tomb. The *Monitor* published eulogies from other newspapers and an account of her funeral, but nothing directly about her death. Because the Christian Science Publishing Company trustees were not identical with the Church's board of directors, a lengthy power struggle began in the courts.

Frye, threatened with loss of his position, reminded the authorities that he knew many secrets better left untold; he was kept at the Chestnut Hill mansion and provided with a generous pension. On his deathbed a few years later he disowned the Church.

Edward VII (1841-1910)

The eldest son of Queen Victoria did not succeed his mother until he was fifty-nine years old. He was an affable man-about-town with a taste for personal diplomacy on his country's behalf. At the end of April 1910 he traveled from London to the royal residence at Sandringham in Norfolk and, though the weather was cold and wet, attended the village church and inspected his home farm and pedigree stock. He was coughing and wheezing on his return to Buckingham Palace on 2 May. Though he dined out that evening, he spent a wretched night with severe bronchial spasms; yet his doctors were unable to keep him in bed. Queen Alexandra, returning from a Greek vacation on the fifth, found her husband hunched in a chair, gray and exhausted, barely able to utter a word.

After lunch next day the king collapsed; a series of heart attacks followed and he fought for breath. Still he resisted orders to lie down. Morphine was given; as he lost consciousness he murmured, "I shall not give in. I shall work to the end." In a compassionate gesture the queen summoned Mrs. Alice Keppel, the dying man's mistress since 1898, to make her farewells. Only in his final minutes was Edward lifted onto his bed. The Archbishop of Canterbury said the Commendatory prayers and, at 11:45 P.M. on 6 May 1910, the king ceased to breathe.

The body was left undisturbed for a week while old friends came by. One of them wrote, "No appearance of pain or death. There was even a glow on his face and the usual happy smile of the dead who die peacefully."

A half-million of his subjects filed past the king's catafalque while he lay in state in Westminster Abbey. In the parade to Paddington Station on 20 May, Edward's terrier Caesar followed behind the gun carriage that bore the corpse. At Windsor the carriage was hauled by one hundred Royal Navy midshipmen up the hill to St. George's Chapel. Toward the close of the funeral service the coffin was lowered into the Chancel Crypt below.

Eichmann, Adolf (1906-1962)

The Nazi war criminal escaped to Argentina in 1949 and lived in Buenos Aires under the name Ricardo Klement. Returning from his work at the Mercedes-Benz factory on 11 May 1960 he was captured by Israeli agents near his dismal home in the San Fernando district and flown in a drugged state via a West African country to Israel in the guise of a wealthy invalid.

In 1961 Eichmann sat throughout his four-month trial in Jerusalem behind bulletproof glass. The evidence clearly showed he had displayed fanatical zeal in rounding up every last Jewish man, woman, and child and shipping them off to their deaths. He was found guilty of crimes against the Jewish people and against humanity and, on 13 December 1961, was sentenced to death. In dismissing his claim that he acted only under orders, the appellate court on 29 May 1962 responded, "He *acts,* and his superiors *understand* and *assent.*" On the evening of 31 May Israel's President Yitzhak Ben Zvi rejected his mercy plea.

For this, the first execution in modern Israel, a third-floor room in Ramla prison had been converted. Eichmann was led to the trapdoor at 11:50 P.M. on the thirty-first. Refusing a hood, he addressed the assembled witnesses and officials; he said they would soon meet again and that he died believing in God. "Long live Germany . . . Argentina . . . Austria . . . I greet my wife, my family and my friends. I had to obey the rules of war and my flag." A noose was placed around Eichmann's neck; three men, screened by blankets, each pulled a lever. One was a dummy; the others shot the two bolts of the trapdoor. At 11:58 Eichmann was pronounced dead. The body was cremated three hours later and the ashes were scattered outside Haifa harbor. *See* Moshe Pearlman (1963).

Elgar, Sir Edward (1857-1934)

The English composer, generally regarded as the greatest in the land since Henry Purcell (1659–1695), produced all his most significant works in just twenty of his seventy-seven years, beginning with the *Enigma Variations* (1899) and concluding with the *Cello Concerto* (1919). He was a diffident, self-doubting man, married to a woman with social pretensions and too aware of his own low birth. He was self-taught and dubious of the value of his music, though in later years he could sometimes admire parts of it as though written by another. (Listening to a recording of his *Falstaff* at home, he once remarked to a visitor, "Well, that's a good bit, anyway.") He and his wife often differed (he hated city life; she loved it), yet her death in 1920 marked the end of his active career. Though much of his music is nowadays highly acclaimed, this was not so during his lifetime; when an important music handbook (by Edward J. Dent) was reissued in 1930, Elgar was given only sixteen lines, compared with the now obscure Hubert Parry's sixty-six and Charles Villiers Stanford's forty-one.

The seventy-five-year-old Elgar met the sixteen-year-old Yehudi Menuhin in 1932 to discuss the impending recording of the composer's *Violin Concerto* (1910) and was greatly impressed by the young American violinist's maturity. Moreover, "Your friendship has given me a new zest in life," said the old man later.

In August 1932 the young recording-company executive Walter Legge wrote to the composer upon hearing rumors of a *Third Symphony*; though such a symphony did not exist, Elgar in his reply equivocated and the false reports spread like wildfire. The BBC pricked up its corporate ears and offered a thousand pounds, with a further thousand in four installments over a year, as a commission for the work. Instead of "coming clean," Elgar accepted these terms in December and early the following year told the BBC he hoped "to begin scoring [the symphony] very shortly." A first broadcast was scheduled for October but was put off until May 1934.

From the testimony of friends who visited Elgar at his home, Marl Bank in Worcester, in the English Midlands, it seems certain that the symphony in 1933 existed only in short sections, and that even these derived from old notebooks. In October, as he was about to enter the South Bank Nursing Home in Worcester for surgery, he wrote to the BBC's chairman, Sir John Reith, apologizing for the holdup and offering, if the work "does not materialise the sums you have paid on account shall be returned." By that date Elgar had received all of the promised £2,000; after his death the BBC, learning that the composer had been able to leave only a meager estate to his daughter, refrained from demanding repayment.

For years, Elgar had suffered from "lumbago." It was now being referred to as sciatica and finally, after consultation of his doctor with the eminent specialist Lord Horder, as a malignant tumor pressing on the sciatic nerve. Surgery was ruled out and Elgar continued to weaken. Before losing consciousness on 20 November 1933 he begged his intimate friend W. H. "Billy" Reed not to let "anyone tinker with the symphony, all bits and pieces, no one could understand . . . I think you had better burn it." The dying man's only child Carice Blake was present, and she and Reed were both startled by the request. They did not promise to destroy the work, but undertook to see it was not "tinkered with."

Elgar unexpectedly regained strength enough to return to Marl Bank on New Year's Day 1934 and even to have his bedroom linked by telephone to a London recording studio on 22 January while extracts from his cantata *Caractacus* (1898) were played. As though there were not enough enigmas in his life and works—the two kinds of enigma in the *Variations,* the puzzle behind the *Violin Concerto*'s dedication (in Spanish): "Here is enshrined the soul of . . . ," and the ethics of his acceptance of the BBC's commission, one more was added after his death by the musicologist Ernest Newman, who saw the dying composer early in February. Many years later Newman revealed that Elgar had made a "distressing remark" that "consisted of only five words, but the scope they would give to a 'reading' of him is infinite, so I am determined to keep them to myself. They are too tragic for the ears of the mob." It is impossible now to fathom what the words might be, but in any case Elgar was far gone when he uttered them and heavily sedated with morphine.

In his final days Elgar's great pleasure lay in the phonograph. In the late 1920s, electric recording had replaced the old acoustic method in the production of 78 rpm discs, with considerable improvement in playback quality. From under his pillow on 28 January Elgar produced the music for a short piece, *Mina,* written the previous year as a tribute to his dog. A friend took it to London and by 15 February the composer was not only able to play the record in his bedroom but sufficiently roused up to make a detailed criticism of the performance.

Elgar died at 7:45 A.M. on 23 February 1934. Burial in Westminster Abbey had been suggested by Reith some weeks earlier, but the dean had refused because he understood Elgar was "a Roman." The dead man had never been clear about his religious beliefs and according to Mrs. Blake "always and emphatically expressed his wishes that there should be no memorial service." Without consulting the family, the Dean of Worcester arranged a memorial service in the cathedral there. A Low Requiem was said on 26 February in St. George's Church, Worcester, where both Elgar and his father had played the organ. The composer was then laid to rest next to Lady Alice Elgar in St. Wulstan's Roman Catholic Church in the hamlet of Little Malvern, fifteen miles south of Worcester.

Over the years since, the meager sketches for Elgar's *Third Symphony* have been repeatedly studied with the idea of their somehow being performed, if only on the piano, but such plans have all come to naught; either because in the end it was considered unethical to defy the composer's wishes, or because the sketches were too fragmentary. In 1980 a former head of music and the arts at BBC Television, Humphrey Burton, is recorded as saying, "Whatever Elgar may have told the BBC, he had not got very far with the *Third Symphony*." *See* Michael De-la-Noy (1983).

Eliot, George (1819-1880)

Mary Ann Evans was an Englishwoman who knew her own mind. She abandoned her strict evangelical upbringing, became a freethinker and traveled to London to seek her fortune. After eight years as an editor of the *Westminster Review* she published *Adam Bede* (1859) under the male pseudonym "George Eliot"; in this and later novels, including *Mill on the Floss* (1860) and *Silas Marner* (1861), she portrayed rural life in her native Warwickshire with a sharp eye for intellectual hypocrisy.

Defying the conventions, she lived with the philosopher and critic George Henry Lewes (1817–1878) from 1854 until his death. (Lewes had condoned the birth of two children to his wife by another man and under the laws of the period was thereafter prevented from seeking a divorce when she bore a third to the same father.)

Though Lewes's death in November 1878 desolated her, she determined, by the end of a year's mourning, to marry John Cross, an affectionate friend of the Leweses twenty years her junior. It seems that Mary Ann did the proposing and, though Cross was evidently a reluctant lover, they were married quietly in the fashionable St. George's Church in London's Hanover Square on 6 May 1880.

Their honeymoon tour of Europe was a disaster. Close confinement with the gaunt, gray-haired woman, up till then regarded by him as a revered mother figure, drove the bridegroom to distraction. Disturbed by signs of mental instability, Mary Ann on their arrival in Venice consulted a doctor and told him of madness in the Cross family and fears for her husband's sanity.

During the interview, Johnnie Cross leapt from the hotel balcony into the Grand Canal and, resisting his rescuers, was saved from drowning only with difficulty. (The secret of this suicide attempt was not disclosed until the seven-volume edition of George Eliot's letters, edited by Gordon S. Haight, was published in the 1950s.)

Mary Ann Evans survived the unhappy marriage by less than eight months. The Crosses lived at her country home in Witley, near Haslemere in Surrey, while a house was prepared for them at No. 4 Cheyne Walk in the Chelsea district of London. In October Mrs. Cross was abed with a kidney stone. On 3 December the couple moved into their Chelsea house and on the eighteenth attended a regular Saturday concert in St. James's Hall. That evening Mary Ann caught a chill, followed by laryngitis. At first it seemed she would recover, but a few days later she suffered a relapse. The doctor prescribed cold beef tea jelly and an egg beaten up in brandy. The patient complained of a pain over her right kidney. Early on the twenty-second Dr. Andrew Clark found her lying on her back, eyes closed, her breathing frequent but quiet, her pulse small and irregular. He later recorded that "With the stethoscope a loud to-and-fro friction was heard." Shortly before she died, at 10:00 P.M. on 22 December 1880, she whispered to Johnnie Cross, "Tell them I have a great pain in the left side." The medical report explained: "The cold had traveled down to the pericardium and complete loss of the heart supervened." In other words, George Eliot succumbed to pericarditis, inflammation of the membrane surrounding the heart.

Funeral arrangements were delayed over Christmas. Friends pressed for burial in Westminster Abbey's Poets' Corner, but the dean turned down the request. The influential T. H. Huxley, one of those whose views were sought, wrote, "George Eliot is known not only as a great writer, but as a person whose life and opinions were in notorious antagonism to Christian practice in regard to marriage, and Christian theory in regard to dogma . . . One cannot eat one's cake and have it too."

George Eliot was buried in the unconsecrated section of Highgate Cemetery in north London after a simple service in the chapel there. By skillful selection and editing of his dead wife's writings, Cross was able to publish in 1885 an account of her life from which all unpleasant and controversial matters were excluded. He lived on until 1924. *See* Ina Taylor (1989).

Eliot, Thomas Stearns (1888-1965)

Considered by many the greatest poet of his generation, T. S. Eliot was also an influential critic and editor. He was born in St. Louis, Missouri, but settled in London in 1914 and became a British citizen in 1928, the year after his baptism and confirmation in the Church of England.

Eliot's 1915 marriage to Vivien Haigh-Wood was a tragedy for both.

Friends who observed them during their eighteen years together saw her despair at being shut out from his interests, while he demonstrated what was seen as an exasperated concern for her health; she suffered a blend of physical and mental disabilities he was at a loss to deal with. An Anglo-Catholic, Tom Eliot was at once a shy man of high principles and tender conscience while yet possessing the attribute of "formidable sarcasm" (in the words of a friend) and a mind that a journalist once described as like a steel trap, "all tensile and teeth." When Vivien died in a London mental home in January 1947, fourteen years after he had legally separated from her, his guilt and horror were palpable.

Eliot's second wife Valerie Fletcher was attracted to his poetry while a fourteen-year-old Yorkshire schoolgirl. She succeeded in becoming his secretary in the offices of Faber and Faber, the London publishers, but until the moment he proposed to her she had always addressed him as "Mr. Eliot," and was not at all sure he even liked her. When they married, very quietly, in an Anglican church in Kensington in January 1957, she was thirty, and he was a sixty-eight-year-old in poor health, prone to attacks of bronchitis and emphysema (exacerbated by cigarette smoking) and suffering from congenital hernia. The marriage assured him of a happy existence during his final eight years, despite a worsening of his respiratory problems. The Eliots often escaped London's winter weather in North Africa, Jamaica, or Bermuda, and Tom's occasional lecture tours in America provided them with additional income. By the time of his last U.S. tour in November 1963, when he visited his native St. Louis and dined with the composer Igor Stravinsky in New York, he was a hunched figure, his face ashen and deeply lined. In October 1964 he collapsed in his London home, apparently from a stroke that paralyzed his left side; he spent time in the hospital in a deep coma but was allowed to return home. "Hurrah!" he exclaimed repeatedly as he was carried over the threshold. Too weak to take solid foods and continuously under an oxygen mask, he sat each day for two hours by the fire in a wheelchair while Valerie read to him or played the piano. By Christmas there seemed to be improvement, but Eliot's heart began to fail. He lapsed into a coma, becoming conscious only once as he spoke his wife's name; he died quietly on 1 January 1965.

The poet's 1984 biographer Peter Ackroyd wrote of him, "He was a strange, private and often bewildered man who was raised into a cultural guru, a representative of authority and stability."

Fawkes, Guy (1570-1606)

British children celebrate the Fifth of November ("Guy Fawkes Day"), the anniversary of the planned culmination of the Gunpowder Plot, by dragging Fawkes's effigy through the streets and begging "a penny for the guy" before burning it on a bonfire at nightfall to the accompaniment of fireworks.

The plot was led by Robert Catesby, infuriated by James I's breaking of promises of tolerance toward Roman Catholics. He schemed to kill the king, his family, the privy councilors, and members of Parliament by blowing up the House of Lords on the first day of the new session. Fawkes, a Catholic convert from Yorkshire, was recruited because of his expertise with explosives, gained during his twelve years with the Spanish army in the Netherlands. He moved a ton and a half of gunpowder to a rented coal cellar directly under the Lords on 23 March 1605 and concealed the barrels under faggots and coal.

At the end of October someone tipped off Lord Mounteagle, and on 4 November Fawkes was discovered in the cellar by the king's officers. Next day he was taken to the Tower, where he was tortured for five days before revealing the names of his accomplices. All were arrested or, like Catesby, shot in ambush. After trial and conviction by a special commission, four of the condemned men were executed in St. Paul's Churchyard on 30 January 1606. On the thirty-first Fawkes and the three remaining plotters were dragged on hurdles to the Old Palace Yard, close by the fatal cellar, and hanged amid throngs of spectators while church bells rang out. Fawkes, weakened by torture and captivity, was helped up the ladder to the noose. He knelt, crossed himself, and prayed silently before expressing regret for his treason. Although, like the others, he was cut down, castrated, drawn and quartered, he may have been lucky enough to have had his neck broken by the rope. The heads of all four men were impaled on the spikes of London Bridge. To this day a ceremonial search of the vaults is made before every session of Parliament.

Ferrier, Kathleen (1912-1953)

The greatest British contralto of her generation, a Lancashire woman of simple tastes and remarkable charm, enjoyed only a brief career before her life was cut short.

Her professional life was launched after winning an award at the Carlisle Musical Festival in 1937, and her fame grew during years of difficult wartime travel around the country. Her name was suggested to a dubious Bruno Walter in 1947 when the conductor was seeking a contralto for Mahler's *Das Lied von der Erde* at the first Edinburgh Festival. Of her audition he wrote: "She had the charm of a child and the dignity of a lady . . . I recognized with delight here was potentially one of the greatest singers of our time" with "a voice of rare beauty"; and Rudolf Bing, director of the festival, commented, "It was love at first sight." After Ferrier's death, Walter said his two greatest musical experiences were "To have known Kathleen Ferrier and Gustav Mahler, in that order."

Though fearful of breast cancer for several years, she was slow in recognizing the first sign of the disease. It was only in March 1951 that she felt a lump as she smoothed down her dress and asked her nurse-secretary Bernadine Hammond to take a look at it. Shocked, "Bernie" urged the singer to seek medical help. A mastectomy was performed on 10 April. Thereafter her life was marked by a continual series of radiation treatments and hospital stays interspersed, when she could find the strength, with concerts and recitals. Astonishingly, as her health failed her singing grew ever more glorious.

The only opera that interested her was Gluck's *Orfeo,* of which a series of four performances was planned for February 1953 at the Royal Opera House, Covent Garden, under Sir John Barbirolli's direction. By now, Kathleen's disease had metastasized to the skeleton. During the second performance, on the sixth, she felt a searing pain in her left thigh. Barely able to walk, she leaned against the scenery and in that posture sang the beautiful "Che farò" ("What is life to me without thee") over the body of Euridice (Victoria Dunne). (Moved by this beautiful lament, the God of Love restores Euridice to life.) Dunne helped Ferrier from the stage in as formal a Greek manner as she could muster and the audience remained unaware of the catastrophe. Part of the contralto's femur had separated from the shaft. After a period of off-stage vomiting from the pain, she was able, not only to complete her role but to receive the congratulations of backstage visitors before gasping, "Get me a stretcher." She spent many weeks in the hospital.

In June Ferrier's ovaries were removed in the hope that reduced estrogen levels would inhibit further spread of the cancer. In July, as a last-ditch measure, her adrenal glands were taken out. The patient's courage and resilience amazed the staff of London's University College Hospital, where a plaque now commemorates her and where in 1987 a chair in clinical oncology was established in her name. Only when her strength had gradually ebbed away did she murmur to the head nurse, Sister Rhona Phillips, "Wouldn't it be lovely if I could just go to sleep and not wake up again?"

Kathleen Ferrier, created Commander of the British Empire at the beginning of the year, died peacefully on the morning of 8 October 1953. Her body was cremated at Golders Green. The following month over a thousand admirers attended a memorial service in Southwark Cathedral, where she had so often sung in oratorios. In May 1954 a concert in her honor by the Hallé Orchestra, conducted in turn by Barbirolli and Walter, ended with the solemn prelude from Elgar's *Dream of Gerontius*. As the music died away the orchestra rose and stood with bowed heads; the audience followed suit and for two minutes the silence was absolute. Then Barbirolli quietly left the stage and the Royal Festival Hall slowly emptied. *See* Maurice Leonard (1988).

Feynman, Richard (1918-1988)

The iconoclastic U.S. physicist was something of a whiz kid at Los Alamos, New Mexico, during the construction of the first atom bomb there in World War II. From 1950 he was professor of theoretical physics at the California Institute of Technology. He shared the Nobel Prize in 1965 for discoveries in the subatomic realm of quantum electrodynamics.

When he was quite small, his father Melville, who sold uniforms, taught him to look beyond appearances and disregard titles. ("You can know the name of a bird in all the languages of the world, but when you are finished, you'll know absolutely nothing about the bird . . . So let's look at the bird and see what it's *doing*; that's what counts.") It was advice he never forgot.

In 1977 he suffered a mysterious fever while on vacation with his third wife Gwyneth in the Swiss Alps. Not until October 1978 did he have a checkup, when a malignant tumor, a rare form of cancer, was discovered at the rear of his abdomen. By the time it was removed, it weighed six pounds and had destroyed his spleen, a kidney, and an adrenal gland. In 1984 he again neglected to seek medical help after tripping and striking his head on a building. He behaved oddly for three weeks before a massive subdural hematoma was found and drained.

Feynman's favorite recreations were playing bongo drums and painting. Increasingly fascinated by thought processes, especially his own, he dabbled with what he called "antiscience"—sensory deprivation tanks and est—and experimented with hallucinatory drugs.

After the *Challenger* space shuttle exploded on 28 January 1986 with loss of the crew of eight he was asked to join the commission of inquiry; he told his caller, "You are ruining my life," meaning "I haven't much time left." By then he was afflicted with a second rare malignancy, Waldenström's macroglobulinemia, in which one type of B lymphocyte, a white blood cell, secretes a surfeit of the protein globulin, making the blood viscous, hindering the circulation and promoting clotting. The chance of anyone, in ordinary circumstances, being victim to two such unlikely cancers is vanishingly small. Could it be that their causes lay in the radioactive materials he had worked on at Los Alamos forty-odd years earlier? He had always been the most inquisitive kid on the block; at the Trinity test in July 1945 he had been the only observer to throw aside his welder's goggles and view the blinding light of the first atomic explosion with the protection only of an army vehicle's windshield. Maybe he'd been a little too curious—had gotten a little too close—on other occasions in the presence of uranium 235 or plutonium. Feynman himself refused to think about it.

Even before he arrived in Washington for the *Challenger* inquiry he suspected the O-rings, the thin rubber seals between the rocket sections designed to confine the hot propellant gases. The commission's chairman, William P. Rogers, said he would rely largely on the National Aeronautics and Space Administration's own internal investigation and did not intend "to point a finger." Irritated by Feynman's independence and irrepressible nosiness, he was soon describing him privately as "a real pain in the ass." The physicist was aware that the fatal launch took place with the air temperature at the Florida launch site near freezing, so he did a simple experiment one evening at dinner. The next day he repeated it at the hearings. With television cameras trained on him, he dipped a piece of O-ring material into a glass of ice water and demonstrated that "when you put some pressure on it for a while and then undo it it doesn't stretch back . . . I believe that has some significance for our problem." It was an old problem NASA had repeatedly ignored. Feynman declined to sign the commission's majority report, which effusively praised the space agency. His own minority findings, published as an appendix, were scathing, labeling NASA's decision making "a kind of Russian roulette."

Richard Feynman underwent surgery for another abdominal tumor in October 1987. The previous month the *Los Angeles Times* had sent him his obituary. Thanking the author, Lee Dye, Feynman wrote, "I have decided it is not a very good idea for a man to read it ahead of time; it takes the element of surprise out of it." He was readmitted to UCLA Medical Center on 3 February 1988 with a ruptured duodenal ulcer. His remaining kidney had failed, but he refused dialysis to extend his life. In a decided tone he told his adopted daughter Michelle, "I'm going to die." As uremic poisoning dimmed his consciousness, with Gwyneth, his sister Joan, and cousin Frances Lewine beside him, he murmured, "I'd hate to die twice. It's so boring." His heartbeat ceased shortly before midnight on 15 February 1988. *See* James Gleick (1992).

Flynn, Errol (1909-1959)

The swashbuckling Australian-born movie star of *Captain Blood* (1935), *The Adventures of Robin Hood* (1938), and *The Sea Hawk* (1940) drank heavily most of his life and in his last years further damaged his health with heavy drug use. He lived up to his motto: "I like the whiskey old and the women young." A high-court judge in London said, during a suit over the division of Flynn's property after his death, "In his career, in his three marriages, in his friendships, in his quarrels and in bed with the many women he took there, he lived with zest and irregularity." Until he lost his sparkle, this devil-may-care attitude made him attractive to his many friends, female and male.

A book by Charles Higham, *Errol Flynn: The Untold Story* (1979), charged that the actor was a dedicated Nazi who aided the enemy as a spy during World War II. The accusations were based on some 250 documents obtained by Higham under the U.S. Freedom of Information Act. But Tony Thomas, in his *Errol Flynn: The Spy Who Never Was* (1990), says the main basis for the allegations is Flynn's friendship with an obscure Austrian physician, Hermann Friedrich Erben (1897–1984). "Of 184 documents [listed by Higham] about Erben . . . only five mentioned Flynn," says Thomas, "and in each case he is referred to only as an acquaintance of Erben." Flynn repeatedly defended Erben when questioned about him by U.S. agents, but also described him as a "screwball" with no marked political leanings. According to Higham, Erben was "one of the most important and ingenious Nazi agents of the twentieth century." "He was nothing of the kind," responds Thomas. He "is a figure of no consequence, and had it not been for his friendship with a famous movie star his name would mean nothing." True, the ostentatiously athletic actor's failure to serve in the military did arouse suspicions, but records show that he volunteered for service and was rejected as 4-F because of his history of tuberculosis; he had also picked up malaria and gonorrhea in New Guinea as a young man and later developed a heart condition.

Flynn's physical appearance worsened rapidly during his last years. He played the part of the world-weary souse Mike Campbell in the movie version of Hemingway's *The Sun Also Rises* (1957) and his last major film was *The Roots of Heaven* (1958). He wrote and narrated a short movie titled *Cuban Rebel Girls* (1959), but this is usually dismissed as a "bomb."

Flynn's chief home between 1952 and 1956 was his yacht *Zaca*, which he sailed endlessly around the Mediterranean, but by 1959, short of funds, he decided to sell her. He had left his third wife Patrice Wymore two years before and taken up with a fifteen-year-old part-time actress, Beverly Aadland. When a couple in Vancouver, British Columbia, agreed to buy the yacht, he and Beverly flew north to clinch the deal. But he wasn't in a hurry; for a week the couple toured Vancouver's nightclubs. "I've always been one for burning the midnight Errol," he quipped.

As the couple's hosts, the purchasers of the *Zaca*, Mr. and Mrs. George Galdough, prepared to drive them to the airport on 14 October 1959 for their return trip to California, Flynn complained of back pain. The Galdoughs drove him and Beverly to the home of Dr. Grant A. Gould, where the actor was given a shot of the painkiller Demerol. Feeling better, Flynn began chatting about his Hollywood acquaintances but soon asked to lie down. The doctor suggested his bedroom floor would be best for the sore back. Beverly covered him with a blanket and left him to rest; thirty minutes later she found him lifeless, his skin a blue-gray color. An Adrenalin shot directly into the heart and mouth-to-mouth resuscitation proved useless. Flynn was raced to a hospital and there declared dead of a heart attack. An autopsy revealed myocardial infarction, coronary thrombosis, coronary arteriosclerosis, fatty degeneration and partial cirrhosis of the liver and diverticulosis of the colon. Flynn had taken a drink of vodka before leaving the Galdoughs'; his blood alcohol was found to be .25 percent, at least double the safe driving limit but not enough to incapacitate the actor. His body was shipped by rail to Los Angeles and, after an Episcopal service, buried in Hollywood's Forest Lawn Cemetery.

Fonda, Henry (1905-1982)

The U.S. actor was a difficult man to know—reserved, even remote—especially to those who should have been closest to him. So shut off from him was his second wife, Frances Seymour Brokaw Fonda, that, distraught, she had herself committed to a sanitorium in Beacon, New York, and there slashed her throat with a razor blade. (The cause of her death was kept from her teenage children, Jane and Peter Fonda.) Two more unsuccessful marriages, to Susan Blanchard and Contessa Afdera Franchetti, followed before Fonda, at sixty, made a long, happy match with Shirlee Mae Adams.

Though he made more than eighty films, it was from his stage work in fifteen plays that he derived his greatest satisfaction. Toward the end of the Broadway run of his one-man show *Clarence Darrow* in 1974 he collapsed in his dressing room from heart failure; a pacemaker was implanted in his chest. The heart condition grew progressively worse from then on, but Fonda kept up a steady schedule. In his final two years he appeared in three television movies; these included *Gideon's Trumpet* (1980), in which he convincingly played the part of Clarence Earl Gideon, who successfully fought in the U.S. Supreme Court for the right of everyone facing a prison term to be afforded a defense lawyer.

Jane Fonda bought the movie rights to the play *On Golden Pond* with the idea of her father playing old, grumpy Professor Thayer with Jane herself as his anguished daughter trying to make real contact with him. On and off the set their relations were a continuance of a long-established real-life pattern; the audience sensed that father and daughter were hardly acting at all, but, rather, playing themselves, and this was close to the truth. Earlier roles, Henry Fonda had long explained to interviewers, were quite unlike his real self. He usually played honest, upright characters who were in sharp contrast to his real self—timid, hard to know, ashamed of his many failed marriages ("It's not like me . . . how it happened I don't know. I don't dwell on it.") But here, in his final movie, we see at last something close to the real man.

Rehearsing a scene that depicts the characters' mutual hostility, Jane begged her father to look into her eyes; it would give greater veracity to their acting, she thought. But he rebuffed her: "I don't *need* to look at you. I'm not one of those actors." Fighting back tears, she was comforted by

Katharine Hepburn, who played Mrs. Thayer. Never mind, said Hepburn, she had been subjected to just his kind of putdown for years by her lover Spencer Tracy.

On Golden Pond was a near-perfect finale to the veteran actor's career. Of it, Henry Fonda said, "I thought, that's the peak. I don't have to reach higher than that." Jane Fonda was happy to have helped him win, at last, a well-deserved Oscar. Yet she still found him to be a stranger. In his last days in the hospital she would, as she put it at the time, "sit and watch him and wonder who he is."

He completed work on the movie only with difficulty and in November 1981 was admitted to Cedars-Sinai Medical Center in Los Angeles for observation. Only Shirlee Fonda was really close to her husband at the end. At home in their white brick house in Bel Air, California, she slept in a cot near his bed to help him when his chest pains came. He was readmitted to Cedars-Sinai on 8 August 1982 and died early on the twelfth. Shirlee, Jane, and Peter were at his bedside. His death was quiet and painless, Mrs. Fonda told reporters. "He had a very good night the night before. He talked to all of us and was not unconscious at any time. He woke up this morning, sat up in bed and quietly stopped breathing." He was never in the hospital's intensive-care unit and no extraordinary measures were taken to extend his life.

Henry Fonda willed his eyes to the Manhattan Eye Bank and his body was cremated; he had requested that there be no ceremony. His estate was left to his wife, except for $200,000 bequeathed to his daughter Amy, whom Henry and Susan Blanchard Fonda had adopted. He disinherited Jane and Peter because, as he said, "they know how to take care of themselves." That a token gift might have comforted them never, it seems, occurred to him. See Allen Roberts and Max Goldstein (1984).

Fonteyn, Margot (1919–1991)

The English ballerina began her long solo career at fifteen and continued it beyond her sixtieth birthday. At forty-two she successfully met the challenge of dancing regularly with twenty-three-year-old Rudolf Nureyev. Fonteyn in 1955 married the Panamanian diplomat Roberto Arias, a childhood sweetheart who married and had a family before reentering her life. She was dancing with Nureyev at the Bath Festival in 1964 when she heard that her husband, campaigning in Panama City, had been seriously wounded, as he sat in his car, by a crazed political opponent, a fellow-member of the Panamenista Party. (As he lay in the hospital, recovering from three bullet wounds in the left side, another gunman was foiled as he tried to reach Arias and finish him off.) Thereafter, Fonteyn's chief concern was her paralyzed husband's care, and her retirement was delayed by her need to earn funds for this purpose.

In 1979 she retired to the modest ranch, La Quinta Pata, she shared with Roberto near the village of Higa, along the coast east of Panama City. Confined to a wheelchair, unable to talk above a whisper and totally dependent on her, he was nevertheless able to accompany Margot to England each year, where she was president of the Royal Academy of Dancing and chancelor of Durham University.

Roberto "Tito" Arias died in Panama in November 1989. To suggestions that she should now return to England, Margot replied, "I'm proud to be English, but it is here that I decided to make my life; it is here where my husband is buried. I've chosen to live in Panama, and to die here when the moment comes." When she said this to a visitor in March 1990 she knew she was dying of bone cancer. By then she was almost penniless and under pressure from creditors. Medical bills for treatment in Houston and New York had exhausted her savings but, slow to complain, she had never aired her troubles. At this low point she could perhaps be forgiven for a trace of bitterness when she added, "It is better to leave early if you are going to be left alone without money and far away from friends and family." The faraway friends came to her rescue and arranged a sell-out benefit performance at Covent Garden, London, in May 1990. Attended by royalty, it featured Nureyev and the tenor Placido Domingo and brought in a quarter-million pounds for a Fonteyn trust fund. It was there that her devoted admirers saw her—shrunken, but still erect and bright-eyed—take her final curtain call.

After further treatment at the Nuffield Hospital, Margot Fonteyn left her native land for the last time and, as promised, passed her last difficult days in her adopted country. She died at Paitille Hospital in Panama City on 21 February 1991.

Forbes, Malcolm (1919-1990)

The U.S. multimillionaire publisher and art collector was a shy, bookish man who transformed himself in later life into a flamboyant publicist for his financial magazine *Forbes*, which was founded by his father, a Scottish immigrant. Malcolm took up hot-air ballooning in 1972; he broke six world records and was the first person to fly coast to coast (from Coos Bay, Oregon, to Chesapeake Bay in 1973). He liked to arrive at glitzy charity balls on one of his sixty-eight motorcycles and he intrigued gossip columnists whenever he squired actress Elizabeth Taylor around New York.

But behind the glitter a different Forbes could sometimes be glimpsed: a man who frequented gay bars; a man who sought out new male staff members at the magazine to invite to private dinners. In 1989 a twenty-two-year-old model threatened to reveal their regular sexual encounters; the man was indicted for extortion after Forbes's death. In December 1989 a lowly proofreader at *Forbes* begged the boss to help the gay cause by publicly declaring his sexual orientation; Malcolm, clearly embarrassed, cut short the discussion. It was not until several months later that the scandal sheets (and the gay publication *Outweek*) were able to exploit the story without fear of the libel laws.

As Forbes authored (with Jeff Bloch) his 1988 book *They Went That-a-Way* he may well have wondered whether future editions would add his own death—perhaps in a motorcycle crash, perhaps in a balloon mishap like the one he narrowly survived in January 1975—to those of the other celebrities he describes. But, alas, he died with a disappointing lack of drama. On 23 February 1990, in the old mansion he rented near the Thames, Forbes hosted a charity bridge tournament between coroporate America and British members of Parliament (the British team won). He flew home overnight in his private jet, arriving at his forty-acre estate, Timberfield, in Far Hills, New Jersey, at 5:30 A.M. He told his houseman Dennis Stewart to make a doctor's appointment for that afternoon and went to bed. (Forbes's thirty-nine-year marriage had ended in 1985.) When he failed to waken, Stewart, alarmed, called the doctor, Oscar Kruesi, in Bedminster. Kruesi told reporters, "I raced out of my office for the Forbes home. Mr. Forbes had obviously died in his sleep. He died peacefully, apparently!"

The millionaire was pronounced dead of a heart attack at 4:30 P.M. on the twenty-fourth.

At the private service in nearby Bernardsville, a bagpiper played "Scotland the Brave" in tribute to the dead man's heritage. His four sons and daughter were present again among the two thousand crammed into St. Bartholomew's Episcopal Church in Manhattan for a memorial service three days later. Outside on Park Avenue, Hell's Angels roared by in a noisy salute; Malcolm's own favorite red and gold Harley-Davidson stood outside the church with a small U.S. flag at half-staff mounted on it. Inside, ex-President Richard Nixon and his daughter Tricia sat in the front pew next to Elizabeth Taylor; ex-wife Roberta Remson Laidlaw Forbes was relegated to a seat further back.

In accordance with the dead man's wishes, his ashes were buried on the most remote of all his possessions, the tiny island of Lauthala, east of Taveuni in the Fiji group. A marker on the grave reads: WHILE ALIVE HE LIVED. *See* Christopher Winans (1990).

Forster, E. M. (1879-1970)

The last of the English writer's handful of novels, *A Passage to India,* was published back in 1924, yet his literary reputation continued to grow in his later years. After his death his novel on homosexual themes, *Maurice,* could at last be published, and this and his other novels have produced impressive films in recent years. The man who was called "a liberal moralist" and "the most civilized of novelists" was unimpressive in appearance, with a receding chin, an untidy moustache, and a timid, hesitant manner.

When his mother died in 1945 he lost the home they shared; King's College, Cambridge, came to his rescue and made him an honorary fellow, letting him settle down in rooms there. Volumes published in his final two decades included *Two Cheers for Democracy* (1951)—essays and miscellaneous writing—and *The Hill of Devi*—letters and diary extracts related to his two visits to India—published in 1953, the year he was made a Companion of Honour.

At his ninetieth birthday luncheon, organized by the college in January 1969, Forster sat "silent and slumped," according to P. N. Furbank, his 1977 biographer. He had suffered a heart attack in 1962 and a series of strokes; he was deaf and his sight and speech were affected. When he was ill, his friends Bob and May Buckingham had always welcomed him to their suburban home in Coventry, in the English Midlands, a home the generous Forster had helped them to buy. Bob once confided to May that he was shocked by Forster's confession of love for him, not being aware (he said) of the writer's sexual orientation. May defended him as their dear friend and benefactor.

At 6:00 P.M. on Friday, 22 May 1970, Furbank, who had rooms above Forster's, heard two loud shouts. He went down to find his friend had collapsed in his bedroom and crawled to the apartment door. Forster himself guessed that he had suffered another—and this time fatal—stroke, but as he lay on his sofa he asked that Furbank's evening guests be brought down to talk to him. One of his legs, he said, was paralyzed; it was all right, but "did rather dominate." Until the Buckinghams could come to his aid, he was made comfortable by Furbank and other friends. Taken to Coventry on 2 June, he lay "perfectly serene" but growing weaker. "On 6 June, for most of the morning," writes Furbank, "he held May Buckingham's hand in silence, opening his eyes when she tried to take it away—till at last he fell asleep or unconscious. He died, without recovering consciousness, early the next morning."

Forster had asked that he be "disposed of" wherever he happened to die, and wished for no religious observances. Bob Buckingham, recalling an incident in his friend's 1910 novel *Howard's End* (filmed in 1992), played a movement from Beethoven's *Fifth Symphony* on a phonograph during the secular ceremony.

> Despite this [writes Furbank], it was for the mourners a slightly depressing experience, as all such nonreligious rituals are; but as we filed back towards the cars there was a diversion. The undertaker's men were peering inside the bonnet of the leading Rolls, evidently unable to make it start. The chief undertaker approached, pressing his black gloves to his forehead in a theatrical gesture, protesting that never, never in twenty years, had such an unfortunate thing . . . And at this [Professor W. J. H.] Sprott, who had been gloomy, brightened greatly, remarking that Forster's spirit was clearly at work.

Sprott was Forster's chief beneficiary, and after his death King's College. The ashes were scattered on the rose bed in the Buckinghams' garden.

Fossey, Dian (1932-1985)

The San Francisco–born naturalist, a tall, brawny woman, set up the Karisoke Research Center in 1967 to study the mountain gorilla and became the world authority on the rare primate. The inroads of poachers on the Center, at Mont Visoke in the central African nation of Rwanda, were a serious threat from the first, and Fossey's war against them led to grave tensions with the local population and the national government. By 1978, Dian was being urged by the Rwandan authorities and the U.S. State Department to leave the country. She was offered a visiting professorship at Cornell University, and while there wrote her book, *Gorillas in the Mist* (1983).

She returned to Karisoke in June 1983, to the disquiet of staff members. Her temporary replacement as director, Richard Barnes, says, "We were disturbed by her racial attitudes." She screamed at the African workers, who "were frightened of her and carried themselves like beaten dogs." Her rages were evidently triggered by the depredations of poachers, who by now had killed several of her beloved gorillas, including her favorite, Digit.

On the night of 27 October 1985 Dian Fossey discovered on her doorstep the wooden image of a puff adder—the curse of death. On 27 December her manservant Kanyaragana came to her cabin early to light the stove and make coffee. Her door, bearing a red felt Santa Claus, stood ajar. The living room was a shambles; in the bedroom the mattress had fallen from its frame and the furniture was overturned. Dian's body lay on the floor, face upward, with her automatic pistol and a clip of ammunition (of the wrong caliber) by her side. Her skull was split from the forehead to the corner of her mouth. The weapon had been her own panga. There had been no robbery.

She was buried beside Digit and her other slain gorilla-friends in the yard behind her cabin after a service conducted by the Reverend Elton Wallace, a missionary from Gisenyi. Her tombstone bears her Rwandan name Nyirmachabelli ("the woman who lives alone on the mountain") and an epitaph: NO ONE LOVED GORILLAS MORE / REST IN PEACE, DEAR FRIEND / ETERNALLY PROTECTED / IN THIS SACRED GROUND / FOR YOU ARE HOME / WHERE YOU BELONG

White staff members were certain the assassin was a black poacher seeking vengeance. "She really had it coming to her," said one. "She mistreated everyone around her and was finally done in," said another. But the Rwandan police were sure it was an inside job. They arrested most of the African workers, but all were released except Emmanuel Rwelekana, a tracker, who had been fired by Fossey several months earlier. In August 1986 he and Wayne McGuire, a young research student from Oklahoma whom she had described as "nice" but terribly slow, were charged with the murder. Rwelekana reportedly hanged himself weeks later. McGuire returned to the United States before the charges were made public, probably by arrangement between the two governments. On evidence that Fossey's 1987 biographer Farley Mowat believes was contrived, McGuire was convicted in absentia on 11 December 1986 by a Rwandan tribunal. He was sentenced to death by firing squad if he ever returned to the court's jurisdiction.

Mowat believes Fossey was killed by an African in the employ of powerful interests who found her an impediment to the commercial exploitation of the gorillas. "I believe," he writes, "that the extension of Dian's visa [early in December] for two full years was her death warrant."

Her final letter, typed on her old Smith-Corona portable, was unfinished. A thank-you note for Christmas gifts, it ends: "Camp will be bulging by the time I leave for America in March, but right now it is awfully quiet . . ."

Frank, Anne (1929-1945)

The young victim of Nazi anti-Semitism was born in Frankfurt but moved with her family to Amsterdam in 1933. When her elder sister Margot was summoned to a labor camp in 1942 the family hid for twenty-five months in cramped quarters at 263 Prinsengracht above her father's former offices. The Gestapo found them on 4 August 1944 and they were shipped like cattle to Auschwitz, Poland, where as many as 4 million Jews and other "undesirables" perished. Though the youngest in her group, Anne was made leader and distributed bread and showed other kindnesses to her fellow victims. Her mother Edith died at Auschwitz in January 1945, but by then Anne and Margot had been moved to the squalid Bergen-Belsen camp near Hanover, Germany, where louse-borne typhus was rife. They celebrated Christmas with tiny sandwiches of onions and boiled cabbage. Margot died at the end of February 1945. Anne, half-starved and sickening from typhus, was not told. She died peacefully not long after, feeling, according to a witness, "that nothing bad was happening to her." She was fifteen years old. The bodies of the two sisters lie with thousands of others under the burial mounds of Bergen-Belsen.

Their father Otto Frank, in the hospital when the Red Army liberated Auschwitz, died in August 1980, aged ninety-one in Basel, Switzerland. Anne's diary, published in the original Dutch in 1947 and in English in 1952, aroused the conscience of the world.

Franklin, Rosalind E. (1920-1958)

The British scientist who helped elucidate the structure of DNA, key to the reproduction of all living things, was a shy but aggressive woman who had difficulty in relating to her colleagues at King's College, London. In James D. Watson's frank, often indiscreet account of the DNA breakthrough, *The Double Helix* (1968), Franklin emerges as a truculent, almost sinister character with whom it was impossible to communicate effectively. Watson was persuaded to soften this portrait in an epilogue to his book, but, according to Franklin's American friend and champion Anne Sayre in *Rosalind Franklin and DNA* (1975), he continued to remember her as "impossible" and "stubborn."

Also at King's, working more or less independently on DNA, was Maurice H. F. Wilkins, and it was he who, while barely on speaking terms with his colleague Franklin, maintained a friendly relationship with Watson and Francis H. C. Crick at Cambridge University, and later shared the Nobel Prize with them. Sayre and others believe that without Franklin's unusually clear X-ray diffraction patterns of crystalline DNA, Watson and Crick would have been seriously hampered in their mission to build a convincing model of the deoxyribonucleic acid molecule, whereas Franklin, without Cambridge's contribution, might well have reached the same goal within weeks.

Her difficulties with coworkers were undoubtedly aggravated by her unhappy social position at King's College, denied access to the common room, made the butt of sexist remarks, and otherwise treated as an inferior in a male-dominated profession. A more enlightened attitude had prevailed in Paris, where she made many friends while working in a government laboratory on carbonaceous substances between 1947 and 1950. So the contrast at King's was a sad disappointment, and it was a relief to her to move on to Birkbeck College, London, in 1953. There, in the few years left to her, she did fine work on the structure of viruses, publishing, alone and jointly, no fewer than seventeen papers.

Rosalind Franklin fell ill with ovarian cancer late in 1956, and there were soon extensive metastases. After surgery in 1957 she convalesced with the Cricks in Cambridge. In her final months she took up the challenge of the poliomyelitis virus, despite warnings against handling it. Advised that a Swiss vacation was unwise because a sudden intestinal obstruction might occur, she went ahead anyway and enjoyed her last holiday. She died in London at the Royal Marsden Hospital on 16 April 1958. According to her physician, Mair Livingstone, "She was saddened, not depressed, I would say, since she remained combative till the end." In a 1992 letter, Anne Sayre writes, "She suffered a great deal . . . It is my understanding that Rosalind . . . was by her own wish cremated and that her ashes were not interred. There was no funeral conducted, though there was a memorial service in London shortly after her death, and another in New York arranged by several of her American friends. Although Rosalind's family was observant of religious customs, Rosalind was not a believer, and her family respected her wishes."

Had she lived, the Nobel Prize Committee in 1962 would have been faced with a pretty problem. The prizes, never awarded posthumously, are not shared by more than three laureates. It seems possible, even probable, that the 1962 Nobel Prize for Medicine and Physiology would have gone to Crick, Watson—and Rosalind Franklin.

Gandhi, Indira (1917-1984)

The Indian prime minister (1966–77, 1980–84) was the only child of Jawaharlal Nehru, the country's first premier. Many regarded her in awe to the end as "Mother India," an all-powerful symbol of her nation. But in her last years she made grave mistakes. In June 1975, rather than risk being voted out of office, she declared a state of national emergency. In 1984 the Indian army flushed Sikh separatist extremists from the Golden Temple at

Amritsar; even moderate Sikhs were outraged by this desecration and the resulting heavy casualties. It is possible she knew that by this act she had signed her death warrant. But she was fatalistic; within a day or two of her death she said in a speech in Orissa, "I don't mind if my life goes in the service of the nation." Though she was advised to transfer Sikhs out of her personal security guard, she did nothing. After all, she felt, what was the use? "Those supposed to save me will be the first to run away."

Despite Indira Gandhi's great eminence and power—or because of it—she felt cut off from love and intimacy; she wrote in a confidential 1954 letter to a friend that she was "sorry . . . to have missed the most wonderful thing in life—having a complete and perfect relationship with another human being." Her estranged husband Feroze Gandhi died in 1960. Her younger son Sanjay was killed in June 1980 in the crash of a stunt plane he was piloting. (Seven years after her own death, her elder son Rajiv, who succeeded her as prime minister, was assassinated at a rally near Madras by an unidentified young woman who, apparently with explosives tied to her body, bent in obeisance to touch his feet.)

On the morning of 31 October 1984, Indira Gandhi rose as usual at six o'clock in her New Delhi residence, No. 1 Safjardung Road, and was served piping-hot tea by her valet. She did yoga exercises, bathed and donned a bright orange sari. For once she left off the bulletproof vest that might have saved her life, probably because she was due to be interviewed for television a few yards away on the lawn of her office next door by the playwright and actor Peter Ustinov.

At breakfast she was joined by her Italian-born daughter-in-law Sonia, wife of Rajiv, and two grandchildren. At 9:15, with a policeman holding a sunshade over her head and her aide R. K. Dhawan, her valet, and another policeman following, she walked briskly along a path toward a garden gate in the hedge and smiled at the tall bearded Sikh policeman, Beant Singh, 28, who stood there; he had been in her security guard for six years. He moved toward her, whipped out a pistol and fired three times into her abdomen. Another Sikh guard, Satwant Singh, 21, emerged from behind the hedge and, as she crumpled, opened up with a Thompson automatic carbine. The prime minister's small entourage scattered or dived to the ground. Beant Singh stood with hands raised. "We have done what we set out to do," he said. "Now you can do what you want to do." But for a whole minute everyone froze, paralyzed. An ambulance stood ready, but the driver was nowhere to be found. Sonia ran out of the residence. "Get a car," she cried.

Mrs. Gandhi's body, torn by thirty-two wounds, was lifted into an Indian-made Ambassador car and driven through heavy traffic to the All-India Institute of Medical Sciences; the two-and-a-half-mile trip took an incredible forty minutes and because no one thought of calling ahead there was further delay before the institute's gates were opened.

Meanwhile, the two assassins were arrested. Twenty minutes later, shots were heard from the guardhouse; on the pretext that they were trying to escape, both were shot. Beant Singh died instantly. Satwant Singh was injured in the spine and kidneys; he and a third conspirator, Kehar Singh, were tried and, after long-drawn-out appeals, hanged in New Delhi on 6 January 1989.

The fight to save Indira Gandhi's life was hopeless from the first. There was virtually no sign of life when she was rushed into the emergency room. Though her heart was intact, her spine was severed and the loss of blood was grievous. "She was probably dead by the time she hit the ground," said a surgeon. Nevertheless, eighty units of blood were transfused and a heart-lung machine was hooked up. The BBC announced her death to the world long before it was officially confirmed at 2:30 P.M.

Various faiths were represented at Indira Gandhi's ceremonial Hindu cremation at Shantivana, near where Mahatma Gandhi and Nehru had been cremated and where Rajiv would follow his mother seven years later. The United States was represented by Secretary of State George Shultz; a tearful Margaret Thatcher came from the United Kingdom, and a host of other world leaders were present, including even President Zia ul-Haq of Pakistan, India's mortal enemy. Indira Gandhi's flower-swathed body was placed on a bed of sandalwood logs. Her son Rajiv and his son Rahul circled the body and then dropped water pitchers to the ground to represent a shattered life. Ghee (clarified butter), cloves, pine nuts, and fruits were placed around the corpse as final gifts. Rajiv Gandhi walked around the pyre nine times before setting it alight with a joss stick. Later it was his duty, distasteful to many who watched, to crack his mother's skull with a bamboo pole to complete the immolation.

Rajiv scattered some of the ashes from a plane; the rest were immersed in the sacred Ganges River. *See* Pranay Gupte (1992).

Garbo, Greta (1905-1990)

The Swedish-born actress became a U.S. citizen in 1951. After the last of her twenty-five movies, the unimpressive *Two Faced Woman*, she retired at the age of thirty-six. Unlike another famed recluse, Howard Hughes, her whereabouts were not secret; she lived alone in a seven-room apartment on the fifth floor of a cooperative apartment building overlooking the East River at 450 East 52nd Street in Manhattan. As the years passed, she was often seen by fellow New Yorkers, a solitary figure walking a regular four miles a day while window-shopping in the East 50s and 60s, her famous eyes hidden behind spectacles, her long gray-blond hair falling below a large hat, wearing little or no makeup.

Garbo never married, but there were reports of affairs with the actor John Gilbert, whom she jilted in 1926, the conductor Leopold Stokowski, and others. She was close, for many years before his death in 1964, to George Schlee, a financier who lived at the same address and who was married to the couturiere Valentina.

In her last years, the actress escaped the city's heat for several months every summer in the Swiss resort of Klosters. She enjoyed speaking her native tongue to a Swedish couple who vacationed there, and confided to them her deep-seated desire to be left alone. "I would have liked to be a countess . . . to live in the country, to be protected and sheltered." Sometimes she would stay in bed all day, but when she was up she had to walk. Of Aristotle Onassis's yacht, she shrugged, "It was too small; I couldn't go for my walks." She enjoyed quiet retreats: the churchyards around Klosters and Napoleon's tomb in Paris, which she visited again and again.

Even in her Hollywood days, Garbo was often unwell, and later in life she was plagued by diverticulitis, arthritis, and inflammation of the ovaries. Cigarette smoking was her only vice, and probably triggered her attacks of bronchitis. At Klosters in 1988 she complained of weakness: "I can only walk a few steps . . . I spend most of my time in my room . . . I can't eat anything . . . I am in a daze . . . the life around me no longer seems real . . . I feel I am dying bit by bit." And about death she confessed, "I really wish I could believe, but I can't. For me it's over when it ends. Maybe I am too prosaic."

In New York, death gradually robbed her of her few friends. Her visitors were limited to her doctor and nurse, her niece Gray Reisfield, Gray's husband Donald (a gynecologist in Passaic, New Jersey), their four children, and a very few others. When she tripped over a vacuum cleaner and sprained her ankle her precious walks were interrupted.

During her final eleven months, Garbo needed kidney dialysis sessions three afternoons a week. On 11 April 1990 she was able to walk across to the taxicab as usual, wearing slacks and bedroom slippers. But this time, on arrival at New York Hospital's Ralph Bunche Pavilion, she was admitted for treatment under Dr. Stuart Saal. She died four days later, at 11:30 A.M. on Sunday, 15 April. The cause of death was not announced, but evidently kidney failure was largely responsible. The following day her body was cremated in New Jersey. If her known wishes were adhered to, her ashes have been sent to her beloved Sweden.

The sole executor and beneficiary of her estate, estimated at $20 million, was her niece. Her art collection and furnishings were auctioned by Sotheby's late in 1990 in sales that drew national attention.

Gardner, Erle Stanley (1889-1970)

The U.S. mystery writer, creator of the Los Angeles attorney Perry Mason, was proud of the fact that of 151 detective and mystery books selling over a million copies in the years 1895–1965, ninety-one had been written by him. Gardner wrote 131 works of fiction, of which eighty-two were Perry Mason novels and twenty-nine were Bertha Cool/Donald Lam mysteries written under his pseudonym A. A. Fair. All told, they sold 325 million copies. In association with *Argosy* magazine Gardner helped run the Court of Last Resort, a committee of experts who investigated possible miscarriages of U.S. justice. In the decade up to 1952 the court, he claimed, demanded four-fifths of his time. Gardner also wrote nonfiction books about his explorations of Baja California and California's Sacramento River delta, and he was a proficient archer and an enthusiastic stargazer.

The writer had several hideaways around rural California where he could park his trailer and write undisturbed, but his most permanent home in later years was at Rancho Paisano outside Temecula, sixty miles north of San Diego. His first wife Natalie died in February 1968 after a separation of over thirty years; he married his longtime secretary Jean Bethell six months later. Shortly after their Mexican honeymoon Gardner fell and fractured two ribs, hindering work on his final nonfiction book, *Drifting Down the Delta*.

Early in 1969 the Gardners went on a whale watch in an airship (the Goodyear blimp). The last of the Perry Mason novels, *The Case of the Fabulous Fake,* was dictated and transcribed by mid-February. (Two more, written previously, were published posthumously.) There were sessions in a Palm Springs, California, hospital during the year, for Gardner had been diagnosed with cancer some time previously but kept the fact secret. As his eightieth birthday approached, he kept up his regular writing pace—on a Mexican book (*Host with a Big Hat*), his last A. A. Fair mystery (*All Grass Isn't Green*), which would be published posthumously, and speeches in Stockton, California, and Houston.

His birthday celebration, a big one, was celebrated at Rancho Paisano on 17 July 1969. Late in the year he had cobalt treatments over a four-week period in a Riverside, California, hospital, and by Christmas was too ill to spend the holiday as usual in Baja; he stayed quietly at the ranch instead. He was back in the hospital on 12 January, and Jean stayed nearby. It was a habit of Gardner's when under stress to recite to himself the 23rd Psalm ("The Lord is my shepherd, I shall not want . . .") and he needed this comfort frequently now. But he could be playful, even belligerent, with visitors. One day his friend Cornwall Jackson drove the eighty miles from Los Angeles to see him. "How are you feeling?" asked Jackson when he arrived. The sick man was incensed. "Why didn't you pick up the phone in Hollywood and call me here and ask me? . . . Jesus, when in hell are you going to get organized and do things the simple way instead of the hard way?" He went on like this for some time, reported Jackson. But as he left, Gardner said, "Thanks for caring, Corney."

When no further treatment was possible, Gardner returned to the ranch, where Jean and her two sisters, Peggy and Honey, cared for him. It was Honey who was holding his hand when he died on 11 March 1970. A funeral service was held at the Garden of Prayer Chapel in Riverside, where his friend and colleague on the Court of Last Resort, Marshall Houts, delivered the eulogy. At Jean's suggestion, his ashes were scattered over his beloved Baja California. *See* Dorothy B. Hughes (1978).

George V (1865-1936)

The king of Great Britain succeeded his father Edward VII in 1910. He was thrown by his horse while inspecting troops in France in October 1915 and sustained a fractured pelvis and other injuries. In 1928 he fell seriously ill from a streptococcal infection of the right lung, resulting in an abscess that was successfully drained by his doctor, Lord Dawson of Penn. But at that date, before the introduction of sulfa drugs and antibiotics, recovery hung in the balance for several weeks. The king's 1984 biographer Kenneth Rose observes that "Four successive [British] sovereigns, all heavy smokers, died of ailments caused or aggravated by the habit." (They were Edward VII, George V, Edward VIII [Duke of Windsor], and George VI [qq.v.].)

George V's final two years were overshadowed by his elder son's infatuation with a divorced woman, Wallis Simpson, and by his dread of approaching war. At the time of the Italian-Abyssinian crisis he declared, "I will *not* have another war . . . I will go to Trafalgar Square myself and wave a red flag sooner than allow this country to be brought in." After the stress of the Jubilee celebration of May 1935 he was increasingly liable to fall asleep during the day. Breathing difficulties during the night were allayed by oxygen administration. At Christmas he continued a practice begun in 1932 by broadcasting a message to the Empire, but it was noticed that his voice had lost much of its strength.

His physician was summoned to the royal residence at Sandringham in Norfolk on 15 January 1936 and again two days later. By then the king was confined to his room. It was on the seventeenth also that he made the final entry in his diary, which he had kept since 1880: "Dawson arrived this evening. I saw him and feel rotten." A cardiologist, Sir Maurice Cassidy, was called in and the first of six bulletins was issued; it mentioned "bronchial catarrh . . . not severe . . . but [also] signs of cardiac weakness." When the Prince of Wales arrived he observed with irritation the Archbishop of Canterbury, who had invited himself to the house, slipping in and out of the sickroom, "a noiseless spectre in black gaiters." After two days of only partial consciousness the king was found by his private secretary on Monday, 20 January, sitting up reading *The Times.* "How is the Empire?" he muttered before drifting off to sleep again. He would not survive the day.

Three members of the Privy Council arrived from London to have him sign a warrant permitting that body to assume the royal functions. Though paralyzed on the right side, he made valiant attempts with first one hand and then the other to initial the document while apologizing for the delay. It has been long a popular rumor that in the king's final moments the physicians attempted to rally him by referring to Bognor, a favorite resort of his, and promising he could go there again to convalesce. "Bugger Bognor," the sovereign is said to have replied. Rose writes, "The tale carries a certain plausibility. The King was always emphatic in his language, not least when being fussed by his medical advisers."

It was from a bulletin scribbled on a menu card by Dawson on the evening of the twentieth in the Sandringham House dining room that the king's subjects first learned that death was near: "The King's life is moving slowly towards its close." The family clustered around the bed and the archbishop read the 23rd Psalm and a prayer for the dying. The final bulletin was broadcast just after midnight; it ran, "Death came peacefully to the King at 11:55 P.M."

Queen Mary begged that the funeral be delayed no longer than a week, rather than the fortnight that preceded Edward VII's interment. After lying thirty-six hours in the village church, the coffin was taken by rail to London. Borne on a gun carriage and surmounted by the Imperial Crown, it was followed on foot by the king's four surviving sons. As it turned into Palace Yard on its journey to Westminster Hall, the jeweled Maltese Cross atop the crown tumbled into the street.

The king had requested that no religious service be held, but the archbishop held out for a single hymn. Then the late sovereign lay in state for four days. Large crowds watched the procession as the coffin was taken to Paddington Station. George V joined previous British kings and queens in the crypt below St. George's Chapel, Windsor.

George VI (1895-1952)

The Duke of York succeeded his elder brother Edward VIII as king of Great Britain in December 1936. Edward (who became Duke of Windsor) abdicated the throne after only eleven months so that he could marry the twice divorced Mrs. Wallis Warfield Simpson. Though nervous, shy, and handicapped by a stammer, the new sovereign was conscientious in the performance of the royal duties he had so reluctantly assumed. Six years as head of state during World War II seriously undermined his health. Of his physical condition in 1947, a palace secretary recalled that, "As a result of the stress he was under the king used to stay up too late and smoke too many cigarettes—he literally died for England."

Early in 1949 the king's doctors begged him to cut down on his smoking. It was a habit that had helped kill his father George V and grandfather Edward VII and was now exacerbating the progressive arteriosclerosis of vessels in George VI's lower legs and feet; indeed, there was a threat of gangrene in the right leg. A lumbar sympathectomy was performed at Buckingham Palace on 12 March 1949. (Surgeons severed a nerve at the base of the spine on the right side so that constriction of the leg artery, controlled by the nerve, was prevented.) To reduce the risk of thrombosis thereafter, the king used a pony, which he held by a special harness, to help him up the slopes when he went out walking in the grounds of Balmoral Castle.

In May 1951 George retired to bed with a cough and a slight fever; a small area of "catarrhal inflammation" was detected in the left lung and penicillin was prescribed. In September, tomography revealed that the patch was actually a tumor, and bronchoscopy showed it to be malignant. The lung was removed on 23 September; "structural changes," not "cancer," was the term used in the medical bulletins and the patient was kept in the dark regarding the meaning of the phrase. The prognosis was now grave, with thrombosis a serious threat; it seemed unlikely that the king could survive more than a year. At Christmas he was still too feeble to broadcast live to the Commonwealth, and the message on this occasion was recorded in sections beforehand. His listeners worldwide heard that to his usual stammer was now added a noticeable huskiness.

He spent Christmas at his favorite residence, Sandringham House in Norfolk. In London at the end of January 1952 his doctors gave him a clean bill of health and on the thirtieth he attended the musical *South Pacific* at the Drury Lane Theatre. The following day, standing hatless in a cold wind, he saw off his daughter Princess Elizabeth and her husband Prince Philip, who were flying to Kenya on their way to a royal tour of Australasia. Winston Churchill, who was present at the airport, later described the king as "gay and even jaunty, and [he] drank a glass of champagne." But he added, "I think he knew he had not long to live."

George VI returned to Sandringham on 1 February, and on the fifth, a perfect day with a clear blue sky, he was happy shooting hares and rabbits. That evening he dined with his wife Queen Elizabeth and his younger daughter Princess Margaret; he returned to bed at 10:30. A watchman later saw the king fiddling with a latch on his bedroom window. At an early hour on 6 February 1952 a blood clot stopped the beating of the sovereign's heart and he died without waking. His body was discovered by his valet James MacDonald at 7:30 when he took in his master's morning tea.

His daughter became Queen Elizabeth II as she watched rhinoceroses at a waterhole from up a fig tree at Treetops Hotel in Kenya. Hours later she was told the news privately by Philip, whose equerry had heard it indirectly from a journalist. In the United States the House of Representatives passed a resolution of sympathy and adjourned for the day. President Truman wrote in his diary, "He was a grand man. Worth a pair of his brother Ed."

The king's body was placed in Sandringham Church until 11 February.

It lay in state for three days in Westminster Hall as three hundred thousand filed by and was laid to rest in the crypt of St. George's Chapel, Windsor, on the sixteenth. Churchill sent a wreath of winter blossoms bearing a card in his own handwriting, "For Valour." *See* Sarah Bedford (1989).

Gleason, Jackie (1916-1987)

The Brooklyn-born entertainer achieved fame during the 1950s as the blustering bus driver Ralph Kramden in the television series *The Honeymooners*. He was also a movie actor, nominated for an Oscar in *The Hustler* (1961), and claimed—with little reason—to be a composer and conductor. By the early 1960s *Life* magazine was calling him "The hottest performer in all show business."

He aroused very different feelings in colleagues, from anger and disgust to love, even veneration. He was a huge man, often approaching three hundred pounds, so great was his appetite, but as a professional comedian he had little incentive to keep his weight down; early in his career he had been told, "Skinny, you're not funny."

After collapsing in 1978 during a pre-Broadway tour of *The Sly Fox* in Chicago, he underwent triple coronary bypass surgery. His theatrical movies of this period were hardly worthy of his talents, but in March 1983 he teamed up with Lord Olivier in the filming of a fifty-minute cable presentation, *Mr. Halpern and Mr. Johnson,* in which—remarkably enough—he can be said to have outshone the (admittedly ailing) great English actor. This outstanding performance, and his appearance on a *60 Minutes* TV program in 1984 ("I liked him enormously," recalled his interviewer, Morley Safer) gave Gleason's career a much-needed boost in his final years.

His last movie, *Izzy and Moe* (1985), was a lackluster effort with his old partner from *The Honeymooners,* Art Carney; Gleason was credited, falsely, with supplying the music. In 1985 he admitted to having kept in air-conditioned storage over seventy hours of "lost" episodes of *The Honeymooners,* which he was able to sell for almost $6 million, to be spread over seven years.

In April 1987, after feeling uncomfortable for months, he was found to have colon cancer, probably already metastasized to the liver; the comedian refused a biopsy and returned to his Fort Lauderdale, Florida, home. Suffering severe abdominal pain, he was secretly admitted to the Imperial Point Hospital nearby on 21 May and, in a three-hour operation, a large tumor was removed from his colon. But the cancer had indeed spread to the liver and also to the lymph nodes in the groin. Told he had only a few months to live, he insisted on his oxygen supply being turned off so that he could resume chain-smoking. Further intestinal surgery was needed on 3 June to repair his leaking gut and drain the abdomen. Then he went home to die. In his final days he mailed notes and autographed pictures to friends. On *60 Minutes* he had expressed the opinion, or hope, that "God isn't vengeful and if you've committed a sin he's not going to send you to hell for eternity." Not long before the end he said, "If God wants another joke man, I'm ready." On 24 June 1987, after two days in a coma, he slipped off to claim a reservation he had made a decade earlier—when the New York restaurateur Toots Shor died in 1977, Gleason sent flowers with a note attached: "Save a table for me, pal."

Two thousand filed past his coffin in a Miami funeral parlor. Audrey Meadows, his other partner in *The Honeymooners,* was among the mourners at his requiem mass at St. Mary's Cathedral, Miami. He was buried in a marble mausoleum overlooking the water in Our Lady of Mercy Cemetery. His widow Marilyn and other family members later saw a Brooklyn bus depot formally named after him. *See* William A. Henry III (1992).

Grace, Princess of Monaco (1929-1982)

Grace Kelly, the movie actress from Philadelphia who married Prince Rainier III of Monaco in 1956, made her last appearance on film in *Rearranged* (1980), a fluffy tale woven around Monte Carlo's Flower Festival. In August 1982 she and her husband enjoyed a cruise in Norwegian waters and then retired, with their heir Albert, 24, and younger daughter Stephanie, 17, to their farmhouse retreat, Roc Agel, high in the cool hills above Monaco.

Monday, 13 September, dawned bright and warm on the French Riviera. That evening Grace and Stephanie planned to travel to Paris, but first she had an appointment in Monaco with her couturier, who was to alter several dresses for her. These were piled along with suitcases into the back of her favorite brown Rover 3500; around 9.30 A.M. she dismissed her chauffeur, for whom there was no room, and took the wheel herself. With Stephanie on her right she set off down the narrow winding County Highway 53. For five miles she was followed by a truck driven by Yves Raimondo. About two hundred yards before the final and sharpest turn, Raimondo saw the Rover swerve violently, right itself, and run on to the curve without slowing. "The brake lights did not come on," he reported. "She seemed to be going faster and faster . . . she did not even try to turn!" The crash barrier on the outside of the curve might have prevented the disaster, but it extended only halfway around, to permit a narrow dirt road to leave the highway at right angles on the left. The car glanced off the far end of the barrier and tumbled more than a hundred feet through thickets and pines, coming to rest in a market garden near a red-painted house. The right-hand door was crushed and jammed shut. Stephanie, shocked and suffering from a concussion, with a hairline fracture of the spine, was helped by two rescuers out of the driver's door on the left and staggered to the house steps. "You must help Maman," she said in French. "You must call Papa . . . he is the Prince." The car's clock had stopped at 9:54 A.M. Grace was found thrown into the back, her head near the rear window. The *gendarmerie* and two ambulances arrived within ten minutes. They broke the rear window and dragged the barely conscious princess through it; she was taken to the Princess Grace Hospital in Monaco, where her collapsed lung and fractures of the ribs and right femur were attended to. She had a deep wound high in the forehead and her brain was evidently damaged. Because the hospital had no CAT scan machine, the patient was taken that evening to a local doctor's office. The scan showed a small area of bleeding in the temporal lobe, evidence of a possible slight stroke that alone would have brought on dizziness and perhaps a temporary blackout. The accident had caused a massive hemorrhage deep in the brain for which nothing could be done. Princess Grace died at the hospital without recovering consciousness on the evening of 14 September 1982. At her bedside were Rainier and their two elder children, Caroline and Albert.

After lying in state at the palace for several days, she was buried in the Cathedral of St. Nicholas, where she had been married twenty-six years earlier, in the presence of the world's dignitaries.

Various wild rumors circulated: that Stephanie, underage, had been driving the Rover; that a violent argument had caused the crash; even that Grace had killed herself! It seems most likely that she suffered a slight stroke as she approached the dangerous curve, and that Stephanie, too late, made an attempt to apply the emergency brake, which was found half-engaged. An argument, or simply a moment's inattention, cannot be ruled out. Grace was known to be a reluctant driver; Stephanie is reported to have told her father: "Oh, Maman panicked. She didn't know what to do. She lost control."

Grainger, Percy (1882-1961)

Australia's most famous composer settled in the United States in 1914. He is remembered now for his folk song arrangements and lighter pieces, including *Country Gardens* and *Molly on the Shore,* but in his heyday he was a renowned pianist, particularly distinguished for his performance of the Grieg concerto.

His upbringing was unorthodox and probably skewed his lifestyle and sexual practices. His mother Rose disciplined him with a horsewhip and, after discovering her husband had infected her with syphilis, for several years was reluctant to touch her only child. The two left for Europe when Percy was twelve years old to advance his musical training and thereafter she controlled his professional and intimate private relations so closely that rumors (probably unfounded) of incest arose. These may have led to Rose's suicide in 1922 when she leaped from the eighteenth floor of New York's Aeolian Hall.

Percy's sexual partners, including his Swedish-born wife Ella, were subjected to flagellation, often violent, a form of sexual deviance he had discovered as a teenager in Frankfurt. He also practiced self-whipping till his blood flowed. Though aware of possible arrest for his activities, he was not ashamed of them; indeed he produced a series of photographs of the resulting wounds and presented them to the Grainger museum in Melbourne with instructions that they be made public ten years after his death. He told a woman friend he wished he had children he could whip for his own pleasure; as for daughters, he would commit incest with them.

Grainger's cancerous prostate gland was removed in Denmark in 1953, but the malignancy had by then spread to the pelvis. Frequent urinary retention required dilatations of the urethra, and in February 1960 a bilateral orchidectomy (removal of both testicles) was performed in White Plains, New York, where he lived for many years. There was a decline in his mental powers late in 1960. He entered the White Plains Hospital for the last time on 14 February 1961 and died on the twentieth after three days of unconsciousness. His last words were to Ella: "You're the only one I like." The autopsy report, deposited in the Grainger Museum, is discussed in a 1987 study by J. G. O'Shea. Extensive metastatic disease of the brain and skull was found, extending into other parts of the skeletal system. A recent extensive cerebral hemorrhage was also evident.

His last wishes were ignored. His will directed that the flesh be removed from his bones and his skeleton bequeathed to the University of Melbourne for possible display, and that there be no funeral service or other ceremony. Instead, in the only flight he ever took, his body was flown to Australia and buried beside his mother's ashes in the West Terrace Cemetery, Adelaide, after an Anglican service. *See* John Bird (1976).

Grant, Cary (1904-1986).

The English-born Hollywood superstar's only child Jennifer was born in February 1966 to his fourth wife Dyan Cannon at a time when their marriage, after only seven months, was already falling apart and he had just completed work on his last movie, *Walk Don't Run*. He married his fifth wife Barbara Harris in April 1981. At the end of the year the couple and Jennifer attended a Washington ceremony at which Grant and four other Americans were honored for their achievements in the performing arts. He suffered a mild stroke in 1984 but did not slow down in his traveling, his social life, and his promotional work for Fabergé perfumes.

On 28 November 1986 he arrived with Barbara in Davenport, Iowa, for another in a sporadic series of stage presentations he had begun in 1983 titled *A Conversation with Cary Grant*. He felt fine—relaxed, free of the many tensions that had long tormented him. Rumors of his bisexuality had faded; marriage with Barbara had been good for both. They checked into the Blackhawk Hotel and next morning enjoyed a privately conducted tour of the city's attractions, including the municipal art gallery, which houses many of Grant Wood's paintings, and the Palmer College of Chiropractic. They were, reported their guide Douglas Miller, a local businessman, in wonderful spirits.

In the afternoon the Grants ran through the evening's arrangements at the Adler Theater, checking microphone placements for the audience's questions and discussing movie clips with the projectionist. After a while Grant complained of feeling unwell and retired to a dressing room, leaning on Barbara for support. After an hour he gave up plans for the show and was taken back to the hotel. Still he refused medical help until at last Miller took the responsibility of calling his own doctor, Duane Manlove. Arriving around 8:00 P.M., Manlove found Grant had vomited and was complaining of dizziness and a headache; his blood pressure was 210/130. Despite the patient's resistance an ambulance was called. He told the paramedics, "I'm feeling a little pain in the chest; but I don't think it's anything. I don't want to make a big fuss." While being put on a heart monitor, given intravenous medication, and supplied with oxygen, the dying man reached out for his wife's hand and gave it a reassuring squeeze. At St. Luke's Hospital on the way to the intensive care unit Grant murmured, "I love you, Barbara . . .Don't worry," and they clasped hands for a moment. A CAT scan revealed a massive stroke; Cary Grant was declared dead at 11:22 P.M.

Barbara Grant flew back to Los Angeles in a private Learjet with her husband's body in the early hours of 30 November. In accordance with Grant's wishes, there was no funeral service of any kind. His ashes are said to have been scattered by his widow in the hills around their home in Benedict Canyon, Beverly Hills. She and Jennifer shared Grant's fortune, estimated at $40–60 million. *See* Warren G. Harris (1987).

Greene, Graham (1904-1991)

The English novelist embraced Catholicism upon his engagement to Vivien Dayrell-Browning in 1926. The exploration of sin and morality was an essential motif of his works beginning with *Brighton Rock* (1938), but he objected to being described as a Catholic author, maintaining that only a few of his twenty-four novels had a religious emphasis. At best, he said, he was "a Catholic agnostic." (It is significant that he took the confirmation name of Thomas, the doubter.) A world traveler, he opposed U.S. policies in Vietnam and Haiti, as demonstrated in his *The Quiet American* (1956) and *The Comedians* (1966).

After the birth of his son and daughter, he and Vivien separated in the 1960s. Neither married again, but it was revealed after his death that he carried on a passionate romance with the U.S.-born Catherine Walston, wife of a British peer, from 1948 to 1960, begging her repeatedly to become his wife.

For the final third of his life, Greene's companion was Yvonne Cloetta, a French woman twenty years his junior. She lived with her husband Jacques in their Antibes home on the French Riviera, but would drive over daily to the writer's modest apartment five minutes away. They lunched together at an obscure restaurant, Félix au Port, on the harbor and in the afternoon walked her spaniel, Sandy. At seven she drove home after preparing Greene an evening snack. Though they shared no literary interests (even when playing Scrabble her spelling was atrocious) they could be seen to be obviously devoted to one another. He called her HHK (for "happy, healthy kitten") and dedicated *Travels with My Aunt* (1969) to "HHK who helped me more than I can tell."

When Greene's health failed, he and Yvonne moved to her small Swiss apartment overlooking Lake Geneva near Vévey. In his last days he foresaw paradise as an active place, where the dead are able to help the living. He died in Vévey's La Providence Hospital of a blood disorder on 3 April 1991. To Yvonne he murmured his last questions: "Will it be an interesting experience? Will I find out what lies behind the barrier? Why does it take so long to come?"

It was a shock to learn that his estate, estimated at around $18 million, was only $350,000. Evidently he had been more generous to his favorite causes (Trappist monks in Spain, left-wing guerrillas in El Salvador) than anyone suspected. During his long wait for death he had planned his bequests carefully. Everything was divided between Vivien, whom he had never divorced, and his children, Francis and Caroline. Nothing was left to Yvonne, but, as a family member pointed out, "Everything doesn't have to be in the will." At the Swiss funeral and the memorial service in Westminster Abbey Vivien and Yvonne sat far apart. "We have never met," said Yvonne afterward. "I have nothing against her and I don't think she has anything against me."

Guthrie, Woody (1912-1967)

The U.S. folksinger's wandering life was blighted first by alcohol and later by the slow, insidious disease that stole his wits before killing him. To the second of his three wives, Marjorie Greenblatt, he wrote as he turned forty, "I wish you'd grab my next bottle out of my hand and break it over my head . . . To kick me out the door like you do (when I need help most of all) does not help . . ."

The onset of Huntington's disease may already have affected his judgment when he wrote passionate letters to many women in the belief his sentiments were welcomed; in 1948 one of them pressed charges and he was sentenced to imprisonment for mailing obscene material. In 1952 he called on Marjorie unexpectedly and attacked her physically. At Brooklyn State Hospital in September his disease was finally diagnosed; it had killed his mother and probably contributed to her father's death (he fell off his horse and drowned in a shallow river).

Huntington's disease (progressive hereditary chorea) affects, on the average, half the sons and daughters of an affected parent, showing up only in middle age—that is, too late to permit a decision on whether to have children. Psychiatric disturbances and personality changes become evident, caused by progressive degeneration of certain brain cells. Walking, even swallowing, become increasingly difficult, and the limbs exhibit wild, flailing movements. The latter may be controlled with tranquilizers, but the disease has no known cure.

Woody was able to check out of the hospital and by the end of 1952 had run off with his third wife, twenty-year-old Anneke, and in 1953 severely burned his right hand and arm in a barbecue accident in Florida. He returned voluntarily to the Brooklyn hospital in September 1954; Anneke divorced him two years later and their daughter Lorina was adopted.

Woody checked himself out of the hospital in May 1956 and tried to bus across the country; he was arrested for vagrancy in New Jersey and committed to Greystone Park in Morris Plains, where he remained for five years. Marjorie had remarried. Though Woody wrote her anguished letters in almost illegible writing and a style severely affected by mental deterioration ("Six biggy loney somey hard months here since I seed any or alla you . . . "), he found Greystone an improvement on Brooklyn. Marjorie and the children began visiting him. He asked for a guitar, then a typewriter, but was unable to handle them. By the end of the year he could no longer write at all. New friends took him home on Sundays, and looked after him, clipping his nails and hooking his right hand to a belt loop to prevent it flying up with force and tearing his forehead.

By now folk song had eased its way onto the pop charts; other singers were doing well with Woody's songs, notably "This Land Is Your Land," often suggested as a more singable national anthem than "The Star-Spangled Banner." Bob Dylan, much influenced by Woody, went to see him at Greystone in 1960. In 1961 Marjorie had him moved back to Brooklyn State Hospital and brought him to her home at Howard Beach at weekends. By then he could barely speak, but when he did manage to utter something it was usually perceptive or funny. Slowly he lost ground; by 1965 he could no longer speak, but was able to respond to questions by waving his arm wildly toward YES and NO cards.

In 1966 Woody was moved to Creedmore State Hospital in Queens, New York, where Dr. John Whittier was studying Huntington's disease sufferers. Shortly before he died he listened to his son Arlo's popular recording of "Alice's Restaurant." By the time he died, early on 3 October 1967, he weighed less than a hundred pounds, his skin was waxy, almost transparent, his skeleton quite visible, his shaking reduced to a gentle quiver. The previous evening Marjorie thought she detected a flicker of recognition on her final visit. A priest offered a prayer. Well, said Marjorie, we're not Catholic, but Woody had always believed in the validity in all religions. Yes; all right; it would be nice. The priest read the 23rd Psalm. "Then," writes Guthrie's 1980 biographer Joe Klein, "Marjorie got up on her tiptoes [and,] arching over the steel bars of Woody's bed, [kissed] him goodbye."

There was no funeral service. Woody's body was cremated in Brooklyn and Marjorie and the children—Arlo, Joady, and Nora—took the can of ashes to Woody's favorite spot, the jetty separating Coney Island from Sea Gate, intending to scatter them to the wind. They punctured the container with a beer can opener but the ashes just wouldn't pour out. ("It's not coming," said Arlo, waving the can about. "What should I do?") So he threw the can into the ocean; at least it disappeared from sight. Trying to guess what Woody's next move would have been, Marjorie said, "Why don't we go to Nathan's and have a hot dog?"

A memorial concert took place in Carnegie Hall some months later; the proceeds went to the Committee to Combat Huntington's Disease, founded by Marjorie.

Harlow, Jean (1911-1937)

The U.S. movie actress, dubbed "Blonde Bombshell" (the title of one of her twenty-three films), visited Washington, D.C., in February 1937 after completing *Personal Property* and attended Franklin Roosevelt's second inaugural ball. While in the East she caught a chill and needed nursing care during the rail journey back to California on the *Santa Fe Chief*. While convalescing in Palm Springs she developed a gum infection that led to the extraction of several impacted molars.

Harlow was still feeling weak late in April when she began work with Clark Gable, Lionel Barrymore, and Walter Pidgeon on her final movie, *Saratoga* (1937). On 29 May after a week of shooting, she collapsed on the set and was taken to her home on North Palm Drive in Beverly Hills. At first, inquiries about her health were met with scorn by her mother, Jean Harlow Bello, a devout Christian Scientist. Clark Gable asked whether her daughter had been seen by a doctor. Mrs. Bello laughed and said she'd obviously have to introduce him to "Science." When the actress's agent, Arthur Landau, accompanied by Gable and others, forced his way into the house they found Harlow semiconscious and moaning. Dr. E. C. Fishbaugh, an internist, was summoned. He diagnosed gallbladder inflammation and urged immediate hospitalization and surgery, but Mrs. Bello opposed this. Though she reluctantly allowed nurses to be brought in, she refused to leave the sickroom and interfered with their ministrations at every opportunity.

The odor of ammonia on the patient's breath was detected by the nurses on the sixth day after her collapse, a sign of uremic poisoning. Landau recalled that during the star's two-month marriage to Paul Bern (her second husband) several years before, Bern had beaten her severely across the back before killing himself. Ever since, Harlow had complained from time to time of pain around the kidneys.

With Mrs. Bello's resistance to hospitalization undiminished, efforts were made to locate the patient's father, Dr. Mont Clair Carpenter (a dentist) and her stepfather Marino Bello. The head of MGM, Louis B. Mayer, was appealed to and the studio's research staff hunted desperately through the writings of Christian Science's founder Mary Baker Eddy to find loopholes in her ban on the use of orthodox medical resources.

By 6 June, when the twenty-six-year-old actress was spirited out of her home into Good Samaritan Hospital in Los Angeles, it was too late to save her. Two blood transfusions were given overnight but by 9:00 A.M. the ominous Cheyne-Stokes breathing had begun. The city's fire department was called in to provide oxygen. The patient's mother repeatedly shook her in a vain effort to rouse her; the last love of Jean's life, the actor William Powell (q.v.), tried to talk to her, until he broke down and fled from the room. Jean Harlow, still comatose, died at 11:37 A.M. on 7 June 1937 of uremic poisoning.

Wild rumors swept the community about the "real" cause of death: a bungled abortion, cancer from breast implants, ill-advised dieting. The body was dressed for burial in the flower-trimmed pink gown the actress had worn in *Libeled Lady* (1936). In her half-closed hand was a white gardenia with an unsigned note: "Good night, my dearest darling." After a Christian Science service in the Wee Kirk o' the Heather at Hollywood's Forest Lawn Memorial Park Jean Harlow was laid to rest temporarily in a mausoleum near the chapel until a crypt, provided by Powell, was made ready in Forest Lawn's Sanctuary of Benediction. (Mrs. Bello joined her there in 1958.)

The star's net estate, amounting to only $28,000, was left to her mother. The movie *Saratoga* (1937) was completed with Mary Dees, her face usually obscured, standing in for Harlow and Paula Winslowe dubbing her voice. *See* Irving Shulman (1964).

Heine, Heinrich (1797-1856)

The great German lyrical poet published his *Buch der Lieder* in 1827. He settled permanently in Paris in 1831. Because he was a convert to Saint Simonism, a new religion that viewed marriage and the family as repressive instruments, his works were banned in his native Prussia. He was a lover of George Sand, following Alfred de Musset and preceding Chopin, and married an illiterate shop assistant, Mathilde Mirat, in 1841.

Migraine headaches troubled him all his life. The first sign of his fatal disease appeared in 1832, when the fingers of his left hand became irreversibly paralyzed. For several years in the 1830s his vision was sporadically weakened. By 1843 he was suffering from facial palsy and had lost all feeling on his left side. For his remaining eight years he retired to his "mattress-grave," entirely paraplegic, half-blind and with his writing hand partly crippled. In January 1850 he writes of "dreadful cramps . . . lower half of body knotted . . . can only lie on my side . . . constipated 14 days" and complains of the doped condition brought on by the necessary morphine. But this last period saw the publication of many fine poems and prose works, and he toiled sedulously at his memoirs, most of which were destroyed after his death, perhaps by relatives who found themselves viciously described therein.

Heine's final nine months were brightened by the visits of a twenty-seven-year-old admirer whom he called "La Mouche" and to whom he addressed six love poems. She has come down to us under the name "Camille Selden" but her legal name was Elise Krinitz. Acting as his secretary and reading to him, she became very close to Heine. Their intimacy, inhibited only by the dying man's physical disabilities, was viewed rather dispassionately by Mathilde.

In the last weeks he complained of choking; just before the end he began to vomit uncontrollably. Camille visited him on Tuesday, 12 February 1856; his last letter was probably to her, saying he was too ill to see her. On Saturday night she had, she said, a vision of his departing soul. Heine died at 5:00 A.M. on Sunday, 17 February, lucid almost to his final moments. When he was buried without clergy in Montmartre Cemetery, Camille was there; so were Alexandre Dumas and Théophile Gautier.

In a 1990 medical study, E. H. Jellinek challenges the usual diagnosis of neurosyphilis. "Surely the dissemination of lesions in time and in space (optic nerves, brain-stem and cord) makes multiple sclerosis . . . much the likeliest cause." Augustus D'Este, a first cousin of Queen Victoria who was three years senior to Heine, had died eight years earlier after twenty-six years of suffering from the same disease. Jellinek concludes that Heinrich Heine "is the second recorded and certainly the most eminent victim of multiple sclerosis." *See also* J. L. Sammons (1979).

Hellman, Lillian (1905-1984)

The U.S. playwright (*The Children's Hour*, *The Little Foxes*) wrote three volumes of autobiography which are highly regarded. Always a dauntless political activist, she inspired deep loyalty and violent disagreement. She was criticized for never revealing her membership (1938–40) in the Communist Party and for exaggerating—in her *Scoundrel Time* (1976)—her defiance of the House Un-American Activities Committee. There is strong evidence that the "Julia" section of her autobiographical *Pentimento* (1973) is not autobiography at all, but that it is a fabrication based on the exploits of an American, Muriel Gardiner, in the Austrian anti-Nazi underground. Most damning of all to many was her almost total failure to regret Stalin's excesses even after his 1956 denunciation by Khrushchev.

Of Hellman's many lovers, Dashiell Hammett (1894–1961), father of the hard-boiled "private eye" story, was by far the most influential in her life.

She spent her final winter at the Beverly Hills, California, home of Mrs. William Wyler, widow of the film director. She had worn a pacemaker for three years, was almost blind from glaucoma, and her three-packs-a-day habit had given her emphysema. But she hired a college student to carry her up and down the stairs and drive her around to restaurants and shops. Back home in Manhattan, in the spring of 1984 she was even espied in a crowded discotheque, to which an actress friend had taken her. "I'd go anywhere for Pat Neal," she said.

Almost to the last she worked on a sort of recipe book with Peter Feibleman, thirty years her junior but her closest friend. Hearing she was dying at her Martha's Vineyard home in Massachusetts, Feibleman hurried there and before seeing her was warned she was blind and partially paralyzed, had rage attacks and crying fits, and could neither lie nor sit up comfortably. "How are you?" he greeted her. "Not good, Peter, not good . . . This is the worst writer's block I've ever had."

To a book critic who visited her the day before she died she admitted, "Most of the time I spend trying to figure out how to kill myself." But a moment later she added, "I shouldn't have said that." That evening she was carried to the home of friends, John and Barbara Hersey, for dinner.

When she died on 30 June 1984 the cause was announced to be heart failure. Amid much publicity and in the presence of celebrities from around the country she was buried in Abel's Hill Cemetery in Chilmark on Martha's Vineyard. In one of the eulogies John Hersey said "a few words about Lillian's anger . . . Anger was her essence. It informed her art." It was her rage that may have been in the mind of her friend Milton Gordon when, phoned by Hersey to report Hellman's death, he retorted, "She didn't die; someone reached down from up there and grabbed her by the throat."

Her estate of almost $4 million was shared by two funds, in the names of herself and Hammett, and by many friends, notably Feibleman. *See* William Wright (1986).

Henson, Jim (1936-1990)

The U.S. puppeteer, creator of the Muppets, voice of Kermit the frog, probably died at fifty-three because he was too considerate—too modest and unassuming. The thirtieth anniversary of the Muppets in 1986 also saw his Muppetless movie *Labyrinth* damned with faint praise from the critics. It was then that Henson and his wife of twenty-seven years, after living apart for two years, legally separated. The relative failure of *Labyrinth* and, earlier, *The Dark Crystal* (1983) "were great losses," said Jane Henson, "and *Labyrinth* was a real blow."

In the spring of 1990 Henson began negotiating the sale of those Muppets not featured on public television's highly successful *Sesame Street* to the Walt Disney Co. for around $150 million. In his last weeks he jetted ceaselessly between Los Angeles and New York, with side trips to Orlando, Florida, working on films and a new Muppet show for television. On 4 May 1990 his bearded, six-feet-three-inch frame could be seen slumped in a chair on the Arsenio Hall talk show as he admitted to tiredness and a sore throat. Nevertheless, he maintained his busy schedule, flying off to New York on business as planned.

He and his daughter Cheryl spent the weekend of 12–13 May in Ahoskie, North Carolina, visiting his father and stepmother but sleeping at a motel nearby. He visited a local doctor, complaining of flulike symptoms, on Saturday, 12 May, but there seemed nothing seriously wrong, and the doctor prescribed no treatment beyond aspirin. On Sunday he had to force himself to get out of bed and fly back to New York with Cheryl. She was puzzled when her father, as they left the airport, suddenly sat down against a radiator in the corridor and exclaimed, "Hi ho, Kermit the frog here."

He spent a "rough night," he said, trying to sleep that night in his apartment in the Sherry Netherland Hotel, overlooking Central Park, and canceled a Monday recording session. In the evening Jane came over and "we just talked," she said. "There was no division of broken marriage or anything like that. We were just there together."

A few hours later signs of severe illness were evident. It was 2:00 A.M. on Tuesday and Jim, within twenty-four hours of death, was coughing up blood and barely able to breathe. But he refused to be taken to the hospital. He just didn't want "anyone else to be disturbed by his pain," said Jane. But, she added, it was partly "his Christian Science upbringing." He didn't practice the religion but it had some effect on his thinking. "Not that he distrusted doctors, but he would rather just see it through by himself."

At last, around 4:00 A.M., he said, "I'm breathing too hard. My heart's racing," and agreed that Jane should call for a car. Taken to the wrong door at New York Hospital, he walked around the building rather than bother the driver. Henson was admitted at 4:58 A.M.

X rays showed abscesses in the lobes of both lungs. At 8.00 A.M. he was anesthetized, connected to a mechanical ventilator, and taken to the intensive-care unit. Throughout the day Jane and their five children kept vigil in the corridor, creeping in at intervals to peek at the invalid. He had sought help too late to be saved. Eight hours earlier the result would likely have been very different. As the director of the I.C.U., Dr. David Gelmont, explained to reporters, Henson had been attacked by an especially aggressive type of pneumonia caused by streptococcus Group A. Though the patient was given high doses of six different antibiotics, his body had already been overwhelmed by infection; kidney and heart failure were evident from the beginning, and the blood was no longer able to clot. Death was the direct result of uncontrollable bleeding into the lungs. Immunologists Philippa Marrack and John Kappler have explained that Group A streptococcal infections, often beginning as "strep throat," whip the immune system into extraordinary activity, deluging the body with a surfeit of hormones, called lymphokines, that slow down the kidneys and dilate the blood vessels, causing a calamitous drop in blood pressure.

Jim Henson's death, after two cardiac arrests, occurred at 1:21 A.M. on Wednesday, 16 May 1990. A memorial service at the Cathedral of St. John the Divine in New York City was attended by five thousand admirers, many flourishing handpainted fans. The puppeteer, who left his lucrative business to his five children, had written a letter to them four years earlier to be opened after his death: "I'm not at all afraid of the thought of death and look forward to it. It would be lovely if there were a song or two . . . and someone said some nice happy words about me . . ."

Hess, Rudolf (1894-1987?)

The deputy Führer of Nazi Germany astonished the world when he flew secretly to Scotland in May 1941 at the height of World War II in an apparent bid to make peace with Britain. The bid was ignored and Hess was sentenced at the Nuremberg War Criminal Trials to life imprisonment.

Over the years his six former colleagues in Berlin's Spandau prison were released and from 1966 Prisoner No. 7 was the sole inmate, guarded in rotation by American, British, French, and Soviet personnel. In 1969 he nearly died of a perforated duodenal ulcer, which was tardily handled by the Soviet authorities who were on duty. Thereafter he suffered some of the disabilities of old age: uncertain gait, poor posture, and restricted vision.

The Americans were on duty during August 1987. On the seventeenth, Hess napped after lunch as usual. At 2:30 he walked down to the garden with a warder for his afternoon exercise. A little later the two men sat on a bench in a cluttered summerhouse until the warder was called away briefly to take a phone call. On his return he found the prisoner bent forward on the floor with his knees against his chest, propped against a folding chair. His face was a dark leaden color and around his neck was wound a length of electric cable. Mouth-to-mouth resuscitation and external heart massage were unavailing; so were further measures at the British Military Hospital, where Hess was declared dead at 4:10 P.M.

At the first of two autopsies a note was found in the dead man's pocket: "Please would the authorities send this home. Written a few minutes before my death. Dear Ilse [Hess's wife], Thank you for what you have done for me and what you tried to do." Cause of death was recorded as "Asphyxia; compression of the neck; suspension." The family, dissatisfied, had a second autopsy performed: "Death was caused by a strangling implement around the throat." The Hess family, and many others, suspected murder. Because the cable was a loose piece, not attached to an immovable object, suspension, i.e. hanging, seemed to be ruled out and the deep bruising of the neck was evidently beyond the powers of a feeble old man to inflict by self-strangling. In March 1988 the West Berlin state prosecutor began a homicide investigation, which has so far proved inconclusive.

Because it was feared neo-Nazis would make the burial place a shrine, Rudolf Hess's interment at Wansiedel was delayed until 17 March 1988.

Dr. Hugh Thomas, in his 1979 book *The Murder of Rudolf Hess,* challenges the accepted story of the deputy Führer's flight to Britain and the identity of the man who lived and died in Spandau. As a surgical consultant at the hospital where Hess would later be pronounced dead, he was present when Prisoner No. 7 underwent a routine examination in 1973. He was astounded to find no trace, either as a visible scar on the chest or in X-ray photographs, of the serious bullet wound suffered by Hess on the Romanian front in August 1917, a wound so serious that he spent four months in various hospitals and was unable to resume active service.

Following up on the discovery, he investigated the mysterious 1941 flight in detail. The genuine Hess left Augsburg, near Munich, at 5:45 P.M. on 10 May in a twin-engined Messerschmitt 110D without auxiliary fuel tanks. He told no one where he was headed. Because his own flying suit was missing, he borrowed one from a friend. An apparently bogus Hess (says Thomas) arrived in Scotland around 11:00 P.M. the same night in a 110D (or 110E) with fuel tanks fitted below the wings; they were jettisoned over the Clyde estuary, from which one was recovered next day. And with or without extra tanks, the route claimed by the new arrival was far beyond the Messerschmitt's range. He was wearing Hess's flying suit and was without Hess's identity disc or personal papers.

Thomas believes the real Hess was shot down as part of a plot by Heinrich Himmler, or another rival in the Nazi leadership who knew of Hess's plan, and a Hess-double, standing by at Aalborg, Denmark, flew the much shorter route to the Glasgow area.

According to this theory, Hess's feigned amnesia, maintained for many years, was to disguise his lack of essential knowledge when questioned. Whereas Hess was a vegetarian, the prisoner was omnivorous. Frau Ilse Hess never doubted that the prisoner was her husband, but he refused to see her until 1969 and she then remarked on his unexpectedly deeper voice and the absence of a prior gap between his front teeth.

In his updated book, *Hess: A Tale of Two Murders,* 1988, Thomas joins with the family in believing that the prisoner, whoever he was, did not die by suicide.

To the disinterested observer, it is difficult to determine which version of the facts is the true one. It seems scarcely credible, whatever the threats or inducements, that an innocent man would willingly submit to forty-six years of imprisonment in Britain and Spandau. Thomas's theory has much evidence in its favor, but its author offers no identity for the mysterious double and also fails to present a reasonable motive for a German mission to Britain in 1941.

But until at least the question of the chest scars (confirmed as absent by the two autopsies and as clearly present by Hess's wife) is resolved, rumors of a plot concocted by the Nazis and perhaps covered up for years by the Churchill government can never be quite allayed.

Heydrich, Reinhard (1904-1942)

The Reichsprotektor of Nazi-occupied Czechoslovakia, second only to Martin Bormann in the Hitler hierarchy, was also in charge of the notorious death camps. Within twenty-four hours of his arrival in Prague in September 1941 he launched a terror campaign against the population; by the end of the year the Czech government-in-exile in London were determined he must be killed.

The mission was entrusted to two young Czech commandos, Jan Kubiš and Josef Gabčík, who had been trained in Britain. They parachuted into Czechoslovakia in December 1941, joined up with the resistance movement and painstakingly made their plans.

On 27 May 1942, a warm and sunny morning, Heydrich was being driven from his luxurious residence at the village of Panenské Břežany to his headquarters in Prague, fourteen miles away. Members of the Resistance monitored his progress and signaled ahead. When he reached the northern suburb of Holešovice, just beyond the point where Kirchmayerova Street twists sharply downhill to Troya Bridge on the right, he was ambushed. Gabčík waited just beyond the turn on the right side of the street with a Sten gun hidden under his coat. Twenty yards farther stood Kubiš with a Mills grenade.

It was 10:30 A.M. The open Mercedes-Benz slowed to a walk and made the turn. Gabčík walked toward the hated Reichsprotektor, raised his gun and pulled the trigger at point-blank range. Nothing happened; the weapon had jammed. A startled Heydrich reached for his revolver. By now, the car had passed Kubiš; he lobbed the grenade toward the right rear seat, occupied by the quarry. The blast hurled two spare uniform jackets from the seat onto the trolley wires overhead. Kubiš staggered backward, wounded in the face. The car stopped, its near-side door shattered. The wounded Heydrich rose and fired at Gabčík, who stood a moment in bewilderment before hurling his useless gun to the ground and racing away. He was pursued by the chauffeur but escaped on foot, unhurt. Dodging behind an arriving trolley car, Kubiš grabbed his bicycle and pedaled furiously down the hill.

Heydrich now collapsed. He was taken in a passing truck to the Buvlovka Hospital close by suffering from multiple injuries to the back and side from bomb splinters. After his diaphragm had been repaired and a blood transfusion given, his lacerated spleen was removed. Top German surgeons took charge of the invalid, who for several days seemed likely to recover. On 3 June Heydrich was able to sit up for lunch, but during the meal he suddenly collapsed; he died at 7:30 A.M. on 4 June 1942. Contemporary reports gave the cause of death as mediastinitis (inflammation of the membrane separating the lungs) but the pathologist who conducted the autopsy, Herwig Hamperl, finally believed (according to Richard A. Davis's 1971 medical study) that "anemic shock" was the cause. No postmortem evidence of disease was found, the sudden collapse is better explained as due to a postoperative embolism, as the Paris physician E. Roseau suggested in a 1972 study. Heydrich was buried in Berlin's Invaliden Cemetery after ceremonies attended by Heinrich Himmler, who delivered the eulogy, and by Hitler himself.

It was the Führer who ordered Karl Frank, the dead man's deputy, to wreak revenge on the Czech nation. The village of Lidice, which was in no way connected with the assassination, was razed to the ground; all 173 men and youths were shot on 10 June, the women were sent to concentration camps, where most perished, and the children were "re-educated" in Germany. In Prague a curfew was imposed on 27 May, a house-to-house search was conducted, and thousands of executions followed.

At first the assassins were able to lie low, but two fellow-parachutists, Karel Čurda and Viliam Gerik, betrayed them. On 18 June 1942 their final hideout in the crypt of Prague's Greek Orthodox Church in Resslova Street was besieged by an S.S. battalion. With bullets and grenades, with smoke, tear gas and water pumped from the river, the soldiers tried all day to dislodge them. Kubiš, who had been on watch in the choir loft, died early from shrapnel wounds. Only as their ammunition ran out did Gabčík and three comrades shoot themselves in the flooded crypt. It is now a national shrine.

In 1946, Frank, Čurda, and Gerik were tried by the liberated Czechs and hanged.

Hitchcock, Alfred (1899-1980)

The English-born movie director of *The 39 Steps* (1935), *Psycho* (1960), and over fifty other British and U.S. feature films could show great kindness and patience, be witty and a good companion. But though he was a faithful husband to the petite, frail Alma Reville for more than half a century, colleagues glimpsed a darker side of his nature, exhibited during his later years in unwelcome advances toward more than one of his young actresses, on and off the set.

When he was honored by the American Film Institute with a life achievement award on 7 March 1979 he refused all cooperation with the arrangements. "He looked on the evening as his own obituary," said an associate, "and he didn't want to attend the funeral." Alma managed to attend despite partial paralysis. Hitchcock himself, 150 pounds overweight, racked by arthritis and undermined by heart disease, for which he wore a pacemaker, had to be kept away from the customary brandy and vodka, and for safety his acceptance speech was recorded during the afternoon to permit editing. Throughout the actual ceremony he wore a blank stare.

He had slowed down considerably even before making his final film, *Family Plot* (1976); he would discuss future ventures, but nothing came of them. He spent his days at the office in Universal Studios, complaining to his small staff of illness and loneliness; there were childish rages and obscene approaches to a temporary secretary. In May 1979 he shut down the office without warning, leaving his secretaries without compensation. When Ingrid Bergman called at his home, 10957 Bellagio Road in Beverly Hills, he gripped her hands and, with tears streaming down his face, wailed, "Ingrid, I'm going to die."

In January 1980, when he was created Sir Alfred Hitchcock by Queen Elizabeth II, the papers were presented to him at Universal Studios by the British consul general. In March he was able to tape an introduction for the American Film Institute's tribute to James Stewart. Hitchcock's death was undramatic; his arthritis pains diminished in April and he was able to sleep undisturbed, but his liver and then his kidneys failed. He died quietly at his home at 9:17 A.M. on 29 April 1980.

At least five hundred mourners attended his Catholic funeral service at the Church of the Good Shepherd in Beverly Hills. Many of the actors who starred in his movies were present. The body was cremated. Hitchcock's ashes were scattered over the Pacific Ocean off Los Angeles. *See* Donald Spoto (1983).

Hoffa, James Riddle (1913-1975)

The feisty, controversial president of the International Brotherhood of Teamsters from 1957 to 1971 was kidnapped and almost certainly murdered on 30 July 1975.

Hoffa was convicted of jury tampering and diversion of union funds in 1964 and began a thirteen-year sentence at Lewisburg Federal Prison in March 1967. He held on to the union presidency until early 1971 and, under pressure from Frank E. Fitzsimmons, his successor, the Nixon administration released him late the same year.

Angered to discover that he was barred from all union activities, he began a fight in the courts to have the restrictions set aside. Little by little his popularity with union members dwindled as Fitzsimmons and his allies fought off his threatened return to power. In his autobiography, published posthumously, Hoffa accused the union president of things he had earlier done himself: "selling out to mobsters" and "making vast loans from the billion-dollar Teamster pension fund to known mobsters." To the union bosses and, even more, to the underworld behind it, Jimmy Hoffa was seen as a threat.

On 30 July 1975, Hoffa left his summer home at Lake Orion, north of Detroit, for a rendezvous at the Machus Red Fox Restaurant, nineteen miles away just outside Detroit. His wife Josephine thought he looked nervous as he drove his 1974 green Pontiac hardtop out of the driveway. He had told her he was going to meet two men: his friend Anthony "Tony Jacks" Giacalone, the Mafia's Detroit "enforcer," and Anthony "Tony Pro" Provenzano, a Mafia boss with a reputation for violence who was also head of a New Jersey Teamsters local.

Three books in 1977–78 by Lester Velie, Dan E. Moldea, and Steven Brill are in general agreement about what happened next. Hoffa was picked up by Charles "Chuckie" O'Brien, 41, who had lived with the Hoffas since childhood. With O'Brien in the car, a borrowed 1975 maroon Mercury, were Salvatore "Sally Bugs" Briguglio, 45, and another trusted associate of Tony Pro. (Tony Pro and Tony Jacks themselves had watertight alibis.)

Hoffa was probably stunned with the butt of a gun and, at a location in Detroit, either shot or garroted. The killers raced back to New Jersey by private plane from Pontiac airport the same afternoon. The actual killer was probably Briguglio; he was indicted but gunned down outside a New York restaurant before facing trial.

Brill believes Hoffa's body was destroyed locally at Central Sanitation Services, a mob-controlled business in Hamtramck equipped with a shredder, compactor, and incinerator.

Holden, William (1918-1981)

The U.S. movie actor had his first leading role in *Golden Boy* (1939); he created a box-office sensation playing opposite Gloria Swanson in *Sunset Boulevard* (1950) and won an Oscar in *Stalag 17* (1953). But he was ambivalent about acting, and anxiety over his abilities drove him to alcohol from his earliest years on screen. After his marriage to Brenda Marshall fell apart his name was linked with several world-famous Hollywood stars. But he also expended much time in Africa in aid of endangered animal species, and set up a game reserve in Kenya.

Of Holden's impressive roles in *Network* (1976) and his final film, *S.O.B.* (1981), a critic wrote that in these latter days he had become a "symbol of hard-bitten decency." Flying back to Los Angeles in July 1981 after leading a promotional tour for *S.O.B.,* he talked to a colleague about death; "I've got it all settled," he said. "It cost me twenty-five dollars to join the Neptune Society. They'll cremate my body and scatter the ashes at sea. I'm not going to waste my money on some big monument or a damn Hollywood funeral." Depressed when work on *That Championship Season* was put off until 1982, he drove from his Palm Springs home to a thirteen-story apartment building in Santa Monica, California, the Shoreham Tower, of which he was part owner. Thereafter he was seldom seen, talking—often in drunken tones—with friends and associates on the telephone. When the prospective director of *That Championship Season,* William Friedkin, called him on 2 November, he answered in a slurred voice. "I'm not going to do the picture, Billy," he said, and added repeatedly, "I'll see you in Africa." Calls to the apartment during the following week were unanswered.

The manager of the apartments unlocked Holden's door 16 November 1981 and discovered the actor's body lying beside the bed in a pool of blood. The signs pointed to a fall on a loose throw rug and a blow to the right forehead from a corner of the bedside table; there was no evidence of foul play. Holden had been dead for several days; he had evidently tried to staunch the blood flow from a two-and-a-half-inch cut with a series of paper tissues and had been too drunk to phone for help. He probably lost consciousness within five or ten minutes and died within half an hour. The television set was on and a movie script was nearby; there was an empty quart vodka bottle in the kitchen waste basket and .22 percent of alcohol in the blood, equivalent to at least eight or ten shots of liquor.

There was no memorial service; the Neptune Society fulfilled its twenty-five-dollar pledge. *See* Bob Thomas: *Golden Boy* (1983).

Hoover, J. Edgar (1895-1972)

Sometimes called the most powerful man in America, Hoover ruled the Federal Bureau of Investigation for almost forty-eight years. He served eight U.S. presidents, more than one of whom wanted him gone (the last, Richard Nixon, twice tried to fire him), but fear of the secret Bureau files caused them to back off. To many, Hoover was a guardian of law and order, staunch preserver of all that is best in the American system; to others he was a bully and a menace to freedom of speech and assembly. (A Senate investigation of the Bureau in 1976 found "a pattern . . . of activities that threatened our Constitution.")

Hoover put in a full day at the Justice Department on 1 May 1972, understandably furious with Jack Anderson's column in the *Washington Post,* which quoted verbatim from FBI documents. "Hoover seems to have a hang-up on sex. His gumshoes go out of their way to find out who's sleeping with whom in Washington and Hollywood."

After work, the director's chauffeur Tom Moton drove him to the house of his intimate friend Clyde A. Tolson for dinner and at 10:15 P.M. to Hoover's own home at 4936 Thirtieth Place N.W. There, Hoover let out his pair of Cairn terriers and before turning in called James Crawford to come in the morning to plant some rose bushes. (Crawford was a retired special agent still on call to do odd jobs in the house and yard.)

Next day, 2 May 1972, Hoover's housekeeper Annie Fields was puzzled not to hear the shower as she cooked his usual breakfast of soft-boiled eggs, toast, and coffee. Moton arrived and waited; around 8:15 Crawford came and began work in the yard. A few minutes later Annie, by now quite worried, asked Crawford to go upstairs; she didn't want to go herself, Crawford knew, because Hoover slept in the nude. The handyman knocked on the bedroom door and looked in to see "the Boss" sprawled on the oriental rug beside the bed; the body was cold to the touch.

Because mention of Crawford might raise awkward questions, says Hoover's 1991 biographer Curt Gentry, Annie Fields was given credit, in the official announcement, for finding Hoover dead. What was a *retired* agent doing there? What were his duties? Who paid him for them? What else was going on?

Though Dr. Robert V. Choisser said his patient had suffered only slight hypertension, the death certificate gave as the cause "hypertensive cardio-vascular disease." There was no autopsy; but then, the dead man was seventy-seven, and neither homicide nor accident was likely.

The lead-lined coffin lay in state on 3 May in the Capitol Rotunda on a catafalque built for Lincoln. The FBI director was only the twenty-second person, and the first civil servant, to be so honored. The thousand-pound coffin was carried up the Capitol steps by eight military pallbearers, two of whom suffered hernias during the ordeal.

At the funeral service in Washington's National Presbyterian Church, Nixon spoke of the dead man as having "made the FBI . . . the invincible and incorruptible defender of every American's precious right to be free from fear." But on a White House tape, Nixon can be heard saying later, "He's got files on everybody, God damn it."

By now, Tolson, who knew he would inherit nearly all of his friend's $560,000 estate, had moved into his house and resigned from the Bureau. (He died in April 1975; the nature of his relationship with Hoover still open to speculation.) Hoover's files were being selectively destroyed by his secretary Helen Gandy and others. Patrick Gray was immediately nominated as director of the FBI but later withdrew under pressure.

J. Edgar Hoover was buried in the old Congressional Cemetery in southeast Washington, overlooking the Anacostia River and just a few blocks from his birthplace. His parents lie nearby.

Hopkins, Gerard Manley (1844-1889)

The verse of the English poet and Jesuit priest was not published until long after his death, but it is now recognized, despite its often startling rhythms and frequent obscurities, as belonging to the modern age, far ahead of the time it was written. He was born an Anglican and moved to the Roman Catholic faith in 1867. When he entered the priesthood eleven years later he burned all the poems he had written. His final five years were spent as professor of classics at University College, Dublin.

A slightly built, shy man, burdened by heavy duties—some perhaps self-imposed by an overscrupulous conscience—he suffered from a periodic melancholy that, he feared, bordered on madness. On 29 April 1889, as the onerous task of preparing papers for the summer examinations once more approached, he sent his final poem, the sonnet "To R.B.," to his closest friend, the future poet laureate Robert Bridges. It had been written a week earlier during a rare day of freedom while out sketching on an estate near Dublin. In an accompanying letter Hopkins wrote, "I am ill today, but no matter for that as my spirits are good . . . Now I must lie down."

Within a day or two he was confined to bed, but his illness was not at first viewed seriously. To his father in England Hopkins wrote, "I saw a doctor yesterday, who treated my complaint as a fleabite, a treatment which begets confidence but not gratitude." His illness was an isolated case of typhoid fever, doubtless picked up from the wretched sanitation at his rooms on St. Stephen's Green in Dublin. (After his death the sewers there were found to be full of rats and filth.)

His end came slowly; for six weeks the disease gradually weakened him. By 4 or 5 June peritonitis had set in and his parents were sent for. Final rites were administered on the morning of 8 June 1889; these included the Holy Viaticum (the Eucharist for the dying). He died at 1:30 P.M. on that day. His last words were said to be "I am so happy," whispered several times.

For fear of infection, the body was not taken into the Jesuit Church on Upper Gardiner Street; the coffin at the High Mass was empty. Burial was in the plot reserved for the Society of Jesus in the Prospect Cemetery, Glasnevin, on the northern edge of the city. Individual graves are not identified, and there is doubt about the exact location of Hopkins's.

Obituaries were few, and none mentioned the dead priest's poetic achievements, still unknown to the world; instead, his classical scholarship and art criticism were praised. Bridges was held back from publishing his friend's verses by the difficulty of composing a memoir to accompany them that would avoid picturing the dead man as eccentric. The few poems published in anthologies early in the century met with mixed, even hostile, reviews. At last, almost thirty years after Hopkins's death, Bridges in 1918 published a first edition of the collected verses. Ezra Pound, for one, greeted them as "the useful, but monotonous, in their day unduly neglected, as more recently unduly touted, metrical labors of G. Manley Hopkins." *See* Norman White (1992).

Horowitz, Vladimir (1904-1989)

The Ukrainian-born U.S. pianist married the Italian conductor Arturo Toscanini's younger daughter Wanda in 1933. Though he was bisexual, a hypochondriac, and subject to manic-depressive swings, the couple's relationship grew into a mutually supportive one; nevertheless, they separated from 1949 to 1953 and there were several stormy interludes.

Added to depression brought on by unfavorable reviews in the fall of 1953 were fears that one of his frequent attacks of colitis would beset him during a performance. It was this combination of causes that led to Horowitz's twelve-year withdrawal from public view. Again, in the early 1980s, overdependence on prescription drugs was blamed for a period of sloppy playing followed by a second retirement, this time for only a year and a half.

The virtuoso reemerged in near-miraculous style to make a highly successful television film, *Horowitz: The Last Romantic,* shot in his Manhattan living room on East 94th Street in April and May 1984. But the highlight of his life was his return, after nearly sixty years, to the Soviet Union in 1986. His wildly acclaimed Moscow recital was broadcast live by CBS Television on Sunday morning, 20 April.

In March of the next year he traveled to Milan to make his last concerto recording; again it was filmed for television and again the videocassette was a best-seller. Because of his newfound love of Mozart, an enormously challenging composer ("In five days I can memorize and play the *Funérailles* of Liszt but I could not play a sonata by Mozart," he once wrote), he performed that composer's *Concerto in A major,* K.488, and *Sonata in B flat,* K.333. The conductor of La Scala orchestra was Carlo Maria Giulini, and there was obvious tension between the two Mozart specialists. They disagreed over tempi and over the nature of a grace note: "It's an acciaccatura," said the conductor. "No, it's an appoggiatura," said the pianist; "you play it your way and I'll play it mine." Giulini finally gave way.

Horowitz's final public appearance was at a Manhattan record store on 11 October 1989 to sign his albums, but he continued to make recordings at his home until four days before his death. Six sessions of Haydn, Chopin, and Liszt for CBS/Sony ended on 1 November. On the third he awoke feeling nauseated and dizzy but the doctor could find nothing wrong. On Sunday, 5 November 1989, he rose late and had breakfast, then visited

Wanda's bedroom to discuss their dinner menu. Celine Wright, the house-keeper, came in and Wanda turned to speak to her. At that moment Mrs. Wright gasped as she saw Horowitz, apparently stricken by a massive heart attack, slump in his chair and slide to the floor. Wanda looked round and said, "He's dead." Paramedics were called and worked on him for an hour, but the eighty-five-year-old pianist showed no sign of life.

His body was taken to the Campbell funeral home on Madison Avenue as messages poured in from all over the world; Horowitz lay in state for two days while a tape of his playing could be heard in the background. How was it that a Jew, even a nonobserving Jew, could be buried in a Catholic cemetery? "Nobody asked any questions," said Wanda. So her husband lies in the Toscanini family crypt in the Cimitero Monumentale in Milan beside his daughter Sonia, who died—possibly of a drug overdose—in Geneva in 1974.

The musician's estate, valued at $6–8 million, went mainly to his wife, with $300,000 for scholarships at the Juilliard School and $200,000 for Giuliana Lopes, the friend and household companion who helped him regain his health and career in 1984. *See* Harold C. Schonberg (1992).

Hubbard, L. Ron (1911-1986)

The U.S. science-fiction writer introduced the new "science" of dianetics in the May 1950 issue of *Astounding Science Fiction*. It was followed up within weeks by a best-selling book and announcements of five-hundred-dollar courses for would-be practitioners eager to cure insanity and a host of other human ailments. Dianetics was converted two years later into a religion dubbed "Scientology" which in 1984 was to be described by a British court as "immoral, socially obnoxious, corrupt, sinister and dangerous" and by a Los Angeles judge as run by "an organization [that] clearly is schizophrenic and paranoid, and this bizarre combination seems to be a reflection of its founder . . . a pathological liar [about] his history, background, and achievements. The . . . evidence [reflects] his egoism, greed, avarice, lust for power, and vindictiveness and aggressiveness against persons perceived by him to be disloyal and hostile." The judge could have added that he was also an overweight, foul-mouthed bully who tyrannized his adoring followers.

While his "church" was raking in millions of dollars, Hubbard spent many years avoiding prosecution by cruising in and out of the Mediterranean. Meanwhile his agents infiltrated U.S. agencies, stealing or neutralizing documents he deemed dangerous. (In 1983–84 his third wife Mary Sue, abandoned by her husband, served a prison term for her role in this.) During 1976–79, Hubbard lived under cover at La Quinta, near Palm Desert, California, and then for a year at Hemet, about sixty miles away. In February 1980 he disappeared.

On 25 January 1986 the Reis Chapel in San Luis Obispo, California, was summoned by telephone to pick up a body from the Whispering Winds Ranch at Creston, twenty miles to the north. The death certificate bore the name Lafayette Ronald Hubbard. The local coroner had the body photographed and fingerprinted, and the prints corresponded to those in FBI files. The time of death was given as 8:00 P.M. on the twenty-fourth, and the cause as cerebral hemorrhage, but a certificate of "religious belief" forbade an autopsy. It was learned later that Hubbard had lived very quietly at the ranch with a young couple named Mitchell since 1983. Hubbard's ashes were scattered in the Pacific nearby from a small boat. *See* Russell Miller: *Bare-Faced Messiah* (1987).

Hudson, Rock (1925-1985)

The world was shocked to learn in July 1985 that the famous movie actor was suffering from AIDS, a disease that at that date was almost exclusively contracted by male homosexuals. The news spurred the Hollywood community into action to help AIDS research and generate sympathy for its victims. In September 1985, movie celebrities, headed by Elizabeth Taylor, organized an AIDS benefit at which a statement ostensibly from Hudson himself was read by Burt Lancaster. But by then the stricken actor was down to ninety-seven pounds and virtually comatose.

Rock Hudson had not felt well since he filmed *The Ambassador* in Israel late in 1983 with Robert Mitchum. On 8 June 1984 a bump on his neck was diagnosed as Kaposi's sarcoma, usually a telltale sign of AIDS, and other tests confirmed that he was indeed suffering from the full-blown acquired immune deficiency syndrome. But he told virtually no one. Though a tight circle of Hollywood acquaintances knew he was an active homosexual, he had always denied it in the past and, in fact, never did admit it. One man he kept in the dark, according to a suit brought against the Hudson estate, was his last live-in lover, Marc Christian.

For several weeks, as an outpatient, he was given secret treatments of an antiviral drug, HPA-23, by Dr. Dominique Dormont during an August–September "vacation" in Paris, but he cut short the therapy to fulfill a contract to appear in the TV series *Dynasty*. He completed ten shows, of which nine were broadcast; a kiss with Linda Evans in one episode was to cause much controversy months later after the news broke.

His last public appearance was on 15 July 1985 in Carmel, California, near the home of his old costar, Doris Day. Though weak and pathetically thin, he wanted to fulfill his promise to publicize her new annual show, *Doris Day's Best Friends*, on the Christian Broadcasting Network. "This guy's near death" was the reaction of the shocked press corps. Why had he agreed to appear? His rambling explanation of his late arrival suggested he was no longer making sound judgments.

He returned to Paris by Air France on 20 July, but was in such feeble condition that at first he was forbidden by the airline to board. He collapsed as he arrived at the Ritz Hotel and was taken to the American Hospital for tests. The news that Hudson was an AIDS sufferer was broken by *Daily Variety* columnist Army Archerd on 23 July, and was confirmed two days later in Paris. When the press release was read to the patient, he replied—in an obvious reference to the journalists waiting outside—"Go and give it to the dogs."

A jumbo jet was chartered—at a cost of $300,000—to return Hudson, his secretary, and a small medical team to Los Angeles on 30 July. At the UCLA Medical Center it was deemed essential that the dying actor have nourishment and rest; the few permitted visitors were shepherded through checkpoints to see the confused, comatose invalid for brief periods. On 24 August, Rock was allowed to return home to "The Castle," his sprawling hacienda in the hills above Beverly Hills; there, he was cared for by Tom Clark—who had lived with the actor for seventeen years until he moved out in 1983—and a relay of nurses. Marc Christian was deemed a nuisance; he lived in The Castle's theater-annex and was kept away from the sickroom.

There were bizarre attempts to bring Hudson, an apostate Catholic, back into one fold or another. Toni Phillips, a night nurse and born-again Christian, claimed to have brought him to accept Jesus on 14 September. Father Terry Sweeney, a Jesuit, was summoned by his friends from Loyola of Marymount to anoint him and give him Communion. The actor Pat Boone, his wife Shirley and a mysterious woman, the tall, stately "Eleanor," held prayer vigils and on 1 October visited the sickroom, claiming afterward to have evoked some response from the semiconscious Hudson.

Early on 2 October, a nurse, excited by what she thought were signs of improvement during the previous day's prayers, dressed the barely sentient Hudson and sat him up in a chair. Clark, horrified, returned him to bed, where he fell asleep instantly. An hour later, at 8:30 A.M., a hospital bed was delivered. Around 9:00 A.M., Tom Clark looked in and found the nurses standing by the bed, weeping. Rock Hudson's breathing had stopped; he had died quietly in his sleep. His last words, minutes earlier, were to Clark: asked if he would care for a cup of coffee, Hudson replied, "No, I don't believe so." The death certificate gave the immediate cause of death as "cardiopulmonary arrest," and the underlying causes as "lymphoblastic lymphoma, 4 months; Acquired Immune Deficiency Syndrome, 16 months."

Somehow, news of the death leaked out before the body could be removed (in an unmarked van) to the crematory at Grand View Memorial Park in Glendale, and there were desperate attempts by press photographers to sneak a final shot. There was no funeral service. The ashes were scattered in the Pacific off Marina del Rey by Clark on 20 October. *See* Jerry Oppenheimer and Jack Vitek (1986).

Johnson, Lyndon Baines (1908-1973)

The thirty-sixth U.S. president came into office on the day John F. Kennedy was assassinated and was elected to a full term in 1964. He could have run for a second four-year term but, because of rising opposition to the Vietnam War, he announced on 31 March 1968 that "I shall not seek, and I will not accept the nomination of my party . . ."

Johnson was only forty-six when arteriosclerosis led to his first heart attack in 1955. He stopped smoking then but resumed after retirement. "He smoked like a fiend," said a friend. He soon adapted to a quieter lifestyle: "One of the things I [enjoy] most [is] being able to go to bed after the ten o'clock news at night and sleep until daylight the next morning." But he suffered almost constant angina and had to chew nitroglycerin tablets. Though he traveled (to Florida for a sailing vacation, to Acapulco with a party every February), spent time recording his memoirs for the Johnson Library in Austin (dedicated in May 1971), and became head of the Texas Broadcasting Company, it was always his LBJ Ranch that was his chief concern. The ranch foreman once remarked, "Gee, I hope he runs again for President. There I was at six in the morning milking the cows . . . and lo and behold, there's the President standing there in his pajamas and house shoes saying, 'How are the dairy cows? Do the fences need to be fixed?' "

In March 1970 Johnson was hospitalized in San Antonio with severe angina. On a visit to his daughter Lynda in Virginia in May 1972 he suffered yet another heart attack. He is reported to have impulsively left his bed in a Charlottesville hospital after three days of intensive care and said to his wife, Lady Bird, "Bird, I'm goin' home to die—you can come if you want to." His remaining seven months were full of pain; the latest attack had resulted in congestive heart failure. He had an oxygen supply in his bedroom at the ranch and would lie down from time to time and put on the mask. In October he discussed with two specialists from Baylor Medical School in Houston, Michael DeBakey and Henry MacIntosh, the feasibility of undergoing coronary bypass surgery, developed only within the previous six years and still considered experimental; but this surgery would not have regenerated the heart muscle destroyed in the past, and other health problems, notably Johnson's recurring episodes of colonic diverticulitis, rendered the intervention too dangerous.

Two weeks before the end he thanked a friend, Leonard Marks, for help over the years. "Frequently we take these things for granted," said LBJ, "I just want you to know I'm very grateful." The man who, according to Lady Bird, most hated to be by himself, was alone when he died on 22 January 1973, just two days after the second inauguration of his successor, Richard Nixon. He called from his bedroom around 3:45 P.M. for one of the Secret Service agents, Mike Howard; Howard was unavailable and two other agents, Ed Newland and Harry Harris, rushed to him with a portable oxygen kit. Johnson was lying on the floor, apparently lifeless. He was flown to the Brooke Army Medical Center in San Antonio, where he was pronounced dead by Dr. George McGranahan. An autopsy revealed that two of the three major coronary arteries were completely blocked and the third was 60 percent occluded.

Mrs. Johnson was reached while traveling in a car near the Johnson Library. The body lay in the library overnight on the twenty-third as twenty thousand people filed by. Next day, a national day of mourning, the coffin was flown to Washington, where it lay in the Capitol Rotunda until it was taken on the morning of the twenty-fifth to Washington's National City Christian Church for a funeral service attended by, among others, the Johnson and Nixon families.

The same afternoon, Lyndon Baines Johnson was laid to rest next to his parents, with full military honors, at the Johnson family cemetery on the LBJ Ranch outside Stonewall, Texas, 150 yards north of the Pedernales

River. Former Texas governor John B. Connally and the Reverend Billy Graham gave short addresses and Anita Bryant sang the "Battle Hymn of the Republic."

The ex-president's estate was estimated to be at least $20 million, derived largely from a radio station in Austin. It was left equally to the Johnson daughters, Lynda and Luci; Mrs. Johnson was given a life interest in the ranch.

Jonson, Ben (1573-1637)

The English dramatist, poet, and actor, among whose plays are *Volpone* (1606) and *The Alchemist* (1610), narrowly escaped the gallows in 1598 after killing a fellow actor, Gabriel Spencer, in a duel. Jonson, a man of high moral principles and great learning, suffered a stroke in 1628 and from then on became, in his own phrase, "a bed-rid wit." Severely disabled and living in near poverty in lodgings close to Westminster Abbey, he was at any rate able to carry on his writing until the end. When he died on 6 August 1637 he was engaged on *The Sad Shepherd*, a lively and brilliantly written pastoral drama.

His 1953 biographer Marchette Chute records that he was buried in the abbey "with as great a train of mourners as though he had been a nobleman." But he was not interred in Poets' Corner; his grave is in the north aisle of the nave. There is a story, no doubt untrue, that he joked that he could not afford the honor of joining the other great poets, including Chaucer. He didn't need a six-foot space: "two feet by two feet will do." Whatever the reason, Jonson was only afforded a minimal resting place. In the breezy words of New Yorker Helene Hanff, who was taken by a friend to see the grave and who describes the scene in her *Q's Legacy* (1985):

> Do not put off paying for that crypt or grave you ordered for yourself. Consider what happened to Ben Jonson . . .
> Ben knew he'd be entitled to burial in Westminster Abbey and he reserved a grave there for himself and he never paid for it . . . [The] grave-diggers . . . weren't going to waste valuable space on a deadbeat. So they opened the grave and slid Ben in, upright; and propped him in a corner, to keep the grave available for a paying customer . . .
> He had no luck whatever in Westminster Abbey; even the

plaque in his memory has to be hidden away in a side wall where the Abbey hopes nobody will see it because the eulogy on it begins:

"O rare Ben Johnson"

and that ain't how he spelled it.

Joplin, Scott (1868-1917)

In his lifetime the black U.S. composer gained little recognition for his significant contributions to American music, notably his piano rags. The "King of Ragtime" himself often admitted that his compositions would not be appreciated until after he had been dead fifty years.

Joplin spent his last years in Manhattan, where in 1911–12 he tramped the sidewalks vainly trying to have his opera *Treemonisha* produced, while his second wife Lottie, always his greatest admirer and supporter, worked as a domestic. Earlier listed in the city directory as "composer" or "musician," by 1915 he described himself merely as "music teacher." Early that year he managed to stage his opera at the Lincoln Theater on 135th Street with a small volunteer chorus and a piano, on which Joplin himself played all the orchestral parts, but with no costumes or scenery. The performance was a flop, completely ignored by the critics.

His ensuing depression was compounded by a sudden worsening in his already fragile health. The evidence of surviving piano rolls shows his playing to have been erratic for a year or two before this time. Now he developed a facial tic and stumbled over difficult words. In early 1916 the Joplins moved to 163 West 131st Street, where they rented extra rooms that Lottie could sublet to transients; Scott took a room on 160th Street where he could work and teach, but he produced little and neglected his students. At the piano he could no longer remember even his own compositions and when he tried to compose his mind would go blank. On his few good days he worked frenetically, not on the short pieces of which he was a master but on longer works: a "music comedy drama" titled *If*, and even a ragtime symphony. He brooded over the safety of the unfinished manuscripts scattered about the room, but around December 1916 he suddenly reversed course and burned nearly all of them.

On 5 February 1917 he was admitted to Manhattan State Hospital. By then he could not recognize friends who visited him. Paralyzed, lying motionless, he gradually lost his remaining strength. He died on 1 April 1917 of "Dementia Paralytica–cerebral form. Duration: 1 yr. 6 mos. Contrib.

cause: Syphilis—unknown duration." He may have contracted syphilis during the wandering years, 1903–7, between his marriages, when he toured with his Ragtime Opera Company.

After a modest service at the G. O. Paris funeral home on West 131st Street in Manhattan, Scott Joplin was buried in a common grave, shared with two other bodies, in St. Michael's Cemetery in the Astoria district of Queens, New York.

A Joplin revival, begun by a few enthusiasts in the 1960s, blossomed when the young pianist Joshua Rifkin in 1970 issued the first of three recordings to great acclaim. The recordings led to the choice of "The Entertainer" and other Joplin rags for the soundtrack of the movie *The Sting* in 1973. Within a year, two million copies of the soundtrack had been sold on discs and tapes. In October 1974, after fifty-seven years of neglect, the fifth grave in the second row in St. Michael's Cemetery was recognized by a bronze marker inscribed SCOTT JOPLIN, AMERICAN COMPOSER. In September 1975 *Treemonisha* at last reached Broadway, and in 1976 Joplin was awarded a Pulitzer Prize.

Years after her husband's death, Lottie Joplin confessed that he had asked that his "Maple Leaf Rag" be played at his funeral, but when the time came she felt it was not appropriate. "How many, many times since then I've wished to my heart that I'd said yes." *See* James Haskins (1978).

Joyce, William (1906-1946)

During World War II he was detested by the British even more than they detested Adolf Hitler. The Brooklyn native spent his life in Ireland and England, falsely claiming to be a British subject and gaining prominence in Jew-taunting demonstrations as a leader of the Union of Fascists.

He began broadcasting for the Nazis on 11 September 1939 and became a German citizen in 1940. His haughty, sneering "Jairmany calling" signature soon earned him the nickname "Lord Haw-Haw."

Early in May 1945, after an aborted attempt to escape to neutral Sweden with his Lancashire-born wife Margaret, he was shot in the legs and arrested near Flensburg by two British soldiers who were collecting firewood. They had recognized him by his voice and the scar on his cheek, sustained in a London fracas while leading a Fascist squad in 1924.

He was tried at London's Old Bailey in September on three counts of high treason. Two of them were quickly dismissed as inapplicable to a U.S.

citizen. But he was found guilty of treachery while nominally under the protection of the British government. As Rebecca West put it in her *The Meaning of Treason* (1949):

> He died the most completely unnecessary death that any criminal has ever died on the gallows. He was the victim of his own and his father's lifelong determination to lie about their nationality . . .For if he had not renewed his [U.K.] passport, and had left England for Germany on the American passport that was rightfully his, no power on earth could have touched him [because the United States did not enter the war until after he became a naturalized German citizen].

His appeal was dismissed by three judges on 7 November. The final appeal, before five judges in the House of Lords, was heard in Joyce's presence but again dismissed (by a 4–1 decision) on 18 December. His wife, herself awaiting trial in Holloway Prison, was brought daily to see him. On the eve of his execution he handed a defiant message to family members who were visiting him: "In death, as in this life, I defy the Jews who caused this last war," and he added a warning to Britain about Soviet imperialism.

On the morning of 3 January 1946, three hundred of the curious gathered outside the walls of Wandsworth Prison in south London. The condemned man received Holy Communion and wrote letters (ending in a repeated *"Sieg Heil"*) to Margaret and a close friend.

Three masses were arranged—two in England, one in Ireland—to reach their climaxes in the Consecration at precisely 9:00 A.M., the announced moment of the drop. Britain's leading hangman, the genial pub-owner Albert Pierpoint, greeted Joyce, who was wearing his threadbare blue suit, and led him the few yards from his cell to the execution shed. The British public later heard, with wry amusement, that the doomed man's knee had trembled on his final walk and that he had looked down at it and smiled, but the tremor was very likely a consequence of his leg wounds. Pierpoint gently placed a white hood over Joyce's head. The hem of the hood concealed the noose. The trap was sprung and the drop caused instant unconsciousness and almost instant death. The facial scar was said to have been broken open by the shock and makeup was applied before the coroner's jury saw the body. The death certificate on William Joyce, thirty-nine, read: "Injuries to brain and spinal cord consequent upon judicial hanging." He was buried within the prison walls.

Jung, Carl Gustav (1875-1961)

The Swiss psychiatrist, founder of analytic psychology, which classifies humankind into introverts and extroverts, split with Sigmund Freud in 1912 over the latter's emphasis on the role of the libido as the basis of neuroses.

According to his friend, the writer Laurens van der Post, Jung's last years were a religious quest, however scientific his approach to it might have been. Dreams and visions were of the greatest importance. As he turned seventy he wrote to a friend, "Death is the hardest thing . . . as long as we are outside of it. But once inside you taste of such completeness and peace and fulfillment that you don't want to return." This was written a year after he had broken his leg in February 1944 while on a hike. During his hospital stay he suffered a heart attack that brought him near to death for several weeks. It was at this time that he experienced a vision of himself far out in space, with the earth a globe remote but distinct below him.

Jung's wife of fifty-two years, Emma, died in November 1955 and her loss desolated him. During his final six years he was cared for efficiently and devotedly by the Jungs' English friend Ruth Bailey. He was kept busy, indeed overloaded, with work to the end. A biography, largely an autobiography, written by Jung and his secretary Aniela Jaffé took up a lot of time; his voluminous correspondence grew so unmanageable that he would sometimes hide a bundle of incoming letters behind a shelf of books.

He was confined to bed when he received a Chilean visitor, Miguel Serrano, on 10 May 1961. Jung had been reading a book by a Chinese Zen Buddhist and he told his visitor that "I felt as if we were talking about one and the same thing and were simply using different words for it." After his final drive in the country on the seventeenth he suffered a cerebral embolism; from then on Mrs. Bailey needed to read to him. A final stroke on the thirtieth confined him to his bedroom. Two days before his death he had a dream that enchanted him. "Now I know the truth down to a little bit that is still missing," he told Ruth Bailey. "When I know this too, then I will have died." On the evening of 5 June 1961 he asked her, "Let's have a really good wine tonight."

Jung died around 4:00 P.M. next day at his home in the village of Küsnacht on the eastern shore of Lake Zurich. Van der Post on that day was sailing from his native South Africa toward Europe, and he believes he experienced a vision at precisely the moment of his friend's death. For days he had suffered from sleeplessness; now, in a half-waking state, he found himself in a deep valley "among steep, snow-covered mountains . . . Suddenly, at the far end of the valley . . . Jung appeared. He stood there briefly, as I had seen him some weeks before at the gate at the end of the garden of his house, then waved his hand at me and called out, 'I'll be seeing you.' " Van der Post says he then fell into a peaceful eighteen-hour slumber. He read of Jung's death next day in the ship's daily news sheet.

Carl Gustav Jung was buried, after a service in the village church, in Küsnacht Cemetery. The rectangular gravestone bears the names of his parents, sister Gertrud, wife Emma and finally Jung himself. *See* Gerhard Wehr (1987).

Kerouac, Jack (1922-1969)

The "King of the Beats," a U.S. writer of French-Canadian origin, became a leading voice, in his *On the Road* (1958) and other books, of a post–World War II generation alienated from its parents' values and traditions and searching for a new identity. Other representatives of the movement, including the poet Allen Ginsberg and the novelist William Burroughs, avoided the alcoholic self-destruction that was Kerouac's fate. By 1960 he was having attacks of delirium tremens and admitting to being an incurable alcoholic. In his cups his conversation soured and, despite his long friendship with Ginsberg, took an anti-Semitic tinge—the critics hated him because, unlike Malamud and Bellow, he wasn't Jewish.

With two fleeting, unsatisfactory marriages behind him he lived his last years with his mother Gabrielle ("Mémère") in his native Lowell, Massachusetts, and St. Petersburg, Florida. After his third marriage, to Stella Sampas, in November 1966, the three shared a home together, Stella caring for the by-now-paralyzed Mémère. After the final move to St. Petersburg, in November 1968, Stella went out to work as a seamstress at $1.70 an hour. At home in their cinder-block bungalow she tried frantically to keep Jack in the house, away from his favorite bar crawling; but he was never without an emergency case of Johnnie Walker Red tucked away.

In a final attempt to make money at his typewriter, he completed a story begun eighteen years earlier about a nine-year-old black boy in North Carolina; it was published under the title "Pic." His last published work was an essay, "After Me the Deluge," in which he agonized over his true position; he felt lost in contemporary America, alienated alike by the hypocritical establishment and the irresponsible irrelevant likes of Prankster Ken Kesey and acid guru Timothy Leary.

When not writing he would try to make drunken calls to old friends, often in the middle of the night, but there was often no answer, or the call was refused. In October 1969 he was paler than usual; the local liquor-store owner thought he looked like a bum. Though drinking as much as usual he had lost twenty pounds over the past several months. Early in the month he was beaten up in a black bar, not for the first time; after that he never left the house. On the seventeenth Kerouac was infuriated to find a favorite Georgia pine being cut down in a neighbor's yard. According to Kerouac's 1983 biographer Gerald Nicosia, "he began to shake violently, and the vein in his forehead bulged so that Stella feared it would burst. He rushed out and began hysterically shouting that the neighbor was a 'murderer,' that she was 'killing his brother.'"

At 4:00 A.M. on Monday, 20 October, Kerouac wandered into his mother's room and talked to her for hours. At breakfast time he nibbled tuna from an open can and sat in front of the TV set with a notebook and a small bottle of whiskey, planning a new novel. Suddenly he rushed to the bathroom, and Stella heard him call for help. He was kneeling in front of the toilet bowl, vomiting blood. "I'm hemorrhaging," he groaned. At St. Anthony's Hospital he received thirty units of blood over twenty hours. He died at 5:30 A.M. on 21 October 1969 of loss of blood from esophageal varices, a common destiny of alcoholics. (Cirrhosis of the liver leads to increased pressure in the portal circulation and rupture of blood vessels in the gullet.)

Kerouac's body was returned to Lowell and the funeral service took place at St. Jean Baptiste Church, where he had once trained as an altar boy. He was buried in the Sampas plot in Edson Cemetery. After several years a marker was placed there, bearing under the name JOHN L. KEROUAC the words, HE HONORED LIFE.

Kierkegaard, Søren (1813-1855)

The Danish philosopher and theologian is regarded, along with Nietzsche and Dostoievsky, as the father of existentialism, a philosophical movement that was systematized a century later by Jean-Paul Sartre (q.v.).

Keys to Kierkegaard's complex personality may be found in his close relationship with his melancholic father, which robbed him of a normal childhood, and his love affair with Regine Olsen. He was engaged to the eighteen-year-old Regine for a year in 1840–41; then, inexplicably and to her great despair, he broke off the relationship. Their age difference of ten years was too much; that was his argument. The true reason is harder to fathom; looking back on his actions, he wrote, "When I left her, I chose death."

In his later years Kierkegaard took the extreme position that human sexuality is a sin; from this it follows that God desires the human race to die out. Because "human egoism is concentrated in the sexual relation," this must be given up. "And that is why Christianity upholds celibacy." Not only women ("woman is egoism personified") but all worldly issues must be forsworn. "To love God is to hate the world." "To become a Christian according to the New Testament is to become 'spirit.' To become spirit . . . is to die, to die off from the world."

When Denmark's Christian Primate, Bishop J. P. Mynster, died in 1854, Kierkegaard, who had respected him most of his life, felt liberated. He attacked Mynster's successor, H. L. Martenson, in a series of articles that extended his criticism to the entire Danish church; "The Established Church is, Christianly considered, an impudent indecency . . . an apostasy from the Christianity of the New Testament . . . an effort in the direction of making a fool of God."

Late in September 1855 Kierkegaard's health, never robust, broke down. In the past he had often coughed up blood; now he collapsed at an evening party with a sudden feeling of weakness. A few days later he crumpled in the street and was carried to his modest rooms on Copenhagen's Klaedeboderne. On 2 October he was taken by ambulance to Fredriks Hospital. He was able to shuffle downstairs on the arm of the driver, tipping his broad-brimmed hat and summoning up a last smile for his landlady, Fru Borries, who watched from across the corridor.

At the hospital he told the admitting doctor he was aware he was dying, the causes being "the enjoyment of cold seltzer water during the summer," his exhausting work schedule, and his apartment's bad air. But Joslah Thompson, in his 1973 biography, believes Kierkegaard succumbed to a staphylococcal lung infection, a disease which even nowadays, in the age of antibiotics, kills one in seven of its victims.

Over forty days he faded away gradually, but enjoyed brighter intervals during visits from friends. Of a gift of flowers, which he immediately shut away in a drawer; "It's the fate of flowers to bloom and give scent and die," he said. Would he modify his attacks on the Church? Oh, no; that "doesn't do any good. It has to burst like a bombshell." Would he receive Holy Communion? Yes, but not from a priest. That would be difficult. "Then I'll do without it . . . The clergy are state functionaries, and functionaries have nothing to do with Christianity."

Kierkegaard felt that much in his life had turned out happily. "That's why I'm very happy, and very sad that I cannot share this happiness with anyone." He died at 9:00 P.M. on 11 November 1855. At his funeral service in Copenhagen's Frue Kirke, clergy were entirely absent, except for his brother Peter Christian Kierkegaard and the disapproving dean, E. C. Tryde, who was obviously ill at ease. Peter Christian delivered a short speech, explaining that his brother had gone astray in recent years, then led the congregation in a prayer begging forgiveness for Søren's "bewildered and perplexed soul." An honor guard of students and a large crowd accompanied the coffin to Assistens Cemetery. At the graveside ceremony a burly young man protested that the state church had profaned itself by taking Kierkegaard's body by force and burying it as one of their own, thereby becoming guilty of a kind of rape. As for himself, the speaker said he would follow the dead man's advice: "Whosoever does not take part in the official worship of God has certainly one sin the less."

Kipling, Rudyard (1865-1936)

The British writer, born in Bombay, India, married an American, Caroline Balestier, in 1892 and lived several years in Vermont. He won the Nobel Prize for Literature in 1907. His poems, including "If," "Boots," and "Gunga Din," have always been popular, and his *Just So Stories* have won him a wide audience among young readers. But his posthumous reputation suffered gravely from the jingoistic imperialist message to be found in his works and the vulgar, even brutal terms in which he sometimes expressed himself. But in personal relations he was a shy, often timid man, unusually generous to young writers; in his last, invalid years he felt dominated by his wife.

From 1915, Kipling suffered almost constantly from digestive ailments—gastritis, colitis, and especially duodenal ulcer—that kept him in great pain, but about which he seldom complained. In 1933 he worked on the proofs—"the size of a small hay-rick," he said—of his collected poems and concluded the volume with a plea to future biographers to treat his private life tenderly: "And for the little, little span / The dead are borne in mind, / Seek not to question other than / The books I leave behind."

The Kiplings lived from 1902 mainly near Burwash in Sussex at a house called "Bateman's," but when in London had, ever since their honeymoon, used rooms at Brown's Hotel in Dover Street. In 1935, though virtually retired, he wrote one more *Just So* story ("Ham and the Porcupine") for the nine-year-old Princess Elizabeth's Gift Book. He and his wife traveled that year to Marienbad in Germany to seek a cure for Caroline's rheumatism and spent a few months on the French Riviera.

On their return Kipling set to and rapidly completed his autobiography, published after his death as *Something About Myself*; about personal matters it is disappointingly discreet and about painful memories completely silent. Not a word is to be found about his six-year-old daughter Josephine's death in 1899, or of his seventeen-year-old son John's tragic end in World War I. Kipling had gone to great lengths to have the lad enlisted in the Irish Guards, and consequently felt enormous guilt at the outcome.

He thought much of his own death during his final months and wrote reassuringly to an aunt, "He who puts us into this life does not abandon His work for *any* reason or default at the end of it . . . So there is no fear!" The autobiography ends with a description of his study; the last sentence reads: "Left and right of the table were two big globes, on one of which the great airman [W. G. H. Salmond (1878–1933)] had once outlined in white paint those air-routes to the East and Australia which were well in use before my death." Of this passage, Lisa Lewis of the Kipling Society in London comments, "The look towards the future, followed by a double-take and a shudder, is typical late Kipling."

On 12 January 1936, very early in the morning, Kipling was rushed in great pain from his hotel suite to Middlesex Hospital, London. His physician, Sir Alfred Webb-Johnson, who knew him well, was called to see him. "What's the matter, Rud?" he asked. "Something has come adrift inside," replied Kipling. "This brilliantly summarized the matter," said the doctor later, for the writer had suffered a perforated duodenum, a serious medical emergency that can quickly lead to peritonitis and death.

Caroline's diary, kept faithfully during the forty-four years of her marriage, ends with these entries: *Jan. 9 London*. Rud signs his Will. *Jan. 12* Rud taken ill and to hospital in the early morning for an operation. Webb-Johnson sees him at 3 a.m. and later operates. *Jan. 18* Rud died at 12:10 a.m. Our Wedding Day.

Rudyard Kipling was cremated secretly at Golders Green in north London. On 23 January, the day King George V's body was brought to London to lie in state in Westminster Hall, the writer's ashes, in a marble casket, were laid to rest in Poets' Corner in Westminster Abbey, near the remains of Charles Dickens and Thomas Hardy. The funeral service included Kipling's "Recessional" ("Lord God of Hosts, be with us yet / Lest we forget—lest we forget!"). One of the pallbearers was Kipling's distant cousin, the British prime minister Stanley Baldwin. The grave was covered by a purple slab, later replaced by a tombstone reading simply, R.K. 1865–1936. *See* Lord Birkenhead (1978).

Kobbé, Gustav (1857-1918)

The *New York Herald's* music critic was putting the finishing touches to the manuscript of an impressive reference book at the time of his death. While spending the summer with his daughter on Long Island he indulged in his favorite pastime of sailing in Great South Bay. On 27 July 1918 he was out alone in his single-masted catboat when an officer, viewing the scene through binoculars from the naval station at Brightwaters, saw a navy seaplane skimming over the water toward the boat. Kobbé, unaware of the danger until too late, scrambled to his feet and prepared to dive overboard just as the plane struck the mast. The upper part broke off and fell with great force, splitting Kobbé's skull and killing him instantly. The pilot's name was not divulged; he claimed to know nothing of the collision until he returned to base.

Kobbé's *Complete Opera Book,* published after his death, was an instant success, and three-quarters of a century later, in succeeding editions, is perhaps the favorite reference work of opera lovers throughout the world.

Koestler, Arthur (1905-1983)

The Hungarian author, a British citizen from 1948, showed his disillusion with communism in his novel *Darkness at Noon* (1941). He disappointed many admirers by abandoning his hard-headed skepticism to dabble in mysticism and telepathy with books like *The Roots of Coincidence* (1972).

Though in some ways a shy, self-effacing man, he was nevertheless proud of his reputation as a polymath. He amused Albert Einstein by lecturing him after a party in Princeton, New Jersey, "God Almighty knows everything, but Arthur Koestler knows everything better," Einstein observed later. "He explained to me what relativity is . . ."

Koestler was a relentless pursuer of women, whom he treated as chattels. His third wife, South African–born Cynthia Jefferies, née Paterson, began as his secretary. "There was the customary seduction," writes Woodrow Wyatt, "and the star-struck, naïve . . . girl became a willing slave in a harem which changed frequently . . . She broke away from Koestler briefly, but, following the failure of a short-lived marriage, she was adoringly grateful to be put condescendingly on the strength again and eventually to marry him in 1965, not complaining of his unrestrained unfaithfulness."

Parkinsonism began to affect Koestler in 1978 and later he was diagnosed as having leukemia. As he grew increasingly dependent on his wife, his behavior toward her improved and her self-confidence increased. But the dependence was mutual; she made no friends of her own and lived entirely through him. He wrote a suicide note in the summer of 1982 and in a will drafted around the same date he named Cynthia as chief beneficiary; her decision to die with him evidently came later. (The final will left more than a half-million pounds to endow a chair of parapsychology; this was later established at Edinburgh University.)

After a lump in Koestler's groin was diagnosed as metastatic cancer and he was ordered to the hospital, the couple made their decision. When their servant Amelia Marino had left their London house on Tuesday, 1 March 1983, Cynthia took their eleven-year-old dog David to the vet for humane disposal. On her next visit to the Koestlers' home in Montpelier Square, Knightsbridge, on Thursday, Miss Marino found a note warning her not to go upstairs but to call the police. Koestler was sitting in his usual armchair, a brandy glass in his hand; Cynthia was seated near him on the sofa. They had been dead about thirty-six hours, killed by a large overdose of barbiturate. An empty vial that had contained capsules of Tuinal (a mixture of secobarbital and amobarbital) was on the coffee table in front of Koestler, beside a half-bottle of whiskey, a jar of honey, and two empty wine glasses with a residue of white powder in them.

Public discussion centered not on Koestler's suicide but on his decision to "take with him" his wife, twenty-two years his junior. But her decision, however misguided, seems to have been entirely her own. To the suicide note, dated eight months earlier, she had appended a few words of her own: "I cannot face life without Arthur." *See* George Mikes (1983).

Lacks, Henrietta (1920?-1951)

On 1 February 1951 a young black woman, the mother of five children, was admitted to Johns Hopkins Hospital in Baltimore with symptoms of frequent and irregular vaginal bleeding. A soft, ragged lesion, purple in color and measuring about one inch in diameter, was discovered on the cervix of her uterus. A specimen was taken of this uncharacteristic cancerous tissue, and from it Dr. George O. Gey was able to establish the first successful human-cell culture, to which he gave the acronym "HeLa," derived from the patient's first and last names.

Despite radium therapy the disease, diagnosed as an epidermoid carcinoma but reevaluated in 1971 as a "very aggressive adenocarcinoma of the cervix," spread rapidly throughout the body, causing death about eight months later. But the culture continued to thrive and within a few years could be found, in the form of pale sheets adhering to the inner walls of glass vessels and bathed in nutrient media, in biological laboratories throughout the world. Every twenty-four hours, on average, every cell divides to become two. So aggressive is the HeLa cell line that other, subsequent, human tissue cultures are supplanted by it when contamination occurs and great care must be exercised to avoid this. HeLa cells are now the universal standard, employed in testing human tissue response to drugs, poisons, and pathogenic microorganisms.

Though her cells have become immortal, the name of the Baltimore housewife is all but unknown, even to biologists. An unlucky guess probably led to her being known in the 1950s as "Helen Lane," a name that still persists. But a 1971 medical study by H. W. Jones Jr. and others on the occasion of Gey's death included a photograph of the HeLa patient and supplied her real name, Mrs. Henrietta Lacks.

Lamb, Charles (1775-1834)

The English man of letters is best known for the essays he wrote under the pseudonym Elia for the *London Magazine*. Much of his life was devoted to the care of his sister Mary (1764–1847), with whom he wrote *Tales from Shakespeare* (1807) and two other books for young readers.

In September 1796, in the family's London home in Lincoln's Inn Fields, the twenty-one-year-old Charles was present at the murder of his invalid mother. Mary, in a fit of madness, stabbed Mrs. Lamb to the heart with a carving knife while the young man and his senile father, wounded in the forehead by a fork hurled by his daughter, looked on helplessly. Mary was committed to a lunatic asylum. Only if someone would take responsibility for her actions could she ever be released. In 1799, when her elder brother shrank from this duty, Charles assumed it, thereby dooming himself to bachelorhood and a continuance of his dull career as a clerk in the East India Office. He never repented this decision; at least once a year, as Mary felt herself descending into madness, they could be seen, walking hand in hand and often in tears, toward the madhouse, where she would stay until she was restored to temporary sanity.

Lamb achieved some fame in 1823 when the first collection of his *Essays of Elia* was published. Two years later, after thirty-three years of service and in failing health, he was able to retire with a generous pension. He was ill with a "nervous fever," and his disability greatly destabilized Mary's mental state; her episodes of insanity grew more frequent and more violent. In 1823 the pair had moved north beyond the suburbs to the quiet town of Enfield, but after his retirement from regular work Charles missed his old friends and often suffered from boredom. A rare hostile view of him at this period has been left by Thomas Carlyle; he was, according to the Scots writer, a "pitiful, ricketty, gasping, staggering Tomfool" who "is now a confirmed, shameless drunkard." He certainly did have a stammer and was unusually affected by small amounts of alcohol, but most of his friends declare he was seldom tipsy.

In 1833 the Lambs moved for the last time from Enfield to the neighboring town of Edmonton, where Charles had discovered a private home that took in mental patients. Here, shut away with Mary, he was more isolated than ever. His sister's company satisfied him during her lucid periods; they played piquet and read to one another. Her madness had grown more frequent but less violent and Charles was resigned to caring for her. To a friend he writes, "Have faith in me! It is no new thing for me to be left to my sister. When she is not violent her rambling chat is better to me than the sense and sanity of the world . . . I could be nowhere happier than under the same roof with her."

In July 1834 Charles's best friend, the poet Samuel Coleridge, died. They had not seen one another often, but it had been to Coleridge that Lamb turned in times of crisis for sympathy and support, notably after the murder of Mrs. Lamb. The effect of his friend's death was severe; in his remaining five months of life, Charles would suddenly stop in the middle of a conversation and remark in shocked tones, "Coleridge is dead!" William Wordsworth, for one, believed that Lamb's death was hastened by the loss of his confidant.

On the morning of 22 December 1834, Charles Lamb was walking toward a favorite tavern in Edmonton when he tripped and fell on a stony path. With his face bruised and bleeding, he was taken home. After a day or two his condition suddenly worsened. Evidently he was infected with erysipelas, caused by a hemolytic streptococcus and marked by rapidly spreading redness and swelling of the skin accompanied by pain and fever. Before the advent of antibiotics it was a common cause of death. A London friend who hurried to his bedside found Lamb half-conscious and incoherent; he fell into a coma and died on 27 December 1834.

Mary, brought into the room to see her dead brother, remarked on how beautiful he looked but seemed quite unable to take in the catastrophe. She lived on for thirteen years, more or less out of her mind, and until she moved back to London was fond of visiting Charles's grave in the Edmonton Parish Churchyard, but did not noticeably grieve for him. Perhaps Charles would not have minded her indifference. As his 1983 biographer David Cecil percipiently concludes: "Perhaps . . . though neither had been aware of it, he had, in fact, always needed her more than she needed him."

Laurel, Stan (1890-1965)

The comedy team of Laurel and Hardy made their last movie for Hal Roach in 1940, the undistinguished *Saps at Sea*. British-born Stan Laurel (the thin one, five feet nine inches tall) and Oliver ("Babe") Hardy (the portly one, two hundred fifty pounds and six feet one) said good-bye to Hollywood after nineteen years with MGM's disappointing *Nothing But Trouble* (1945), around the time that Stan, plagued by fatigue, irritability, and depression, was found to have diabetes.

In April 1946 Ruth Laurel (née Rogers) and Stan were divorced after five years together (they had been married to one another twice previously). Stan had already met the movie actress Ida Kitaeva Raphael, and they were wed in Yuma, Arizona, in June 1946. It was the last of Laurel's eight marriages to four women.

The Laurel-and-Hardy partnership enjoyed a renewed lease of life on stage; the comics were highly popular in Britain, where they made tours of the music halls in 1947 and twice in the early 1950s. A film they made in France, *Atoll K* (1950), was by far their longest, but it was a dismal failure that was never widely distributed.

Stan realized their career as a duo was over when, in 1955, Babe after two heart attacks was forced to lose weight. After shedding half of his (by then) three hundred pounds, Hardy was no longer recognizable. It was at this time too that Laurel suffered a stroke that left him with a noticeable limp. He was devastated when Babe Hardy died in the North Hollywood home of his mother-in-law, after almost a year of semiconsciousness, on 7 August 1957. But Stan could not bear to attend funerals, especially this one. Ida attended; so did Ruth, and there was a noticeable coolness between the two Mrs. Laurels.

The rights to reruns of the comedy team's movies were tightly controlled by Hal Roach; the two actors received no continued income from them. The Laurels, not rich but comfortably off, moved to a two-room suite in an apartment house (more or less a motel called the Oceana) in Santa Monica, California, overlooking the Pacific. Stan missed Babe and would reminisce on his years with him. "Funny, we never really got to know one another personally until we took the tours together . . . But whatever I did was tops with him. There was never any argument between us, ever . . ." The Laurels were listed in the phone book and many visitors came by. One of them was the television comedian Dick Van Dyke, who had been inspired by the old black-and-white films; also Dick Cavett, Jerry Lewis, Danny Kaye, and the French mime Marcel Marceau. Laurel accepted their tributes modestly, like an old-style English gentleman.

He was awarded a special Oscar in 1961 but, afflicted by an eye problem, he had Kaye accept it for him. He suffered a heart attack at home in April 1965 and died there a few days later on the twenty-seventh. Aware that his time was running out, he said to the nurse who had been engaged, "I'd rather be skiing than doing this." "Do you ski, Mr. Laurel?" "No, but I'd rather be skiing than doing this."

Arthur Stanley Laurel (né Jefferson) was buried in Forest Lawn Cemetery, Glendale, California, after a service in the Church of the Hills there. Fellow comics Harold Lloyd and Buster Keaton attended and Van Dyke gave the eulogy: "The halls of Heaven must be ringing with divine laughter." *See* Fred Lawrence Guiles (1980).

Lee, Bruce (1940-1973)

Born in San Francisco of Chinese parents, Lee first gained recognition of his martial-arts prowess in the comic-book television series *The Green Hornet*. During the Hong Kong filming of *Enter the Dragon* (1973), which was to prove an enormous success at the box office after his death, Lee's temper tantrums were often evident as he endlessly rehearsed his kung-fu routines, cut himself badly in a fight with broken bottles (real ones) and suffered the bite of a (devenomed) cobra.

On 10 May 1973, dubbing in the sound for the movie in a hot, unventilated studio in Kowloon, Lee collapsed. At Baptist Hospital, unconscious and breathing with difficulty, he had a series of convulsions, evidently caused by cerebral edema (swelling of the brain) of unknown cause. Lee and his wife Linda flew to Los Angeles after his release from the hospital and after tests there he was diagnosed as having suffered a "grand mal—idiopathic."

Back at his large, secluded home in Hong Kong, Bruce worked on a projected film, *The Game of Death*. On 20 July 1973 he drove across town with a colleague, Raymond Chow, to the apartment of a young Taiwanese actress, Betty Ting-pei, who was billed to be in the movie. According to Linda Lee, who was not present that afternoon, Betty and the two men discussed future work until, around 7:30 P.M., Bruce complained of a headache and the actress gave him a tablet of Equagesic (a prescription medication, produced by Wyeth Laboratories of Philadelphia, useful in the treatment of tension headache). Lee went to lie down and Chow set off to have dinner at a restaurant. Two hours later, Chow returned to find Bruce lying peacefully on a bed. When he failed to rouse him a doctor was called.

Bruce Lee was declared dead at Queen Elizabeth Hospital, Hong Kong. Traces of cannabis were found in his stomach; though quite insufficient to cause death, its presence—combined with the delayed revelation that he had died in the home of a woman with whom his name had sometimes been previously linked—caused a stir in the local media. The brain was greatly swollen and weighed 1,575 grams but no hemorrhage was found. Much expert testimony was sought in Britain and elsewhere; at the inquest the jury found a verdict of accidental death caused by hypersensitivity to one of Equagesic's three ingredients.

For the funeral service in Kowloon, Bruce Lee's body was dressed in the Chinese suit he had worn in his greatest role, in *Enter the Dragon*. At his burial in Seattle's Lake View Cemetery, the pallbearers included fellow actors Steve McQueen (q.v.) and James Coburn. *See* Linda Lee (1975).

Lennon, John (1940-1980)

After years of seclusion, the English-born rock star was back at work; his album *Double Fantasy* was released in mid-November 1980. During the final two weeks of his life he was working on a "single," his wife Yoko Ono's

"Walking on Thin Ice." His face looked gaunt and ravaged, the effect of too much cocaine sniffing, which had led to a perforated nasal septum.

Lennon's assassin, Mark David Chapman, was a fat, bespectacled Jesus freak from Decatur, Georgia, with a poor self-image. There were several famous people—Ronald Reagan and Elizabeth Taylor among them—he had thought of killing as a way to public recognition; an article in the October 1980 issue of *Esquire* seems to have diverted his attention to Lennon. Chapman, a former counselor in youth camps who married a Japanese woman in 1979, was now a security guard in Honolulu. He bought a five-shot, snub-nosed revolver—a Charter Arms .38-caliber Special—in a gun shop and two days later flew to New York, where he stayed in a hotel near the Lennons' home, the Dakota apartment building at 1 West 72nd Street in Manhattan, and spent several hours during his ten-day stay haunting the sidewalk outside, taking time for a side trip to Atlanta to obtain ammunition. Suddenly he changed his mind and flew back to Honolulu, only to reverse course again and return to New York on Saturday, 6 December. Next day he hovered near the Dakota for hours; amateur photographer Paul Goresh was also there, and he captured a shot of Lennon signing an album for Chapman as John and Yoko left for the studio at 5:00 P.M.

At 10:49 P.M., when their limousine returned, Chapman was still there. As the Lennons walked toward the windbreak in front of the Dakota entrance, Chapman heard a voice: "Do it . . . do it . . . do it!" He dropped into combat stance, aimed at John and fired all five bullets. The first two hit Lennon in the back and spun him around; two more hit his left shoulder; one went astray. There was a splintering sound as the bullets went through the rock star's body and shattered the glass and wood of the windbreak.

John was able to open the door and stagger up the half-dozen steps to the office before collapsing, bleeding heavily. The young nightie, Jay Hastings, pressed the emergency bell and tried to use his necktie as a tourniquet before running outside. Chapman was standing there under the gate light; he had dropped the gun and was reading a paperback volume. When two squad cars arrived he pleaded with police officers who seized him, "Don't hurt me, please!" and, sobbing, added, "I acted alone."

Without waiting for an ambulance, officers lifted Lennon, barely alive, into a third squad car and sped him to Roosevelt Hospital. His condition was hopeless; one of the bullets from behind had pierced a lung; most serious, another through the left shoulder had severed the aorta. "It wasn't possible to resuscitate him by any means," reported Dr. Stephen Lynn. "He had lost about 80 percent of his blood volume."

Despite Lennon's aversion to the practice, his body was cremated at Ferncliff Mortuary in Hartsdale, New York; there was no funeral service. On Sunday, 14 December 1980, a worldwide ten-minute vigil was held; huge crowds assembled in New York's Central Park at 2:00 P.M. that day.

Chapman was never tried; on 22 June 1981 he pleaded guilty to murder and was sentenced to twenty years to life in prison; he is incarcerated at Attica, New York. *See* Albert Goldman, 1988.

Lewis, Clive Staples (1898-1963)

The English professor of literature is best remembered for his books on popular theology, including *The Screwtape Letters* (1942), and the Narnia fantasies for children.

A confirmed bachelor, C. S. ("Jack") Lewis nevertheless secretly entered a legal but platonic "marriage" in April 1956 with a devoted American admirer, the Jewish ex-Communist Helen Joy Davidman Gresham, to enable her to remain in England with her two young sons. After she was stricken with terminal cancer the couple were united in a bedside religious ceremony in March 1957. A remission occurred and they were able to visit his native Ireland and also tour Greece. She died after a sudden deterioration in Radcliffe Hospital, Oxford, on 13 July 1960, aged forty-five. Her body was cremated, her ashes were scattered in the Oxford Crematorium grounds. Their romance is the subject of William Nicholson's television and stage play *Shadowlands*, filmed in 1993.

Lewis, who took over the care of the boys, suffered prostate and kidney ailments during his last three years. In July 1963 he had a heart attack but was able to leave the hospital and return to his home at The Kilns, Headington Quarry, near Oxford, which he shared, even during his marriage, with his elder brother Warren ("Warnie"). "I am now an extinct volcano," Jack Lewis wrote to a friend. He put his affairs in order and revised the proofs of his latest book, *The Discarded Image*. He enjoyed visits from friends but tended to fall asleep during conversations.

Four o'clock tea was taken in to him by Warnie as usual on 22 November 1963. At 5:30 Warnie heard a crash and found his brother lying unconscious at the foot of his bed. He died a few minutes later. In Dallas, Texas, President Kennedy was beginning a motorcade.

C. S. Lewis was buried in Headington Quarry Parish churchyard, where his faithful Warnie joined him ten years later.

Lewis, Meriwether (1774-1809)

The young U.S. Army captain who, with William Clark, helped open up the Northwest died mysteriously at the age of thirty-five. He was governor of the Upper Louisiana Territory when, traveling back to Washington in 1809 by way of the Natchez Trace, he stopped for the night of 10 October at Grinder's Stand, a rude hostelry in a clearing seventy-two miles southwest of Nashville. He was found dead next morning and was buried beside the trail a few hundred feet north of the cabins.

First accounts from Mrs. Grinder and Lewis's slave were that he muttered to himself and behaved erratically throughout the evening and that two shots and the sound of a falling body were heard around 3:00 A.M. The slave, Pernia, rushed in and heard Lewis's dying words: "I have done the business, my good servant. Give me some water." Mrs. Grinder, a totally unreliable witness, gave different accounts later. In 1811 she said the wounded man crawled to her door after the shots but she was afraid to open it until morning; he was found on his bed and expired as the sun rose. She told a visiting schoolteacher in 1839 that after two or *three* shots Lewis crawled across the trail and disappeared; that the dying man, garbed in tattered clothes, was found trying to cut his throat with a razor; and that Pernia was later seen in his master's garments.

It is not impossible that Lewis killed himself while demented, but robbery and murder are at least as likely. The money (around $120) the dead man was carrying has never been accounted for. Robert Grinder, supposedly away, may have been lurking nearby; Pernia is also a suspect, but many nameless assassins prowled the Natchez Trace at that period.

The novelist Vardis Fisher in his book *Suicide or Murder?* (1963) weighs the competing theories and can come to no certain conclusion, but if "forced . . . to choose, the choice would be murder." A Tennessee legislative committee in the 1840s also plumped for murder, and Lewis's biographers John Bakeless (1947) and Richard Dillon (1965) feel the same way.

In 1848 Tennessee erected a broken limestone column at the spot (to symbolize a broken life). The site, seven miles southeast of Hohenwold, Tennessee, was enclosed in 1925 as the Meriwether Lewis National Monument; it attracts few sightseers.

Liberace, Wladziu Valentino (1919-1987)

The pianistic showman from Milwaukee emerged in the 1950s as television's first matinee idol. Critics scoffed at his flamboyant presentations, his giant candelabra, sequined costumes, full-length ermine coats and mirror-tiled grand pianos. And then there were his jewel-encrusted fingers. "To shake his hand is to flirt with laceration," wrote *New York Times* reporter Bill Geist. But if his permanent, ingratiating grin could seem inane, at least it was not deceitful. On stage or off, this privately shy man aimed to please, to put those around him at their ease. The tributes from fellow entertainers on his death were evidently deeply felt.

His brother George (1911–1985), a violinist, was estranged from him for years on account of the younger man's unrestrained homosexual behavior at his Palm Springs home, a converted hotel called The Cloisters. The pianist successfully sued a London newspaper for a critical 1956 review that spoke of him as a "deadly, winking . . . giggling . . . mincing . . . heap of mother love" and was awarded £8,000.

Liberace's longest relationship was with Scott Thorson, aged eighteen, who came to live with him when he was fifty-seven. After the affair soured and he was forcibly ejected from the Los Angeles penthouse on Beverly Boulevard, he brought an unsuccessful "palimony" action for $380 million; some minor claims were settled in December 1986 for $95,000. On the fourteenth of that month, concerns about the entertainer's health were first expressed at his preChristmas party. But then, only a few weeks earlier he had completed twenty-one shows in only fourteen days at New York's Radio City Music Hall; no wonder he was tired. That he had only seven weeks to live was foreseen by no one.

In January 1987 he sent an unusually formal letter from The Cloisters to his Christmas guests: "Please don't enquire about my health . . . I am on the road to recovery . . . When I feel better I will call you." On the twenty-second he made his will, bequeathing his estate to an attorney acting as trustee (the bulk would ultimately go to the Liberace Foundation for the Performing and Creative Arts). Next day he entered the Eisenhower Medical Center in Palm Springs. A Las Vegas newspaper headlined: LIBERACE VICTIM OF DEADLY AIDS; this was denied: he was being treated for pernicious anemia, emphysema, and heart disease. He spent his last days secluded at The Cloisters, seeing no one but a few very close friends. In the parking lot opposite, a death watch began; television vans were brought in; loyal fans drove in from all directions. As his pulse weakened and his breathing slowed, the dying entertainer was moved from his bedroom to the bright, airy sitting room, where he watched his favorite sitcoms, notably *Golden Girls*, on videotapes.

Liberace died quietly, with a final long sigh, at 11:02 A.M. on 4 February 1987. The last rites of the Catholic Church had been given six days earlier. The body was removed in a large station wagon to Forest Lawn Cemetery, Glendale, before the death was announced; it was attributed to acute encephalopathy (degenerative brain disease).

The Riverside County coroner, Raymond Carillo, two days later ordered the body, already embalmed, to be released for tissue sampling, and hospital records were subpoenaed. Liberace had been found to be HTLV-III-positive three weeks before his death; that is, the human immunodeficiency virus that causes AIDS was present. But had Liberace suffered from the full-blown disease? Carillo, relying on the tissue findings, challenged the wording on the death certificate. He announced on 9 February that "Mr. Liberace did not die . . . of cardiac arrest . . . brought on by subacute encephalopathy. He died of cytomegalovirus pneumonia due to . . . human immunodeficiency virus disease . . . In layman's terms, Mr. Liberace died of an opportunistic disease caused by acquired immune deficiency syndrome." And the coroner accused Liberace's doctors of attempting a cover-up.

Dr. Ronald Daniels, who had signed the death certificate, protested that there was enough doubt concerning the AIDS diagnosis to justify his decision to protect his patient's privacy by reporting the cause of death as heart failure. As Liberace was not an intravenous drug user, he presumably contracted his fatal disease from one of his numerous lovers, possibly many years earlier.

Memorial services were held in Palm Springs and Las Vegas. His body joined those of his mother Frances and brother George in a white marble sarcophagus at Forest Lawn's Court of Remembrance. A brass inset depicts the dead entertainer's trademark, a musical symbol and a piano. *See* Bob Thomas (1987).

Lincoln, Mary Todd (1818-1882)

The wife of Abraham Lincoln was a troubled woman given to strange fears and erratic conduct. She was also a victim of cruel circumstance: four times bereaved, branded by her only surviving child as a lunatic and, after her husband's assassination, doomed to a procession of empty years.

Of the Lincolns' four children, only the eldest, Robert (1843–1926), reached manhood. Edward, 3, died of tuberculosis in 1850; William, 11, probably of typhoid in 1862; and Thomas ("Tad"), 18, of pleurisy and its cardiac complications in 1871.

Even as First Lady, with her husband present to restrain her, Mary Lincoln was a spendthrift. Appalled when told she had overspent a $20,000 appropriation to furnish the White House, he said he would sooner settle the bills out of his own pocket than have the American people know they were paying "for flub dubs for this damned old house, when the [Union] soldiers cannot have blankets."

Restless and unhappy after the president's death in 1865, Mary traveled constantly and found consolation in spiritualism. Lincoln's estate was shared by her, Robert, and Tad, but she complained bitterly that the interest ($1,700) on her portion was insufficient to live on and she went out furtively, trying to sell her clothes and jewelry. By October 1867 Robert was telling his fiancée that "my mother is on one subject not mentally responsible."

Soon after her return from a three-year sojourn in Europe in 1871 she was devastated by Tad's death. By now Congress had voted her a $3,000 pension, but she still brooded about poverty; visual and auditory delusions also beset her. Robert, after consulting medical men, brought her before a Cook County court for a sanity hearing in Chicago in 1875. Tales of her spending sprees, her secreting $57,000 in securities in her petticoats, and behaving irrationally persuaded the court to commit her to a nursing home in Batavia, Illinois. She attempted suicide the same evening by swallowing what she thought was laudanum. After four months she was permitted to go live with her sister in Springfield, Illinois, and in June 1876 was adjudged by a jury to be restored to sanity.

Still at bitter odds with Robert, she traveled to Europe again in 1879 and settled in Pau, the French resort near the Spanish border, where she was able to lose all her considerable excess weight. Apparently diabetic, she was constantly thirsty, had painful boils, vision problems, and backache. Her spine was damaged when a stepladder collapsed while she was hanging a picture.

Reduced to a hundred pounds and half-blind from cataracts, she was returning to the United States on *L'Amérique* in October 1880 when a high wave struck the ship and she was thrown across the wet deck. A fellow passenger, the actress Sarah Bernhardt, grabbed her skirt and saved her from a serious fall down a stairway. Bernhardt wrote in her memoirs, "I had just done this unhappy woman the only service that I ought not to have done her—I had saved her life."

The president's widow lived her remaining year and a half with her sister's family in Springfield, in a darkened upstairs room surrounded by her sixty-four trunks and crates. She restricted herself to one half of the bed, believing Abraham to be lying beside her. Twice she went to New York seeking relief for her partial paralysis. Congress raised her pension to $5,000 and gave her a lump sum of $15,000. By the time of her death she was reconciled with Robert. She suffered a stroke on 15 July 1882 and lapsed into a coma. She died the following day.

Her coffin lay in the parlor, the scene of her marriage forty-one years before, as friends called to pay respects. At her funeral service in Springfield's First Presbyterian Church, the Reverend James A. Reed said, "With the one that lingered it was only slow death from the same cause . . . When Abraham Lincoln died, she died."

Mary Todd Lincoln lies beside her husband and children in Oak Ridge Cemetery, Springfield, Illinois, underneath a 120-foot obelisk.

Lindbergh, Charles Augustus (1902–1974)

The U.S. aviator achieved world fame as the first person to fly solo across the Atlantic (in a single-engined craft, *The Spirit of St. Louis,* from Long Island, New York, to Paris) in May 1927. The kidnap and murder of his and Anne Morrow Lindbergh's two-year-old son in 1932 was called "the crime of the century." There was much criticism of Lindbergh's isolationist and pro-German pronouncements in the late 1930s; when he was labeled "a defeatist" by President Franklin Roosevelt, Lindbergh resigned from the Air Corps Reserve in April 1941. His fifty combat missions as a civilian in the Pacific during World War II drew little public attention. In 1953 his book *The Spirit of St. Louis* won the Pulitzer Prize.

At seventy, Lindbergh was slightly stooped and a little hard of hearing, but his step was vigorous and his appearance hale. He spent some time in 1972 with the primitive Tasadays on Mindanao in the Philippines, trying to preserve them from civilization's inroads. He jumped from helicopters and scaled cliffs like a man half his age. But he was soon telling friends he wanted to settle down and asked them to stop inviting him to formal events. By now the Lindberghs had built a quiet seaside retreat on the southeast coast of the Hawaiian island of Maui, a simple A-frame house with no electricity, no air-conditioning, where they were spending a few weeks every year.

In 1973 Lindbergh showed signs of winding up his life. He wrote to people he hadn't seen for thirty years. To an Englishman hurt by the American's remarks in World War II (that, for example, the British were decadent and, without Yankee aid, sure to be defeated by the virile Germans), he admitted, "Everyone used to call me Silent Sam, but I guess there were times when I said a damn sight too much for my own good."

Several times in his last year he traveled to Washington, D.C., and slipped unnoticed into the Smithsonian Institution, there to lurk behind a showcase, gaze at his beloved *Spirit of St. Louis* hanging above, and no doubt dream of past glories.

His only known previous illness was chicken pox, but returning from an Asian trip in 1973 he was laid low with fever and a rash, probably shingles. His enormous appetite deserted him and by early in 1974 he had lost twenty-four pounds. In May he resigned his longtime directorship of Pan Am and cut back on other business activities.

Back that summer in their seashore home at Scott's Cove, near Darien, Connecticut, after convalescence on Maui, Lindbergh began to cough and sweat. It was announced that he had pneumonia and was admitted to Columbia-Presbyterian Medical Center in New York. Two weeks later his doctors told him he had cancer of the lymphatic system; it had reached an advanced stage and he had only a short time to live.

Lindbergh had written in 1938 that he "would rather, by far, die" flying into a mountain in the fog "than in bed . . . What kind of man would live where there is no daring?" But he had left it too late; he no longer had the strength to seek a hero's death. Still, he didn't need to stay in a hospital bed awaiting the end. He was determined to die on Maui, and was flown there secretly on 18 August. The United Airlines pilot who flew him into Honolulu, William J. Picune, happened to have served as a stand-in for the aviator during the making of the 1957 movie *The Spirit of St. Louis,* which starred James Stewart. Lindbergh, lying on a stretcher on the left side of the commercial jet, was positioned so that he could see out the window. Picune asked him if he'd like the plane to circle Maui as it made its approach. "Oh, no, Captain," said the dying hero. "I don't want to inconvenience the other passengers."

Lindbergh used his remaining week, between periods of pain and coma, to call four of his five surviving children (his wife Anne and son Land were with him), arrange his papers, revise his will, and plan his funeral in detail (he would wear a drill shirt and pants, he decided). He said good-bye to Anne and Land as he lost consciousness on the evening of 25 August 1974. His 1976 biographer Leonard Moseley writes:

> Next morning, at 7:15, he took off on his final flight. He had made a lot of mistakes in his lifetime, but not on the journeys he had made into the unknown. No word came of his safe arrival. But those who knew how carefully he prepared all his flights were pretty certain that he made it.

Lindbergh had already chosen his final resting place, overlooking the ocean not far from his home, and a United Methodist minister was standing by. Ranch hands in Hana, a few miles up the coast, had constructed his coffin. The funeral took place the day of his death behind locked gates at the Hoomau Congregational Church, north of Kipahulu. The inconspicuous grave in the churchyard was filled in, as Lindbergh had wished, with lava rock and beach pebbles.

Lipatti, Dinu (1917-1950)

The legendary Romanian pianist is commemorated by a handful of superb recordings made during the lengthy course of his fatal illness. Swollen lymph nodes first troubled him eight years before his death. Beginning in December 1943, shortly after settling in Switzerland, he was confined to bed for months at his home near Geneva. In April he was told his malady was "a glandular infection of a nontubercular nature." On 16 May 1944 he wrote in a letter, "I started X-ray treatment on 1 May to burn away the famous gland that first appeared like a button on the radiograph taken in 1942, then like a nut in January 1944, and which was as big as a pear by April. Today I had my tenth session of X-rays and I feel much better."

The wonder is that he achieved as much as he did. Concerts throughout

Europe had to be canceled more than once, along with a projected tour of the United States. The radiation brought on headaches, vertigo, and vomiting. When World War II ended, Walter Legge, the Columbia record company executive, was able to invite Lipatti to London. The pianist "had enormous and powerful hands," reported Legge, "the 'little' finger as long as its neighbor—and the shoulders of a wrestler, quite disproportionate to his frail build." The conductor Arturo Toscanini, though he was the father-in-law of the great Vladimir Horowitz, called Lipatti at this time "the greatest living pianist." Mysteriously, Lipatti wrote to a friend in March 1947 that "my illness does not help the technical side of my playing but artistically it is of great help." Apparently he was referring to his need to limit his arm movements—to play, as it were, economically—to minimize the pain in his swollen armpits.

At last the doctors were able to agree on a diagnosis. The pianist was afflicted with malignant lymphogranulomatosis, a condition now usually named Hodgkin's disease. In recent years, controlled amounts of X-irradiation and chemotherapy with a combination of drugs have improved the survival rate to above 90 percent. Lipatti was not so lucky.

In May 1950 he began a course of the newly introduced cortisone therapy. The improvement was astonishing, but it was known that the steroid treatment could not be continued more than a few weeks. The necessary funds were supplied by fellow musicians, including Yehudi Menuhin and Igor Stravinsky. Legge was urged to send a recording crew from London to capture Lipatti's glorious playing. Between 3 and 12 July he recorded in Geneva all Chopin's waltzes, a Mozart sonata, Bach's *Partita in B-flat* and one or two other pieces, including his great favorite, Bach's *Jesu, Joy of Man's Desiring* in Myra Hess's transcription.

Several of these works were repeated in his final recital, just eleven weeks before his death. He arrived in the French town of Besançon, near the Swiss border, in a state of near-collapse, barely able to try out the piano in Parliament Hall. His doctors begged him to cancel his appearance, but, "I promised, I must play," he replied. He was driven to the hall the next day after several injections were given to strengthen him. "Once there," wrote his wife Madeleine in 1957, "it was a real Calvary for him to climb the stairs, for he could not breathe; one could sense that he was close to fainting." The performance, recorded by French radio, reveals no sign of the pianist's physical state. Only at the end did his strength fail him and, rather than play the last of the fourteen scheduled Chopin waltzes, he substituted a Bach chorale—his swan song.

Dinu Lipatti died quietly on 2 December 1950 at his home in Chêne-

Bourg, southeast of Geneva, shortly after a final blood transfusion, in the presence of Madeleine and his mother Anna. During his dying moments he listened to a Beethoven quartet and murmured, "To write music like that you must be a chosen instrument of God." *See* D. Tanasescu and G. Bargauanu (1988).

MacArthur, Douglas (1880-1964)

The U.S. general who commanded Allied forces in the Pacific throughout World War II accepted the Japanese surrender in September 1945 and supervised Japanese reconstruction. He commanded the United Nations action against North Korea from June 1950. After the intervention of Chinese Communists five months later, UN forces were driven back south of the 38th parallel. MacArthur recommended a widening of the war by bombing bases in China, but this was rejected. His public disclosure of disagreement with the Truman administration led to his dismissal from command in April 1951.

MacArthur was a complex man. His 1978 biographer William Manchester saw him as "noble and ignoble, inspiring and outrageous, arrogant and shy . . . with great personal charm, a will of iron, and a soaring intellect . . . the most gifted man-at-arms this nation has produced . . . His paranoia was almost certifiable. [Immersed in Asian affairs, he believed that] Europeans in general, and the English in particular, were conspiring against him." A right-wing Republican, he opposed postwar economic aid for the continent he hated.

After retirement (though he was kept on the active list for life) he addressed Congress brilliantly, the 1952 Republican Convention not so effectively. He and his second wife Jean Faircloth MacArthur settled in Manhattan's Waldorf Towers behind tight security and surrounded by Oriental objets d'art in a huge opulent apartment that was in marked contrast to ex-President Herbert Hoover's on the floor below. He doted on his son Arthur, who felt so suffocated by his parents' affection and intimidated by the MacArthur name that after his father's death he lost no time in seeking anonymity.

The general revisited the Philippines, scene of his greatest triumph, in July 1961 and sadly announced that "the deepening shadows of life cast doubt upon my ability to pledge again, 'I shall return.'"

The MacArthurs' apartment was within easy walking distance of the

First Army headquarters on Church Street, where the general maintained rooms and where he read the cable traffic every morning. Always armed with a derringer while out in the streets, he shopped at Saks Fifth Avenue and attended the theater with Jean and Arthur.

Never seriously ill until 1960, in that year he was hospitalized with a kidney infection and again when a nonmalignant tumor was removed from his prostate. He completed his *Reminiscences* shortly before his eighty-fourth birthday in January 1964; by then he was appreciably shrunken in appearance and may well have delayed seeking medical attention until the manuscript was completed. On 2 March, President Johnson had him flown to Walter Reed Army Medical Center in Washington, D.C., because of moderately severe jaundice. No malignancy was discovered, only gallstones and liver damage. His gallbladder was removed and he rallied, only to be stricken within days by multiple breakdowns, including intestinal obstruction and esophageal hemorrhages. His spleen was removed on 23 March, part of his intestines on the twenty-ninth. Thereafter pneumonia set in. He was a good patient, happy to entertain the nurses and physicians with his recollections while his strength lasted, always grateful for anything that could be done for him. As his kidneys and his liver failed, he sank into a peaceful coma on 3 April.

General of the Army Douglas MacArthur died at 2:39 P.M. on Sunday, 5 April 1964. On his final visit to West Point he had told the corps of cadets that "when I cross the river my last conscious thoughts will be of the Corps . . ."

Late the same day a twelve-car motorcade bearing his body arrived in New York. After a private interfaith funeral service at the Seventh Regiment Armory, the public were admitted to file past the open coffin, in which the dead man could be seen to be dressed modestly in his faded suntans, without ribbons. There was an impressive procession to Pennsylvania Station. In Washington, MacArthur lay in state below the Capitol rotunda and a third time in Norfolk, Virginia, his mother's hometown, before an Episcopal service in St. Paul's Church on 11 April. There was a brief burial ceremony before he was laid to rest below the Norfolk courthouse, which was dedicated as a MacArthur memorial and shrine, housing a vast collection of memorabilia.

McCullers, Carson (1917-1967)

The five novels of the controversial U.S. author, who wrote *The Heart Is a Lonely Hunter* when only twenty-two, have been compared to William Faulkner's. During her Georgia childhood she suffered from "growing pains" and bouts of pneumonia and pleurisy. At fifteen she was afflicted with what has since been diagnosed as rheumatic fever; blood clots from the damaged heart were probably responsible for a series of strokes that began in 1941. In March 1948 she was treated in New York's Payne Whitney Psychiatric Clinic after a suicide attempt.

Though sexually ambivalent, she was twice married to Reeves McCullers; Reeves's violent temper and Carson's vitriolic tongue produced a stormy marriage. When her husband late in 1953 suggested a suicide pact, Carson fled from him; he was found dead of alcohol and barbiturate poisoning in a Paris hotel in November 1953.

Carson McCullers lived thereafter in her Victorian house at 131 South Broadway in Nyack, New York, on the Hudson River. Incredibly thin, with a paralyzed left hand and arm that were operated on four times in 1959 and 1961, she chain-smoked cigarettes and turned for help and companionship to a psychiatrist, Dr. Mary Mercer. Her final novel, *Clock Without Hands*, was published in 1961. In 1962 she underwent a mastectomy and further hand surgery, and in September 1963 an operation on her swollen left leg. In the following year she fell in the bathroom, breaking her hip and elbow. In a rare happy period she was able to enjoy, in the spring of 1967, a sixteen-day sojourn at the Irish home of film producer John Huston.

On 15 August 1967 she suffered a massive cerebral hemorrhage; after a tracheotomy at Nyack Hospital on the nineteenth she improved temporarily. On 8 September her friend Tennessee Williams thought she recognized him; thereafter she was comatose until her death on 19 September 1967.

A memorial service, attended by her many theatrical, literary, and artistic friends, was held at St. James's Episcopal Church in Manhattan. She was buried in Nyack beside her mother in Oak Hill Cemetery, on a slope overlooking the river. *See* Virginia Spencer Carr (1975).

McPherson, Aimee Semple (1890-1944)

The Canadian-born evangelist, a woman of enormous charm and energy, opened her Angelus Temple in Los Angeles in 1923 and founded the Church of the Foursquare Gospel, based on joy with no hint of hellfire. She was a genuinely warm, friendly person, but she was not without human frailties. In 1926, the year of another famous disappearance—that of the English detective-story writer Agatha Christie—she vanished from a beach in Venice, California, in an attempt to hide her affair with a radio man at her Temple. Three months later, when the liaison could no longer be hushed up, she reappeared south of the border with an unconvincing tale of kidnaping. There were grand jury hearings, but charges against Aimee were dropped in January 1927.

Thereafter her evangelistic powers were less effective; she was now a notorious woman, a dubious tourist attraction rather than a holy messenger. There were foreign tours, interspersed with lawsuits against her and her church, numerous bitter quarrels with her feisty mother, Minnie Kennedy, and a third (short-lived) marriage.

But she was never anything less than a colorful figure who could draw a crowd. On the evening of Tuesday, 26 September 1944, she drove a horse and buggy to the municipal auditorium in Oakland, California, to preach on "The Foursquare Gospel" to ten thousand people. Afterward, perhaps because of her warm reception, she seemed to her son Rolf to be very "keyed up" and excited. The next evening she was scheduled to give "The Story of My Life," always guaranteed to be a crowd pleaser. She chatted with Rolf in her room at the Hotel Leamington before retiring. The wartime blackout was in force and the room was dark behind them as they stood at the open window. The sound of airplanes could be heard flying overhead. "I wonder, when we die, if we will be riding around in airplanes." These were her last words. She kissed her son and he went to his room.

At 10:00 A.M. next morning Rolf found his mother lying in bed breathing stertorously. Medical aid was summoned, but Aimee McPherson was declared dead at 11:45 A.M. The tentative finding by the doctors was a heart attack, but barbiturate capsules were found scattered on the pillow and beside the bed. In her purse a vial containing similar capsules was half-full. Her Los Angeles physician denied having prescribed them, and there was no pharmacy label on the vial.

At the inquest, Rolf described his mother's mood in her final hours as essentially normal, with no hint of depression. She had been taking sedatives because of recent laryngitis that had disturbed her sleep. The idea of suicide was preposterous, he said. The pathologist who conducted the autopsy agreed that "A person could get in such a state of forgetfulness that he might not remember how many he had taken of those pills." The capsules on the pillow were moist, as though they had fallen from the somnolent woman's mouth after a previous dose. The coroner's jury found death to have been caused "by shock and respiratory failure due to an overdose of barbital compound and a kidney ailment."

Aimee McPherson was buried in Forest Lawn Memorial Park, Los Angeles, after lying in state in the Angelus Temple and a motorcade of one hundred cars. The cemetery was closed to the public but two thousand people were admitted, including seventeen hundred Foursquare Gospel ministers who had been ordained by Aimee herself. It was her fifty-fourth birthday, 9 October 1944. Her marble tomb stands on Sunrise Slope with a guardian angel on either side. *See* Lately Thomas, 1970.

McQueen, Steve (1930-1980)

The U.S. movie actor with the bright blue eyes and cheeky grin gained fame in half a dozen films, including *The Great Escape* (1963) and *Bullitt* (1968), before insisting on widening his range by playing Stockmann in Ibsen's *An Enemy of the People* (1977), which disappointed many critics and was never widely distributed to theaters.

He was divorced from the Eurasian dancer Neile Adams in 1972 and from the actress Ali MacGraw in 1977. By then he had met his third wife, Barbara Minty, a young fashion model who had a horse ranch near his hideaway in Ketchum, Idaho. His hobby was racing dune buggies, cars, and motorcycles, of which he owned a large collection, but around the time he filmed *Tom Horn*, the tale of a legendary gunslinger, early in 1979 he found a new love, flying vintage biplanes out of the airfield at Santa Paula, fifty miles northwest of Los Angeles, where he also bought a fifteen-acre ranch.

His health began to break down while working on *The Hunter* (1980), perhaps the worst of his twenty-eight movies, in Chicago; "he lacks zip," wrote one critic, and "a tired daredevil" was another's opinion. He caught a cold he couldn't shake off, and it was followed by chills and fever; he collapsed at the ranch and spent ten days in Cedars-Sinai Hospital, Los

Angeles, over Christmas 1979. Tests revealed a malignant tumor of the right lung, a rare, inoperable cancer called mesothelioma. Nevertheless, he and Barbara went ahead with their belated wedding at the ranch in January. A month later he was told there was virtually no chance of his living beyond a year.

Offered no hope by conventional medicine, McQueen searched around for alternatives. He read an article in the obscure *Journal of Health Science* by a Texas dentist, William Donald Kelley, who claimed to have cured his own cancer with pancreatic and hepatic enzymes while "detoxifying" his body with coffee enemas. In a 1969 book he had reported that this regimen, together with doses of vitamins A and C and thymus extract, boosted the body's immune system.

McQueen met Kelley but postponed treatment until after a honeymoon cruise to Acapulco, during which he lost twenty pounds. At Cedars-Sinai he was told the cancer had engulfed his lung and spread to his neck; he was now given just two months to live. After throwing a lavish party for his friends he checked into a Mexican treatment center on 31 July 1980. It was the Plaza Santa Maria Clinic near Rosarito Beach, a few miles south of Tijuana, where Kelley was a consultant. Here, in one of the bungalows on the one-hundred-acre grounds, he was put on Kelley's treatment, with the addition of laetrile and dimethyl sulfoxide prescribed by the clinic's doctors.

When news of McQueen's whereabouts broke in the tabloids, there was much controversy and great skepticism. Directors at the clinic made remarkable claims: that the actor's tumors were shrinking and that he was putting on weight. Steve's first wife Neile tells a different story. She and their son and daughter, Chad and Terry, had always kept in close touch with him and now visited him at the clinic. She writes in her 1986 book, *My Husband, My Friend,* that she is "convinced the treatment did nothing for him except to [cause him] unnecessary pain. And, of course, it gave him hope. The 'clinic' wouldn't (or couldn't) prescribe painkilling drugs for him." He told her, "I'm actually feeling better. Praise the Lord. They say I'm gonna make it." To which Neile responds, "His raspy voice, the shortness of breath, and the tumors that were visible on his body gave the lie to that opinion." A nurse told her there was no emergency equipment at the clinic, no X-ray machine, no laboratory.

Worn down and impatient, McQueen checked out on 24 October for a short break and spent a few days at the Santa Paula ranch. There the pressure from a large abdominal tumor caused severe urination difficulties and he was flown to Juárez, Mexico, across the border from El Paso, Texas, for emergency surgery. "He walked in with a cane," said the surgeon, Cesar Santos Vargas, at the Santa Rosa clinic, "and he looked more pregnant than a fully pregnant woman." In a forty-five-minute operation a five-pound tumor was removed. McQueen gave the thumbs-up sign to Barbara, Chad, and Terry before and after the surgery. Fourteen hours later, early on 7 November 1980, he died of a sudden heart attack. Chad, summoned from his hotel and alone with his father's body, said his good-byes and closed the bright blue eyes with his fingertips. Steve was clutching the Bible Billy Graham had given him. His hands and feet were cold. "And then, you know," said Chad, "I touched his heart. And his heart was still warm. I was surprised. I leaned over and kissed his heart, and then I said, 'So long, Pop. I love you.' "

Public reaction on both sides of the medical controversy was heated. "Don't victimize [your] families by choosing unproven therapies which may, indeed, hasten [your] death" was the advice of the Los Angeles County Medical Association's president. "Cancer therapy in America is a scandal," responded Kelley. "It's a swamp of politics, greed and fear . . . Steve lived three full months longer than his Los Angeles doctors claimed was possible . . . A heart attack killed him, not the cancer. We had it beaten." A director at Rosarito said the tumor removed in Juárez "did not seem to be growing" and the operation was unnecessary. Dr. Santos Vargas disagreed: "Somebody should have operated on that man immediately" when the tumor was discovered.

Steve McQueen's ashes were scattered over the Pacific. All three of his wives attended a funeral service in the garden at the Santa Paula ranch two days later; Ali and Barbara had not previously met. The pastor of the Ventura Missionary Church presided, and vintage biplanes flew over in cross formation. The ranch was bequeathed to Chad and Terry. McQueen left $200,000 to the California Junior Boys Republic in Chino, California, a reform school where long ago he had spent eighteen months as a troubled teenager. See William F. Nolan (1984).

Mahler, Gustav (1860-1911)

The Austrian composer and conductor completed his ten years as artistic director of the Vienna Opera in 1907 amid complaints of his demanding harshness, which were tinged with more than a hint of anti-Semitism. It was a year that also saw the death of his elder daughter from scarlet fever and his physician's warning that both he and his wife Alma had cardiac problems that must not be ignored.

In the spring of 1910 he ended the second of three seasons as conductor of the New York Philharmonic and Metropolitan Opera orchestras. Back in Europe and distressed by worsening marital relations, he sought a lengthy meeting with Sigmund Freud. The great psychoanalyst, it is said, instantly diagnosed Mahler's mother fixation and thereby brought about domestic harmony.

On 21 February 1911, Mahler conducted his final New York concert, the forty-eighth of the season, and collapsed a few hours later, suffering from tonsillitis and general weakness. Bacteriological tests showed a streptococcal septicemia. With his American doctors uncertain about how to proceed, the invalid and his wife decided to set off immediately for Europe, where the prospects seemed brighter. On board ship he was too weak to walk more than a few yards, but on arrival at Paris's Hotel Elysée he seemed to stage a miraculous recovery, dressing and shaving himself and ordering a drive through the streets. On his return he collapsed and was rushed to a nursing home. There, a certain Dr. Chantemesse proved he lacked the ideal bedside manner. "Come and look," he said to Alma as he bent over his microscope. "Even I have never seen streptococci in such a marvelous state of development." She wired for a Viennese specialist; on arrival he was able to calm his famous patient but warned Alma there was no hope. "May the end come quickly. Were he to survive the whole nervous system would go . . . You don't want a senile idiot on your hands." But he arranged for a speedy journey to Vienna and the Löw sanatorium.

At first, Mahler, delighted to be home, was keenly aware of his surroundings and the bouquets that filled his room. But soon his consciousness faded; as with Beethoven, he died during a thunderstorm. Almost to the end he was aware of Alma's presence, but his last word was "Mozart." It was 18 May 1911; he was buried in Grinzing next to his daughter. Only the single name MAHLER appears on his tomb; he had said more would be superfluous. "Anyone who comes to look for me will know who I was, and the rest do not need to know." See Egon Gartenberg (1978).

Malcolm X (1925-1965)

Before becoming the most powerful voice of the Black Muslims he had been a convicted pimp and narcotics dealer in New York's Harlem. He was expelled from the Nation of Islam, founded by the aged, arthritic Elijah

Muhammad, in December 1963 and in his final months formed a rival organization.

On 21 February 1965 at 2:00 P.M. he strode—lanky and bespectacled—to the flimsy, plywood lectern in the Audubon Ballroom on West 166th Street in uptown Manhattan and addressed his audience in Arabic: "*As-salaam aleikum*" (Peace be unto you). Someone complained loudly of his pocket being picked, and a smoke bomb at the back of the hall created a second diversion as security guards moved away from the platform to investigate. A man near the front pulled a sawed-off double-barrelled shotgun from under his jacket and fired a dozen buckshot pellets, each the diameter of a .32-caliber bullet, into Malcolm's chest. As he toppled backward, another Muslim, Talmadge X Hayer from Paterson, New Jersey, and a third conspirator moved forward, firing automatic pistols into their victim even after he fell.

Across the street at the Columbia-Presbyterian Medical Center a team worked on Malcolm X until 2:30, but it was hopeless: of twenty-one shots that hit him, seven had punctured the heart. Over twenty thousand filed past his open coffin in the Unity Funeral Home in Harlem.

The twenty-two-year-old Hayer, wounded in the thigh by a guard's bullet, was arrested at the street door as he fled. Norman 3X Butler, 26, and Thomas 15X Johnson, 30, two Muslims from the Bronx who were out on bail after a similar shooting six weeks earlier, were arrested within a few days. All three were found guilty of murder after an eight-week trial and a twenty-hour jury deliberation. They were given life sentences and judged ineligible for parole for almost twenty-seven years.

Hayer admitted his guilt but denied the other two were his accomplices. Instead, he named four other New Jersey Black Muslims. Peter Goldman, in his *The Death and Life of Malcolm X* (2nd edition, 1979), is inclined to believe him.

Having much earlier dropped his "slave name" (Little), Malcolm adopted the Muslim appellation of el-Hajj Malik el-Shabazz after a 1964 pilgrimage to Mecca, and it is this that is carved on his tombstone in Ferncliff Cemetery, Hartsdale, New York.

Mansfield, Katherine (1888-1923)

The New Zealand–born short-story writer's poverty-stricken years in London laid the foundations of her chronic ill health. Her Bohemian lifestyle, which included affairs with both sexes, a stillbirth and an abortion—as well as a strange one-night marriage—preceded her long relationship with the critic and essayist John Middleton Murry, which began in 1911. She was probably even then suffering from tuberculosis. In a 1955 medical study, Brice Clarke concludes that after her health completely broke down in 1917 "toxemia and the knowledge of impending death heightened her perceptions and enabled her to achieve the artistic perfection for which she had striven all her life."

In October 1922 Mansfield began unorthodox treatment at G. I. Gurdjieff's institute near Fontainebleu in France. There were, according to her 1953 biographer Antony Alpers, "Exercises—dancing—out in the garden in galoshes and around the pigsty . . . " Gurdjieff decreed that she work in the freezing-cold kitchen until 2:00 A.M. scraping carrots and peeling onions. During the day she was directed to lie on a shelf above the cattle in the cowshed to "benefit" from their exhalations.

Murry, whom she had married in 1918, visited her on 9 January 1923. After dancing in the evening they were walking upstairs together when Katherine was seized by a violent fit of coughing. There was a sudden hemorrhage from her mouth and she whispered that she was going to die. Doctors arrived quickly and set to work with hot-water bottles, but by 10:30 P.M. she had expired.

She was buried in the Protestant cemetery at Avon, Fontainebleu; on the slab of stone that covers her grave are some words of Shakespeare's chosen by her for the title page of her 1920 short-story collection, *Bliss*:

BUT I TELL YOU, MY LORD FOOL, OUT OF THIS
NETTLE, DANGER, WE PLUCK THIS FLOWER, SAFETY.

Mao Tse-Tung (1893-1976)

The former Beijing library assistant founded the Chinese Communist Party in 1921 and ultimately became one of the century's most influential leaders. With the failure of the Great Leap Forward he withdrew from the presidency of China in 1959 but retained the party chairmanship. In the Cultural Revolution of 1966–69 he launched the Red Guards, mainly university students and their cohorts, in often capricious attacks against authority; even some of Mao's old comrades in the Long March of 1934–36, including Deng Xiaoping, were not immune to attack.

In his final half-dozen years, Mao Tse-tung (reformed spelling: Mao Zedong) cooperated with the more moderate prime minister Chou En-lai (Zhou En-Lai) in an opening to the West. By the time U.S. President Ford met with Mao in October 1975 it was clear that the frail old man had only a few months left. But it was the much-loved and respected Chou who died first (in January 1976 of cancer, aged seventy-eight). In the struggle to name Chou's successor, Mao chose the second-rate Hua Guofeng over the able vice-premier Deng Xiaoping. A bloody riot resulted in April after wreaths and poems placed on a Beijing monument to honor the dead Chou were summarily removed, apparently on the orders of Mao and, it was widely suspected, his ultra-leftist wife (since 1949) Chiang Ching (Jiang Qing). The precise relations between husband and wife were at that time a puzzle. It was known that they lived apart, but only in 1990 was it revealed that Chiang had to apply to the Communist Party General Office whenever she wanted to see Mao and that he did not always assent.

His last foreign visitor was Singapore's Prime Minister Lee Kuan Yew in May. Parkinsonism had afflicted the chairman for a decade, and now his spoken words were an unintelligible sequence of sounds that had to be deciphered by a niece before translation. There was no agreed procedure to choose Mao's successor, hence he was obliged to shuffle on and off the stage to grunt his lines. Suspicions of the ambitious Chiang's machinations deepened as Mao retired from affairs and took to his bed in the summer. He was sufficiently aware of events to take in the enormity of the midsummer earthquake that killed a quarter-million people in Tangshan.

There were bedside conclaves with the Politburo, at one of which the chairman was understood to say, "Not many live beyond seventy. I am over eighty. I should be dead already. Didn't some of you hope I should have gone already to meet Marx?" But no one present was willing to voice such a thought.

As he lay, steadily losing consciousness, in his Ming-dynasty pavilion in Beijing, diverse rumors of Chiang Ching's plotting circulated: that she was trying to squeeze a last pronouncement favorable to herself from the dying lips, that she was searching for documents to aid her cause, that she was on the contrary far from Beijing, playing bridge.

Death came to Chairman Mao Tse-tung early on 9 September 1976 and was announced over the radio sixteen hours later. A week of mourning was proclaimed, at the end of which all nine hundred million Chinese were called on to stand, at three o'clock in the afternoon, for a silent three minutes while sirens sounded across the immense land. Mao's body lay in state in Beijing's Great Hall of the People while three hundred thousand mourners filed past the catafalque. Years earlier Mao had chosen a burial site for himself and his wife in Papaoshan Cemetery, but he had also been heard to ask that his remains be returned to his native Hunan province. (Chou En-lai had elected for cremation and the scattering of his ashes "on the rivers and mountains of China.") Of all possible methods of disposal the one least likely to have had the dead man's approval was the one adopted: to have him mummified and exhibited, like Lenin, in a mausoleum. Perhaps Hua and his colleagues felt in need of the chairman's presence, even in death.

The Vietnamese embalmers who had preserved the corpse of Ho Chi Minh were called in to work on Mao, and construction began in November on a white marble mausoleum in Tiananmen Square. It was opened on the anniversary of Mao's death, and he could be viewed, dressed in a light gray suit draped with China's red flag, lying in a crystal sarcophagus.

Within a month of his death, Chiang Ching and three associates (the "Gang of Four") were arrested and tried in 1980–81 on treason charges; in particular they were accused of responsibility for the excesses of the Cultural Revolution. Chiang was sentenced to death, but the punishment was commuted to life imprisonment two years later. From May 1984 she lived "out of custody," presumably under house arrest, and was rumored to be a victim of throat cancer. On 14 May 1991 she killed herself (according to a news-magazine, by hanging). *See* Ross Terrill (1980).

Marx, Groucho (1890-1977)

In old age, Groucho was the most visible member of the Marx Brothers, the U.S. comedy team. (Chico had died in 1961, Harpo in 1964.) He was famous for his wicked antiestablishment ad-libs on television's *You Bet Your Life,* which made the transition from radio in 1950 and ran until 1961.

As he turned eighty, he lived a lonely, unhappy life on Hillcrest Road in Beverly Hills, California, sometimes dating his third wife Eden Hartford, from whom he had been recently divorced. After he suffered a stroke in 1971 she offered to return to nurse him, but he was too proud to accept. Late that summer he was introduced to a red-haired Canadian actress, Erin Fleming, and she soon moved in as his manager-secretary-companion.

The relationship undoubtedly worked wonders on the old man; visitors were quick to notice how he brightened when she entered the room. That they loved one another could hardly be doubted; he proposed to her more than once but, wanting children, she said no. She could be autocratic, and her tantrums grew more frequent with time. She once told Hector Arce, the comedian's 1979 biographer, "When I first started with Groucho, I was sweet and agreeable and everyone walked all over me. Now I'm a bitch, and they listen."

Groucho had another stroke in 1972 and the following year was hospitalized twice with heart, lung, and urinary problems. In 1974 he and Charles Chaplin were presented with special Oscars, and the Marx Brothers' movie *Animal Crackers* was rereleased with great fanfare.

Groucho's brothers Zeppo and Gummo attended his eighty-fifth birthday party in October 1975. During 1976, Hollywood executives and others found Erin increasingly difficult to deal with, and Groucho was more and more isolated. Several household employees were fired, and they made accusations that she was tyrannizing Groucho, even giving him unauthorized tranquilizers. She canceled his scheduled appearance in aid of the Ralph Nader organization, citing his medication-induced incontinence.

In early 1977 Groucho suffered another stroke, and this time his peripheral vision was affected. In March he had hip-replacement surgery, and his physician told Arce that his arteries looked like those of a one-hundred-five-year-old. Arthur Marx, Groucho's only son, who distrusted Fleming, applied to the Superior Court in Santa Monica, California, to have himself appointed conservator of his father's estate. Many of Groucho's friends, alarmed at the threatened removal of his close companion, took Erin's side in the dispute. On 21 April, Gummo died but the news was kept from the failing old man.

As feelings between the feuding parties grew more heated, Erin Fleming asked detectives to check the house for listening devices; instead they stumbled on what was probably a red herring: syringes containing traces of barbiturates dumped in a storm drain in front of the house. A criminal investigation came to nothing. Groucho's former writer Nat Perrin, appointed temporary conservator, tried to keep the Arthur- and Erin-sympathizers apart when they came to see Groucho.

By the time Andy Marx, Groucho's twenty-seven-year-old grandson, was chosen as permanent conservator late in July, Groucho had been back in Cedars-Sinai Hospital, Los Angeles, for several weeks with pneumonitis and other ailments, and Andy's appointment was completed in a bedside court session.

After years of uncertain relations with his three children, Groucho made his peace with them. Miriam for years had had a drinking problem but was now a fervent supporter of Alcoholics Anonymous. Melinda came from northern California to visit regularly.

Groucho's final collapse was sudden; he succumbed to pneumonia at 7:25 P.M. on 19 August 1977. Erin had left his bedside just a few minutes earlier; Miriam was on her way to the hospital. A small intimate memorial gathering took place two days later at Arthur's home. Many were not invited—even Zeppo, who had been excluded because, he claimed angrily, he had sided with Erin in the family dispute. Arthur and Andy prayed at private services in Temple Beth El in Hollywood.

Groucho was cremated; his ashes were placed in Eden Memorial Park in Mission Hills, Los Angeles, with a six-inch-square bronze plaque inscribed GROUCHO MARX / 1890–1977, with a Star of David between the dates. The urn containing the ashes was reported stolen in May 1982. The bulk of his $1.8 million estate was left to his children; Erin Fleming received $150,000 and control of Groucho's film and television rights, but this was challenged in court. In 1983 a jury awarded Bank of America, executor of the estate, a $450,000 judgment against Erin Leslie Fleming, whom the bank accused of undue influence. This award was finally reduced to $221,000.

Maximilian (1832-1867)

After President Benito Juárez of Mexico was ousted by the French in 1864, conservatives invited the tall, blond Austrian archduke to establish a monarchy. The French in 1867 withdrew their forces under pressure from the United States, but Maximilian, believing in his destiny as protector of the Mexican people, refused to leave. He withdrew from the capital with a ragtag force of nine thousand men, intent on forcing back Juárez's troops at Querétaro, one hundred miles to the north. After a seventy-two-day siege, Maximilian and General Tomas Mejía were captured on 14 May 1867, along with one of their few European comrades, Prince Felix zu Salm-Salm of Prussia. Later they were joined by the wounded General Miguel Miramón. An escape plan failed when Maximilian, weakened by dysentery and perhaps fearful of a trap, refused to go.

At 10:00 A.M. on 16 June, after a four-day trial, Maximilian and the two generals were sentenced to be shot on the Hill of Bells five hours later. Their confessions were heard, but the stated hour passed without incident; at 4:00 P.M. a three-day postponement was announced to give a Prussian diplomat time to visit the emperor. Mass was celebrated for the doomed men at dawn on the nineteenth, after which three closed vehicles, one for each man and his confessor, made their way through the silent streets of Querétaro to the foot of the hill.

The men walked slowly to the summit and stood against an adobe wall, while four thousand men formed three sides of a square. There were fifteen men in the firing squad, four for each of the condemned and three in reserve. To his quartet of executioners, Maximilian awarded each a gold piece and, pointing to his heart, said, "Muchachos, aim well, aim right here." He concluded a short speech with the cry, "Viva México! Viva Independencia!" After a few rapid words of command twelve rifles were raised, followed immediately by the deafening sound of shots. Maximilian pitched forward and was heard to murmur, "*Hombre*"; the officer in charge turned his body over and a soldier fired point-blank into his heart. Miramón was already dead, but two more bullets were needed to kill Mejía.

The bodies were wrapped in coarse sheets and placed in deal coffins; Maximilian's was too short and his feet protruded from the end. The first embalmment of the emperor was badly botched; newly appointed practitioners attempted to preserve the body by ancient Egyptian methods of desiccation. In November the remains were placed in a new coffin of granadilla wood and conveyed in Maximilian's old flagship, the *Novarra*, to Trieste, from which port Maximilian and his wife Carlota had departed Europe with such high hopes three and a half years before. On the snowy, bitterly cold morning of 20 January 1868 the coffin was placed in a marble sepulchre in the resting place of the Hapsburgs, the Capuchin Crypt of the Augustiner Church of Vienna.

Maxwell, Robert (1923-1991)

The Czech-born British media tycoon, who died at sea in mysterious circumstances, began World War II as a refugee and ended it as a British army captain who took part in the Normandy landings. By 1991 he owned or controlled newspapers throughout the world, including the *Daily* and *Sunday Mirrors* in London and the New York *Daily News*. But it was clear, even before his death, that the edifice he had built was falling apart. Swiss banks were demanding repayment of huge loans, and it was discovered later that he had plundered his employees' pension funds—and investments in his company by outsiders—of over $1 billion to provide collateral for fresh loans.

On Thursday, 31 October 1991, Maxwell flew in his private jet at short notice from England to Gibraltar to join his yacht there. For once he took no guests as he sailed in his *Lady Ghislaine* six hundred miles west-south-west to Madeira, planning to fly home from there at the weekend. But after visits ashore he changed his mind and ordered the skipper to head three hundred miles south to the Canary Islands. Maxwell swam off Tenerife on 4 November and dined ashore. He would fly home next day, he said, and directed the yacht to be put to sea so that the motion would help him sleep.

He was last seen alive looking over the stern rail at 4:10 A.M. on 5 November. He exchanged a few words with a crew member and asked that the air-conditioning be turned on, as it was warm below. He was heard from one last time when he phoned the bridge to order the fans turned off. He was reported missing at 11:05 A.M. and an air-sea rescue search was launched. Maxwell's naked body was spotted at 5:50 that afternoon off Grand Canary and at 6:15 P.M. it was winched aboard a helicopter.

Two autopsies were performed, the first by Spanish authorities, another by a British pathologist before the dead man's burial in Israel. This second examination, by Dr. Iain West on behalf of insurers holding a £20-million policy on the tycoon's life, was hampered by the earlier dissections and partial embalming. The three-hundred-pound man, reported West, had "undoubtedly suffered from a degree of ischemic myocardial damage, but there is no evidence to indicate that this is more than a potential cause of death." Moreover, if Maxwell had collapsed while standing at the ship's rail he would not have rolled into the sea. The torn muscles behind his left shoulder pointed to his having climbed over the rail, hung by one hand and then let go. West concluded that other possibilities, including homicide, could not be entirely ruled out, but that suicide by drowning was the most likely cause of death.

The dead man's behavior was consistent with this. He was unusually indecisive, more than usually pleasant to the yacht's crew, and, as for the head cold he had cited as the reason for the sudden cruise, he evidenced no sign of it.

Robert Maxwell was buried in Jerusalem on the Mount of Olives. Israel's president, Chaim Herzog, delivered the eulogy. Over the grave lies a huge concrete slab. Why did the tycoon choose to rest here? A gravedigger at the cemetery answered a reporter's question by reminding her that Jesus, Mary, and Muhammad had all ascended to heaven from this spot. To the "bouncing Czech" it must have been "like an international airport—just Maxwell's style."

Meir, Golda (1898-1978)

Israel's foreign minister for ten years from 1956 and prime minister (1969–74) was a lifelong Zionist who was born in Ukraine and lived in Milwaukee, Wisconsin, from 1906 to 1921.

She retired from public office after the inconclusive "Yom Kippur War" of 1973. When, reluctantly, she agreed to write her autobiography, *My Life* (1975), it was an instant best-seller. In November 1977, she sat, uncomfortable and stony faced, through the first-night Broadway performance of *Golda* by William Gibson. The play's text was confusing and complicated, but when it closed after only ninety-three performances the reason had much to do with the health of Anne Bancroft, playing the title role of a heavy smoker. Bancroft, a nonsmoker, said afterward, "I had planned not to inhale on stage" but in her nervousness she "inhaled 17 cigarettes in the two hours of performance. Golda had chronic bronchitis from smoking and I developed acute bronchitis from smoking." Performances were suspended when the bronchitis led to influenza. "Two or three nights in a row," said her physician, "a doctor was in the wings. She was like the walking wounded."

A television movie, *A Woman Called Golda* (1980), was more successful. It starred Ingrid Bergman with Leonard Nimoy as Morris Meyerson, Mrs. Meir's estranged husband, who died in 1951. As in the stage version, Golda's romantic attachments were barely referred to.

When Egypt's president Anwar Sadat visited Jerusalem in November 1977, the ex-prime minister stole the show. She presented Sadat with a bracelet for his newborn granddaughter as from "grandmother to grandfather" and referred to herself as "the Old Lady"; "I know, Mr. President," she added with a chuckle, "that you have always called me that." Sadat was delighted, and hopes for a permanent Middle East harmony were suddenly brighter than ever before.

But the health of Israel's "Stalwart Lioness" was clearly failing. Only after her death was it revealed that she had suffered from leukemia since 1972. For years, pain and exhaustion had taken their toll, yet between hospital stays before and after her eightieth birthday in May 1978 she kept to an active lifestyle. Early in September she was admitted to the hematology ward of the Hadassah Hospital in Jerusalem, and except for a four-day respite at her Tel Aviv home she spent her final fifteen weeks there.

Almost to the end she was in charge of events. Her hospital room was made comfortable for the few permitted visitors and she herself directed the flow of conversation and distribution of refreshments. "Menahem," she would request her son, "see if someone needs milk." But gradually her strength ebbed. The leukemia could be kept in check, but not the subsequent viral hepatitis and consequent jaundice. She was always precisely aware of her condition. "See," she said to a nurse, "even steel weakens sometimes." She lost consciousness early on 7 December 1978 and died next day at 4:30 P.M. In her final hours of consciousness her grandson Danny came to tell her of his success in the high school exams. Golda was unable to speak, "but," writes his father Menahem in a 1983 memoir, "her eyes opened and shone for him before they closed again."

Golda Meir lay in state in a flag-draped wooden coffin in the forecourt of the Knesset (the Israeli parliament). At the funeral service in the Knesset's Chagall Hall, the last paragraphs of *My Life* were read by an Israeli actress: "I believe that we will have peace with our neighbors, but I am sure that no one will make peace with a weak Israel . . . " The United States was represented at the ceremonies by Secretary of State Cyrus Vance and the president's mother, "Miz Lillian" Carter. The president himself said in a message, "Golda's gift was extended beyond the bounds of her people. She spoke to all humanity." Sadat cabled a salute to "an honest adversary." Her tombstone in the national cemetery on Jerusalem's Mount Herzl records only her name and date of death.

Golda Meir left a note that read: "I forbid any eulogies and want nothing to be named for me." This instruction has been strictly obeyed in Israel, but the University of Wisconsin's library in Milwaukee is dedicated to the woman who arrived in the city as eight-year-old Goldie Mabowehz.

Mengele, Josef (1911-1979)

The infamous Nazi physician at Auschwitz performed painful and often fatal experiments on countless thousands of prisoners. He was held for several days under his own name in 1945 by liberating U.S. forces. After working on a Bavarian farm he escaped with family help via Genoa to Argentina and, in 1959, to Paraguay. Scared by the capture and forced extradition of Adolf Eichmann (q.v.) in May 1960 by Israeli agents, he moved on to Brazil. He lived for thirteen years with Hungarian-born Geza Stammer and his family north of São Paulo. As a withdrawn but authoritative intruder, always obsessed by the danger of capture, he began to threaten the Stammers' marriage. They helped him to buy his final home, a small bungalow at 5555 Alvarenga Road in the Eldorado suburb of São Paulo, where he lived alone, increasingly unhappy and often suicidal, suffering from high blood pressure, a spinal weakness, and an enlarged prostate. In May 1976 he suffered a stroke that affected his left side. Newspaper reports usually placed him in Paraguay, but he could never relax. He wrote frequently to his family in West Germany by way of a Swiss post-office box and in 1977 his son Rolf visited him for two weeks, their first meeting in twenty-one years, but the son could obtain no rational account of his father's wartime actions; the old man expressed not a shred of remorse.

On 5 February 1979 Josef Mengele traveled by bus to Bertioga, twenty-five miles south of São Paulo, to join friends, the Bosserts, at their rented beach house. At 4:30 P.M. on the seventh he had a second stroke while swimming near the beach. Wolfram Bossert brought him to shore with great difficulty and the rescuer himself was hospitalized for several days. Mengele died on the beach within a few minutes. Liselotte Bossert arranged a hasty burial under the name of Wolfgang Gerhard, a former friend who had returned to Europe and whose identity card Mengele had been using. (Gerhard had arranged for his own burial in the plot next to his mother's.)

The hue and cry for Mengele intensified during the 1980s. A careless remark, in his cups, by one Hans Sedlmeier in 1984 began the unraveling of the secret. Sedlmeier, an employee of the Mengele family business in Günzberg, Germany, had flown to South America five times to see Mengele secretly. A police raid on his house revealed coded telephone numbers and addresses. The São Paulo police raided the Bosserts' house and the whole story emerged, only to be widely disbelieved.

On 21 January 1985 a team of forensic scientists exhibited Mengele's bones at the São Paulo police headquarters and announced to the world an absolute identification had been established. A lengthy 1987 study by a West German professor of forensic medicine, R. P. Helmer, provides full details of the identification. *See* G. L. Posner and John Ware (1986).

Merrick, Joseph (1862-1890)

The English youth exhibited publicly as the "Elephant Man" was first brought to the attention of the medical profession by the young surgeon Frederick Treves in November 1884. (Oddly, Treves always referred to him as John, but on his birth certificate his name is undoubtedly Joseph Carey Merrick.) The future appendectomy pioneer found the grossly malformed twenty-one-year-old in a "freak" show near the London Hospital in White-chapel Road and arranged for a private inspection. Merrick was five feet two inches tall; there were huge asymmetric bony masses above the brow and at the side and back of the skull, which measured thirty-six inches around. Heavy folds of flesh hung from the right shoulder and especially from the buttocks, and the skin over most of the body was covered by warty growths, varying in size from pimples to huge cauliflowerlike masses. The right arm and hand were greatly enlarged and useless, one of the fingers measuring five inches around. By contrast the left arm and hand were nor-mal and delicate—almost feminine in appearance. A short "trunk" that had greatly impeded eating and drinking had been surgically removed in Mer-rick's native city of Leicester, in the English Midlands, two years previously. His strange fluting voice was incomprehensible to Treves, who judged him to be an imbecile.

His history only gradually came to light. His mother died when he was ten years old and his father later cast him out. Four years of misery in a workhouse was followed by a round of freak shows. Treves had him pho-tographed and exhibited before the Pathological Society of London but re-ceived no suggestions about possible treatment. For a year and a half he lost track of him. An abortive European tour ended when the promoter stole his lifesavings and abandoned him in Brussels. Penniless and starving, he somehow made his way back to London. Cowering before a mob that pressed upon him there, he produced Treves's visiting card and the benev-olent surgeon rescued him, arranged for his asylum at the hospital and inspired a public appeal for funds.

A two-room suite was specially furnished for Merrick behind the Lon-don Hospital. ("No mirrors," ordered Treves.) Treves discovered that Mer-rick was, after all, "highly intelligent" and "possessed an acute sensibility." With his one serviceable hand he made little cardboard models that he gave as gifts to those who were kind to him. To Treves, who gradually learned how to understand him, he wryly forecast his probable destiny: to be pre-served for all time in a huge bottle of alcohol. (This final indignity was spared him, but his skeleton is still to be seen at the hospital.)

Many visitors came to talk to him: Alexandra, Princess of Wales, took a special interest in him. In his head-to-foot outdoor costume of hood and cloak he was once smuggled by Treves into a private box at a West End theater to see a Christmas pantomime. In 1889 he was able to journey by rail to a gamekeeper's cottage on a country estate, where for once he was able, for six weeks, to be close to nature—"the one supreme holiday of his life," wrote Treves.

In 1882, the Strasbourg professor F. D. von Recklinghausen had described a disorder characterized by pale brown patches of skin and by tumors (neurofibromas) that could be felt under the skin along the course of peripheral nerves. It was not until 1909 that Parkes Weber ascribed Merrick's gross malformations to von Recklinghausen's disease, and it was the same British physician who in 1930 suggested that the bony outgrowths occurred when neurofibroma formation involved the periosteum (the membrane that covers the skeleton). Though it is an inheritable disease, it can arise sporadically, and no other cases have been traced to Merrick's family. There is no cure.

Cases of neurofibromatosis as extreme as Merrick's are vanishingly rare; one-third show no symptoms at all, being discovered only during medical examinations, and in many others the signs are like those described by von Recklinghausen.

During his final half-year Joseph Merrick's health declined and he seldom left his bed before noon. On Easter Sunday, 6 April 1890, he took Communion and attended evensong. At 1:30 P.M. on the following Friday, the eleventh, he was served lunch on a tray. At a few minutes after three the house surgeon found him dead, lying on his back across the bed; his lunch was untouched. The coroner's inquest judged that death was due to asphyxia caused by the great weight of his head having overcome him during natural sleep. But Treves, writing of "The Elephant Man" in his reminiscences shortly before his death in 1923, has what seems to be a more satisfactory explanation. He was, after all, the London Hospital's anatomist, responsible for dissecting the body after a service in the chapel. Normally, he explains, Merrick had to sleep sitting up, arms clasping his knees, with his enormous head resting on them. "He often said to me that he wished he could lie down to sleep 'like other people.' I think on this last night [sic] he must, with some determination, have made the experiment. The pillow was soft, and the head, when placed on it, must have fallen backwards and caused a dislocation of the neck. Thus it came about that his death was due to the desire that dominated his life—the pathetic but hopeless desire to be 'like other people.' " And Treves continues, "As a specimen of humanity, Merrick was ignoble and repulsive; but the spirit of Merrick, if it could be seen in the form of the living, would assume the figure of an upstanding and heroic man, smooth browed and clean of limb, and with eyes that flashed undaunted courage." *See* M. J. Howell and Peter Ford (1980).

Merton, Thomas (1915-1968)

The French-born U.S. Trappist monk and poet, author of over fifty books, was converted to Roman Catholicism when twenty-six years old and at the abbey of Our Lady of Gethsemani in Kentucky took the name Brother Louis. His many health problems were probably worsened by the privations and meager diet at the monastery. He dwelt much on death; after major surgery he wrote to a friend, "The scenario calls for a quiet death among concerned chipmunks, and I'd like it that way." But this was not to be granted.

Merton arrived in Bangkok, Thailand, on 8 December 1968 and on the tenth addressed a religious conference in suburban Paknam, ten miles south of the city. After lunch he retired to his room in a cottage near the auditorium. The weather was hot and he probably showered. Then, standing on the terrazzo with bare wet feet, he reached up to adjust the tall Hitachi-type electric fan, which had been faultily wired. He bellowed loudly as the lethal current surged through his body. In a private communication his biographer J. H. Griffin writes that he "could still perhaps have been saved except [that] two men sharing the house . . . decided he had only had a bad dream, or perhaps [thought] the noise came from outside and refused to invade his privacy."

The current was still flowing through Merton's body when it was discovered several hours later. His chest was badly burned where the fan had fallen on him, but his expression was peaceful. He was flown back to the United States and buried in accordance with his wishes at Gethsemani. A small white cross, inscribed FR. LOUIS MERTON / DIED DEC. 10, 1968 marks the grave under a cedar tree.

Millay, Edna St. Vincent (1892-1950)

The U.S. poet, an early feminist whose lively verses celebrate love and moral freedom, was awarded the Pulitzer Prize in 1922. She married a Dutch coffee importer, Eugen Jan Boissevain, in 1923 and, giving up her bohemian life in Manhattan's Greenwich Village, moved to an old farmhouse in Austerlitz, New York, near the Massachusetts border. Thereafter her work often took on a more somber, political tinge.

Millay, a neurotic and near-alcoholic, suffered debilitating headaches.

She was well taken care of by her husband, but in 1936 she fell out of their car into the pitch darkness as it took a sharp turn. Boissevain found her down a rock gully "with," he reported, "a big bump on her little red head and scratches and bruises all over." Resulting nerve damage gave her long-lasting pain in her right arm and shoulder. At the age of fifty she already looked old. In her final years at their farm, Steepletop, Boissevain protected and babied his "Vincie," keeping away intruders and coaxing her to eat and rest. The rare visitor reported that he talked to her in language close to baby talk and that she responded like a small invalid child; but the moment he left the room she snapped back into her former hearty manner.

Boissevain died after lung-cancer surgery in August 1949 and Millay collapsed after his funeral. Following several weeks in the hospital she returned home to face a bleak future alone, with no resident help and very little money. But she worked sedulously on a new book of poetry, which was to receive an enthusiastic response after her death.

On the evening of 18 October 1950 she began reading the proofs of her friend Rolfe Humphries's translation of Catullus and became so absorbed that dawn was breaking before she finished. She left a note in the kitchen for her neighbor and part-time help: "Dear Lena, This iron is set too high. Don't put it on where it says 'LINEN' . . . It is 5:30 . . . I am going to bed. Goodmorning—E.St.V.M." She had been sipping Alsatian wine while she read. Now, taking the glass and bottle with her, she mounted the first few steps from the hall to a landing where the staircase turned sharply for the long flight to the second floor. It may have been a spasm of pain that caused her to sit down on the step above the landing, placing the bottle and glass beside her. "There on the stair," writes her 1969 biographer Jean Gould, "she swayed forward and died."

Shortly after 8:00 A.M. the handyman, John Pinnie, came in the back door with the milk; he looked into the hall but saw nothing amiss. But when he returned at 3:00 P.M. with firewood he saw her, dressed in nightgown and slippers, sitting with head slumped forward above the landing. The cause of death was a coronary occlusion. Like her husband, she was cremated at Chatham, New York. After a reading of her poetry at Steepletop, the ashes of both were buried in the laurel grove there.

Mitford, Unity (1914-1948)

The fourth of Lord Redesdale's six daughters, sister to authors Nancy and Jessica, was like her parents besotted with Nazism. On a 1939 visit to Hitler's retreat at Berchtesgaden she was disappointed to find Eva Braun ensconced there, but Hitler installed her in a Munich apartment at Agnesstrasse 26 after its Jewish owners had been ousted. Warned to leave Germany before war began she was at first defiant: "I am under the Führer's protection," she declared, and said she would rather shoot herself; later, when it was too late, she was terrified and tearful.

Within an hour of the outbreak of World War II on 3 September 1939 she was sitting in Munich's English Garden. A shot rang out and a college professor who had taught her math saw her slump forward. A bullet from her revolver had entered through the right temple and was lodged at the back of the skull; then and later it was considered best to leave it there. At the university clinic she was provided with a private room and continuous care, paid for by Hitler personally. He visited her on 8 September and told doctors she wished to return home.

Back in England four months later and living at High Wycombe, midway between London and Oxford, she needed constant care; she was incontinent and lacked a proper sense of balance, but was able to walk and even cycle. In July 1944 the government gave her permission to live on Inch Kenneth, a remote island belonging to the Mitfords off the outer coast of Mull in western Scotland which under wartime security regulations had until then been out of bounds.

On 27 May 1948 her physician called for help from the West Highland Cottage Hospital in Oban on the mainland. Unity had a "chill" with severe headache and vomiting. The old gunshot wound was bulging and meningitis was suspected. By motorboat, ambulance, then motorboat and ambulance again she was rushed to Oban by midnight. Penicillin treatment was begun and by next morning arrangements were afoot to have her transferred to a cranial surgery center at Killearn, one hundred miles away. But even as the ambulance waited outside she took a turn for the worse; her pupils became markedly dilated, she suffered an epileptiform seizure and finally Cheyne-Stokes breathing began.

Unity Mitford died at 9:50 P.M. that evening, 28 May 1948; her death certificate reads: "Purulent meningitis; cerebral abscess; old gunshot wound." She was buried near her old childhood home in Swinbrook churchyard, near Burford, Oxfordshire. *See* David Pryce-Jones (1977).

More, Saint Sir Thomas (1478-1535)

The first layman to be appointed Lord Chancellor of England resigned that office rather than countenance Henry VIII's divorce from Catherine of Aragon and marriage to his mistress, Anne Boleyn. His failure to attend Anne's coronation on 1 June 1533 marked him out for royal vengeance. An attempt to convict him of bribe taking failed; so did a charge of misprision of treason for failure to report false prophecies of Elizabeth Barton, a serving maid known as the "Nun of Kent" who was executed in April 1534.

The same month More was brought down the Thames from his Chelsea home to Lambeth to take an oath to the new Act of Succession. He was willing, though with a sad heart, to accept Anne's succession, but not the supremacy of the king as head of the Church in England, which was also entailed by the oath. He was thereupon imprisoned in the Tower of London. A specific Act of Supremacy was passed late in 1534. (Among the bishops, only one, John Fisher of Rochester, was courageous enough to withhold his consent. He was martyred in June 1535 shortly after Henry heard he had been created a cardinal.)

Beginning on 30 April 1535, a commission interrogated Sir Thomas, but he steadfastly refused to incriminate himself. On 1 July he was brought to trial at Westminster, where he faced indictments for refusing to give an opinion on the king's marriage and Supremacy, for conspiring with Fisher, and for having told a visitor, Sir Richard Rich, that it was beyond Parliament's power to make the sovereign head of the English Church.

Though weakened by his long privation, More made a spirited defense. Silence, he claimed, could never be treason; under civil law, indeed, it implied not dissent but assent. In his letters to Fisher he had done no more than advise him to behave as he believed right. As for the perjurer Rich, the chief witness against him, More asked whether it was likely he would mention in inconsequential conversation what could not be dragged from him under prolonged questioning.

This defense made a great impact, but the judges could not allow themselves to be moved. With his life now clearly forfeit, Sir Thomas at last spoke his mind on the Supremacy Act. It was, he said, "directly repugnant to the laws of God and his Holy Church," taking as it did "spiritual preeminence" from Rome, upon whom it had been bestowed by "our Saviour himself, personally present upon earth." He ended with a taunt: "Howbeit, it is not for this Supremacy so much that ye seek my blood, as for that I would not condescend to the marriage."

As More reentered the Tower his daughter Margaret Roper embraced him passionately several times in a scene long remembered by the onlookers. He awaited his execution in prayer and meditation and in writing final letters to his family and friends. His impatience was evident: "I should be sorry if it should be any longer than tomorrow." On 6 July 1535, dressed in a coarse gray robe belonging to his servant, John a' Wood, and carrying a red cross, Sir Thomas More took the short walk to Tower Hill, conversing with one or two of those who lined the route. To a woman who offered him a sip of wine he said, "Christ in His passion was given not wine but vinegar to drink," and declined. To a man whom he had helped in his fits of despair years earlier and who was again in need of comfort, he made a promise to pray for him in the next world; it is said the man had no further trouble.

Too weak to ascend the scaffold, More asked a sheriff's officer for aid, adding, "When I come down again, let me shift for myself." He recited the *Miserere mei* and briefly addressed the throng. His last remarks were for the executioner: "Pluck up thy spirits, man, and be not afraid to do thine office. My neck is very short; take heed therefore thou strike not awry for the saving of thine honesty." Then he lay down, pulling his long gray beard out of the way "lest it be cut." "Thus with a mock," recorded one shocked onlooker, "he ended his life."

The head was parboiled in the customary way and placed on a stake above London Bridge. His daughter Margaret bribed the executioner to let her have it a month later; it lies now in the Roper vault below St. Dunstan's Church, Canterbury. The body was interred in the west end of St. Peter's ad Vincula . . . close by the execution site and close by the body of Bishop Fisher. They were joined within the year by that of Anne Boleyn. Both martyrs were canonized four hundred years later, in May 1935. *See* E. E. Reynolds (1953).

Morrison, Jim (1943-1971)

The lead singer and lyricist of The Doors rock group was a would-be poet whose idols included Nietzsche and Rimbaud and whose drink-sodden days ended far from home after only twenty-seven years. "I am interested in anything about revolt, disorder, chaos," he once wrote.

When July 1971 began he had been living in France for three months with his longtime girlfriend Pamela Courson. The group's latest album, *L.A. Woman,* was climbing the charts, and the three other members were rehearsing new numbers while awaiting the "Lizard King's" return. But, attempting once again to quit the booze after another heavy drinking bout, Morrison sat, despondent, trying in vain to write verse at the dining table in his Paris apartment on the Rue Beautreillis.

What happened next remained a mystery for many years. Rumors of Morrison's death reached the rock group's young manager Bill Siddons in Los Angeles on Monday 5 July. When he called Pamela he obtained only a tearful, vague response. Arriving next day in Paris, he was confronted with a sealed coffin and a death certificate that cited a fatal heart attack, complicated by a respiratory infection. Though the dead man's parents survived him, Pamela told the U.S. embassy he had no living relatives. He was buried quietly in Père Lachaise cemetery in the presence of Pamela, Siddons, and three friends. Two days later Siddons reported what Pamela had told him: Morrison, some time after midnight on Saturday, 3 July 1971, regurgitated a little blood, but, claiming to feel "okay," took a bath. Pamela reawoke at 5:00 A.M. to find him dead in the tub, his arms resting on the sides, his head back, a boyish smile on his face.

This account was received with much skepticism, but Pamela would break down or become evasive if questioned during her remaining three years.

In their 1991 biography of Morrison, *Break on Through*, James Riordan and Jerry Prochnicky claim three sources for a revised account, all based on Pamela's admission to friends. On the night of 2–3 July 1971, Morrison raided her own stock of heroin and overdosed, accidentally or deliberately, presumably by snorting it. When she later found him dead in the tub, at first she could not face the truth, but at last called a friend and a cover-up was planned. A physician, finding nothing unusual in the body's appearance, except for dried blood around the nostrils, was willing to certify a heart attack, and the medical examiner later went along with this in routine fashion.

Pamela Courson was found dead of a drug overdose in her Hollywood apartment on 25 April 1974; like Morrison she was twenty-seven years old.

Mountbatten, Lord Louis (1900-1979)

The British admiral is best remembered as the last Viceroy of India, who by sheer force of personality almost single-handedly organized the independence of the subcontinent in 1947. Earl Mountbatten of Burma was at once the confidant of the royal family and an unswerving champion of nationalist sentiment and democracy throughout the world. A vain man but an approachable, generous one, he grew old gracefully, with few health problems other than a tendency to vertigo.

His wife Lady Edwina died suddenly of a heart attack in Borneo in 1960 while touring on behalf of the St. John's Ambulance; she was buried at sea off Portsmouth.

For many years Lord Louis and his family had taken an August vacation on the west coast of Ireland at Classiebawn Castle in County Sligo. Around 11:30 A.M. on 27 August 1979 he drove down from the castle to Mullagh-more harbor with five relatives and put out to sea in his twenty-nine-foot motor cruiser, *Shadow V*. He was at the wheel; his elder daughter Patricia sat on the port side; her husband, Lord Brabourne, sat in a swivel chair; their fourteen-year-old twin sons, Timothy and Nicholas Knatchbull, stood in the middle of the boat with a fifteen-year-old local lad, Paul Maxwell, who had come to help; Brabourne's mother, the Dowager Lady Brabourne, sat on the starboard side. A plastic tube containing five pounds of gelignite had been secreted below the decking the night before.

After leaving the harbor and turning to port, the boat slowed and Brabourne leaned over to inspect a lobster pot. It was 11:45 A.M. and someone in a car on the coast road set off the bomb by remote control. Mountbatten was hurled into the air and, stunned, landed facedown in the water; most of his clothes were blown off and he was peppered all over by wood splinters. Only his left leg was severely injured, but he drowned before he could be rescued. Nicholas was killed, his twin severely injured. Paul Maxwell was killed too; the elder Lady Brabourne died next day. The Brabourne couple's legs were broken and they had other injuries. The Provisional Irish Republican Army, whose aim is to expel the British from Northern Ireland, claimed responsibility.

Mountbatten had been much preoccupied for years with detailed plans for his funeral: the order of service, who should be invited to attend, and whether the coffin ought to be lead-lined. At dinner the night before his death he had said, "I can't think of a more wonderful thanksgiving for the life I have had than that everyone should be jolly at my funeral." He was buried, with all the pomp he could have wished, close to his home in Romsey Abbey, a few miles north of Southampton, after a service attended by Queen Elizabeth (his niece by marriage) and dignitaries from around the world.

An IRA terrorist, thirty-one-year-old Thomas McMahon, had driven across the Irish Republic from his home late on 26 August and, changing cars on the way, arrived in Mullaghmore in a yellow Ford Cortina. After planting the bomb he was picked up with a companion in a red Ford Escort in a routine road check many miles away and held on suspicion of being an IRA member. When news of the assassination reached the authorities two hours later, the two men were closely questioned. Traces of green paint from *Shadow V* were found on McMahon's clothes and in the Cortina; nitroglycerin and ammonium nitrate were also detected on his garments. He was sentenced to life imprisonment in Dublin in November 1979; his companion was acquitted. The person who touched off the explosion was never found.

Mudd, Samuel (1833-1883)

The U.S. doctor who on 15 April 1865 set the broken leg of Lincoln's assassin John Wilkes Booth during his flight was arrested at his home, Rock Hill Farm, four miles north of Bryantown, Maryland, on 24 April. He was found guilty by a nine-man commission of conspiring to kill the president, Vice President Andrew Johnson, Secretary of State W. H. Seward, and General U. S. Grant; he escaped the hangman's noose by a single vote. Though he is widely believed in recent days to have been innocent of actual complicity in the plot, there is evidence that he and Booth met two or three times in late 1864 and that the future assassin had stayed at the doctor's house overnight. It is therefore doubtful that Booth's false whiskers would have prevented recognition.

Serving a long sentence in the dreaded prison on Garden Key, an island in the Dry Tortugas group sixty-eight miles off Key West, Florida, Mudd took over the prison doctor's duties after his death from yellow fever in

August 1867. The bold measures he called for were effective in keeping deaths from the epidemic to only forty out of three hundred cases. President Andrew Johnson granted him a full and unconditional pardon in February 1869. He arrived home "frail, weak and sick, never to be strong again."

On New Year's Day 1883 he was observed out visiting his patients in heavy rain without an overcoat. He fell sick of a fever and died on 10 January, probably of pleurisy. His tombstone in the family plot at St. Mary's, Bryantown, bears only his name and date of death.

Responding to the pleas of the Mudd family, President Carter in July 1979 sent a telegram to Samuel's grandson, Richard Mudd, expressing his confidence that Andrew Johnson's pardon was fully justified. In an accompanying letter, Carter explained that even a president cannot set aside a conviction. Richard, who had spent fifty years, logged six hundred thousand miles and spent $100,000 in his quest to clear the family name, expressed himself satisfied at last. In 1991 he was promised final disposition of the case by the Army Board of Correction of Military Records.

Murrow, Edward R. (1908-1965)

The pioneering radio and television journalist made history with his wartime broadcasts during the London Blitz and with his taking on of the demagogic Senator Joseph McCarthy in a 1954 telecast. In 1961 he left the CBS network to join the Kennedy administration as head of the U.S. Information Agency. Even then he was not well, taking sleeping tablets at night and "uppers" in the morning. Always a heavy smoker, and with his gaunt frame steadily losing weight, his friends grew worried. When one of them begged him to quit he replied, "By the time I get cancer, they'll have a cure for it." In the fall of 1962 he collapsed in Teheran during a trip and spent a week in an army hospital. Back in Washington at the Bethesda Naval Hospital, a spot was found on his left lung, but it was dismissed as an old scar from the time when, as a student at Washington State College, he had been caught in a forest fire. At a critical time for the USIA during the thirteen-day Cuban Missile Crisis, Murrow was out of it, flat on his back. A year later, during surgery for a suspected blockage of a bronchial tube, cancer of the left lung was discovered. The lung was removed and Murrow, at last, but with difficulty, quit smoking. At the end of 1963 he resigned, pleading ill health.

That winter, Ed and Janet Murrow were welcomed to Southern California by Dr. Jonas Salk, who found them a house overlooking the ocean near the Salk Institute in La Jolla. In his four months there he caught pneumonia and, though he recovered, the old spark was gone. In the fall of 1964, Salk was visiting Murrow at his upstate New York home, Quaker Hill near Pawling, when his host twice lost the drift of his remarks. After a neurological examination, a brain tumor was removed at New York Hospital on 8 November.

Back in the hospital a few months later with a recurrence of brain cancer, Murrow asked for an old CBS Radio colleague, Bob Dixon, to visit him. "He grabbed me by the arm with both hands with incredible strength," said Dixon later. "His eyes were ablaze." Murrow made him promise to get him out of there, "that you'll carry me out on your back if you have to."

Up on Quaker Hill, at the Murrows' Glen Arden farmhouse early in April 1965, Ed Murrow lay dying, heavily sedated, in a gentle haze. His country gave him its highest civilian award, the Medal of Honor. Queen Elizabeth created him Sir Edward; but then England was where "this reporter left all of his youth and much of his heart."

He was unconscious when, with Janet by his side, he died on 27 April 1965, two days after his fifty-seventh birthday; his ashes were scattered in the glen at Glen Arden farm. Speaking of him, fellow TV journalist Harry Reasoner said, "You get a tradition established and you have made it difficult for small people to corrupt it." Marvin Kalb said, "Murrow was a meteor in a fairly empty sky." *See* Joseph E. Persico (1988).

Nabokov, Vladimir (1899-1977)

The Soviet-born writer settled in the United States in 1940 and became an American citizen five years later; he was professor of Russian literature at Cornell University from 1948 to 1959. His most widely known English-language novel, the controversial *Lolita* (1955), portrays the love of the middle-aged lecher Humbert Humbert for a precocious twelve-year-old "nymphet," a term coined by the author. The admitted beauty and technical brilliance of the prose, contrasted with the near-pornography of the subject matter, led to a sharp division of critical opinion.

Nabokov's earnings from *Lolita* allowed him to retire to Switzerland in 1959 with his wife Véra. There he continued to write novels, including *Pale Fire* (1962) and *Ada* (1969). He was a serious lepidopterist, and it was while collecting butterflies on a slope high in the mountains at Davos in June

1975 that he slipped and fell, waiting over two hours for rescuers to reach him.

After surgery for a benign tumor of the prostate in October 1975 Nabokov's health began to decline. His last completed book, published in the spring of 1976, was *Details of a Sunset and Other Stories,* a collection of tales written up to a half-century before. An obscure infection in June 1976 led to his admission, semiconscious, to a private hospital in Lausanne; from there he was transferred to the Nestlé Hospital. A urinary infection was diagnosed and he suffered weeks of high fever.

He did not return to his home until September; since 1961 the Nabokovs had lived in a suite on the sixth floor of the Palace Hotel in Montreux. He was able in the new year to walk with a cane a short distance up the main street. In mid-March his son Dmitri drove to Geneva to hear a friend sing in *The Marriage of Figaro;* he caught a chill that led to influenza. Back in Montreux his mother caught the bug, and then his father. Bronchial pneumonia followed and Vladimir was back in the Nestlé Hospital for seven weeks. After his return to Montreux in May he was shrunken and stooping. His mind was full of *The Original of Laura,* which he had begun three years earlier but which would never be completed. Writing on index cards, he scratched passages for it in his shaky handwriting whenever he could summon the strength, but by now his concentration was diminishing. The once-famous wordsmith could no longer defeat his sister Elena at the Russian version of Scrabble.

Nabokov was taken back to the Nestlé Hospital on 7 June 1977 with a pseudomonas infection. Dmitri was concerned by the doctors' increasingly negative reports; their "manner was changing from bedside to graveside," he said later. His father was resigned. A particular favorite butterfly, he knew, would by now be on the wing; knowing he would never see it again brought tears to his eyes. A chance draft and a sneezing hospital worker, Dmitri believes, hastened his father's final collapse. His temperature rose higher; much fluid was drained from his chest. He was moved to the intensive-care unit on 30 June; at 6:50 P.M. on 2 July 1977 he died with Véra and Dmitri at his side. The cause of his frequent fevers was never satisfactorily determined.

Nabokov's body was cremated and his ashes were interred in Clarens Cemetery, just half a mile from his hotel home in Montreux, Switzerland. A broad unornamented marble slab marks the grave; it bears the inscription: VLADIMIR NABOKOV ÉCRIVAIN 1899–1977. Three weeks after his death several hundred New Yorkers gathered in the auditorium at his publisher's, the McGraw-Hill Company, to pay him homage. Speakers at the memorial service included Dmitri Nabokov and John Updike, one of the few American writers for whom Vladimir had ever had a kind word.

The Russian master's works, long banned in the Soviet Union, were rehabilitated in 1986. On Véra's death in April 1991 her ashes were placed with her husband's. *See* Brian Boyd (1991).

Newton, Isaac (1642-1727)

The great English mathematician and physicist was a mysterious, complex man. On the one hand he was a giant in the advancement of true science, including mathematics (the binomial theorem and "fluxions," i.e. calculus), optics (the separation of white light into its component colors and the construction of the first reflecting telescopes), and cosmology (the universal law of gravitation); on the other he spent at least an equal amount of time and energy on alchemical experiments and biblical speculation. His religious beliefs are the greatest mystery of all; J. M. Keynes has concluded that he was "a Judaic monotheist of the school of Maimonides."

Newton's health, especially his breakdown of 1692–93, has been the subject of much speculation. In September 1693 he wrote two significant letters; to Samuel Pepys: "I am extremely troubled by the embroilment I am in, and have neither ate nor slept well this twelvemonth . . . I must withdraw from your acquaintance, and see neither you nor the rest of my friends any more . . ."; to the philosopher John Locke: "Being of opinion that you endeavoured to embroil me with women [I said to you] 'twere better you were dead.' I desire you to forgive this uncharitableness." He had a year and a half earlier made charges of betrayal against other friends. A longtime acquaintance once described him as "the most fearful, cautious and suspicious nature I ever knew."

In a 1979 medical study, P. E. Spargo and C. A. Pounds conclude that Newton's breakdown was due to mercury poisoning from his alchemical experiments. They found high concentrations of heavy metals in preserved locks of his hair; in particular, they measured 197 parts per million of mercury, against a normal mean of 5.1. However, the authenticity of the hair has been questioned.

Julian Lieb and Dorothy Hershman in a 1983 study point to Newton's lifelong pattern of manic-depressive illness and argue that "Mercury poisoning would not have induced anorexia [loss of appetite] and insomnia without also causing severe gastrointestinal symptoms, gingivitis, chronic fatigue, and neurological deficits. None of these were in evidence during the [1692–93] crisis. Furthermore, his rapid recovery is not characteristic of mercury poisoning. For 2 weeks during the crisis, Newton slept a total of only 9 hours. Such severe insomnia [could] be produced only by an affective [emotional or mental] disorder . . . Anorexia and insomnia, symptoms of both depression and mania, plagued Newton throughout his life, and there is compelling evidence that he suffered from severe fluctuations of mood and behaviour."

Lieb and Hershman detect a biennial manic cycle. As an example, they cite Newton's first recorded "breakdown" in 1664 as being followed by two years of "hypomania" in which he achieved his highest level of creativity.

The story of Newton's enmities, his quarrels, and his tantrums is softened by knowledge of his great generosity toward unfortunates.

Though he showed a decline in creativity in his eighties, his mind lost little of its sharpness, as evidenced by one of his last thoughts: "I do not know what I may appear to the world; but to myself I seem to have been only like a boy playing on the sea shore, and diverting myself in now and then finding a smoother pebble or a prettier shell than ordinary, whilst the great ocean of truth lay all undiscovered before me."

After being stricken with a cough and inflammation of the lungs in January 1725, Newton moved to a house in Kensington, a few miles west of the City, where the air was cleaner. The strain of attending the 2 March 1727 meeting of the Royal Society, of which he was president, brought back his violent cough. His physicians found him also suffering from stone in the bladder and offered no hope of recovery. We are indebted to John Conduitt, husband of the daughter of Newton's half-sister, for the final scenes. He writes that the stone was probably jolted to a less comfortable position during the final visit to London and that "though the drops of sweat ran down from his face with anguish, he never complained, or cried out, or showed the least sign of peevishness or impatience." On 18 March he read the newspapers and "held a pretty long discussion with Dr. Mead [one of his physicians] and had all his senses perfect; but that evening at six, and all day Sunday [the 19th] he was insensible, and died on Monday the 20th of March [1727] between one and two in the morning."

He steadfastly refused to receive the last sacraments of the church, a fact that those present found scandalous and kept secret. He lay in state in Westminster Abbey on the twenty-eighth and with due pomp was interred in the nave. An enormous monument was erected in the Abbey in 1731.

Niven, David (1910-1983)

In ninety movies Niven usually played the debonair, light-hearted English-man; off-screen, he was much the same, kind and charming. He won an Oscar in Terence Rattigan's *Separate Tables* (1958) as an army officer with a shameful secret living in a seaside hotel; after *The Guns of Navarone* (1961) he was offered only a string of mediocre roles. Luckily, he had a flair for storytelling, and his two books of Hollywood memoirs, *The Moon's a Balloon* and *Bring on the Empty Horses,* were runaway best-sellers, earning him close to $5 million.

The first signs of the disease that was to kill him appeared gradually. As he turned seventy he was filming *The Sea Wolves* (1980) in Goa on the Indian coast with Gregory Peck and Roger Moore when he complained of aching arm and leg muscles and his voice tended to slur. "He began to take long fast walks every day," recalled Peck; "he had begun his valiant fight . . . and it was to last three years. Never has a man fought a losing battle with such courage and such an outrageous sense of humor . . . " After one long walk Niven said to Moore, "You know, it's a funny thing but I can't get my bloody heel off the ground properly."

After completing *Better Late Than Never* (1981), in which his defective delivery was a serious problem, the actor embarked on a promotional tour for his novel *Go Slowly, Come Back Quickly.* The tour began with a 3 October 1981 appearance on BBC TV's *Michael Parkinson Show;* many viewers, shocked, called in. Was he ill? Could he possibly be drunk? In America he checked in to the Mayo Clinic, then called his son James in New York with the verdict: "The good news is that I didn't have a stroke. The bad news is that I've got amyotrophic lateral sclerosis. I am going to lose my voice, my ability to communicate, the use of my hands and legs, and then I'm going to die. Maybe in weeks, maybe in months, maybe in years."

The actor managed to appear in *The Trial of the Pink Panther* (1982) and *The Curse of the Pink Panther* (1983), both filmed near his Cap Ferrat home on the French Riviera in the summer of 1982. When news leaked out that his voice had been dubbed by the mimic Rich Little, the truth that Niven had Lou Gehrig's disease could no longer be withheld from the public.

Leaving his second wife, the Swedish model Hjördis Tersmeden, at Cap Ferrat ("he wanted me to stay and have a rest from him for a while") he returned to his beloved chalet in the Swiss ski resort of Château d'Oex, ten miles east of Montreux, in mid-July 1983. With him, to help with his wasted "Gandhi body," went Kathleen Matthewson, an Irish nurse whose services had been engaged nine months earlier. He had lost forty pounds, but could still enjoy a daily session in a neighbor's indoor pool.

During the last two nights of his life, he reminisced with Kathleen about his happy six-year marriage to "Primmie" (Primula Rollo), tragically cut short in 1946 when, aged just twenty-eight, she tumbled down the basement stairs at Tyrone Power's home and fractured her skull.

Around 7:00 A.M. on Friday, 29 July 1983, Kathleen looked in on him and he gave her a thumbs-up sign. "So I went downstairs to make myself some coffee, and just as I got to the bottom of the stairs I heard a sort of noise, as though he'd been trying to get out of bed, and when I got back into his room he had the oxygen mask off and gave me a big smile and held my hand and away he went. As quickly as that."

At the funeral in the Anglican church in Château d'Oex, Yehudi Menuhin and seven pupils from his school at Gstaad played Mendelssohn's *Octet*. (Mendelssohn was chosen, explained Menuhin, because of that composer's love of Niven's native Scotland. The actor, actually born in London, always fostered the erroneous belief that his birthplace was Kirriemuir.) Niven was buried in the churchyard. Among the mourners were Prince Rainier of Monaco, Audrey Hepburn, and William F. Buckley Jr. A memorial service in Hollywood was led by Gregory Peck and Peter Ustinov, another in London by Lawrence Olivier and John Mortimer. *See* Sheridan Morley (1985).

O'Casey, Sean (1880-1964)

The Irish playwright was a natural rebel, a Protestant in a predominantly Catholic land, whose hot temper drove him in 1926 to a self-imposed exile in England. Poverty and malnutrition in childhood left him with badly ulcerated eyes which, throughout his life, required constant bathing with scalding hot water. He became totally blind in his last years, which were spent with his young wife Eileen in a third-floor apartment at 40 Trumlands Road, St. Marychurch, just outside Torquay in Devon. In 1956 O'Casey was hospitalized for over three months with severe bronchitis, which followed surgery for a kidney stone. Always a slender man, he was now gaunt and never without pain or discomfort. A few months later their younger son, twenty-year-old Niall, developed leukemia and died after a short illness. O'Casey was inconsolable; his constant keening and her own grief so unhinged Eileen's mind that she attempted suicide by swallowing sleeping pills.

On 30 March 1960 telegrams, messages, and flowers were sent from all over the world to mark the playwright's eightieth birthday. His last book, *Under a Colored Cap* (1963), is a collection of essays.

In late 1964 O'Casey was back again in Torbay Clinic, a private nursing home in Saint Luke's Road South, Torquay, with acute bronchitis. When his wife visited him he was in low spirits: "Eileen, I don't appear to see so well. The water is not really hot enough to relieve my eyes. These damn trays! I don't know what is what. I spill things. This morning I knocked over my cup of tea . . . the nurse had to come in and change my top sheet. I feel just terrible." Eileen consoled him and had a word with the nurse. After he returned home in August he was continually tired and exasperated at not being able to read, except for an occasional word if he held the book slantwise near his right eye.

On the morning of 17 September 1964 his nose began to bleed profusely; Eileen drove him to Dr. Hugh Doran's surgery and the bleeding stopped. During the morning the old man, who may have realized death was near, reminisced about their penniless but happy life together. Maybe, he thought, he should not have won her away from her lover, the American producer Lee Ephraim, in whose *Rose Marie* chorus line she was performing when she met O'Casey. "You should have stayed with him for the security," he said. At 2:00 A.M. on the eighteenth he suffered a coronary thrombosis and severe pains in his side and chest. Doran's partner Dr. Haskins gave him an injection and called an ambulance. Eileen held her husband's hand on the way to Torbay Clinic and she noticed that his usual firm grip suddenly lessened before they arrived. After Sean had been taken to a room, Eileen said to the doctor, "I do hope you can save him from any more of that agonizing pain." "He will have no more pain," she was told. "He is dead."

After a short Anglican service at the Torquay crematorium, O'Casey's body was cremated. Like Niall's, Sean's ashes were scattered to the wind outside the Golders Green crematorium in London, between the Shelley and Tennyson rose beds. *See* Garry O'Connor (1988).

Offenbach, Jacques (1819-1880)

By the age of fifty, the German-born French composer had at least four of his operettas, including *Orpheus in the Underworld,* running concurrently in Paris theaters. His only grand opera, *The Tales of Hoffmann,* was left unfinished at his death.

As he worked on the opera through the summer of 1880 in a stuffy, overheated hotel room at Saint Germain, his health worsened. He had long been afflicted by gout, a disorder of purine metabolism in which excessive amounts of urate circulate in the blood and may precipitate in joints, causing a painful and destructive form of arthritis. In September, anxious about his living expenses, he moved back to Paris with his wife Herminie. He ate little now but comforted himself with huge cigars as he worked frantically near his piano and a blazing wood fire, his shrunken frame wrapped in a fur-embroidered robe. The sounds of the piano could be heard to break off frequently as the composer was overcome by a racking cough. Occasionally, when quite exhausted, he would relax over a well-thumbed Mozart biography. "Poor Mozart," he was heard to murmur.

On 25 September, with his body stiff with gout, he was unable to get out of bed. Herminie pleaded with him to take nourishment, but no, he would take only a little brandy as he scribbled frantically on the music papers scattered on the counterpane. "Our grandchildren will be rich," he murmured, thinking of the assured success of *Hoffmann.*

On 4 October 1880, Offenbach clutched at his chest. "I'm not well; it's here," he moaned. "I think the end will come tonight." The children were summoned and a Catholic priest administered the last rites (the composer had abandoned Judaism at the time of his 1844 marriage). A little after 3:00 A.M. on the fifth, Offenbach touched his head, then his heart, sighed deeply and ceased to breathe. After she had stopped weeping over his body, Herminie cut off a lock of hair to be sealed up in her ring.

A comedian who played in *Orpheus* called later that morning. "Monsieur Offenbach is dead," the concierge told him. "He died very gently, without realizing it." "Ah, how annoyed he'll be when he finds out," replied the caller.

There was a lavish funeral service at which excerpts from *Hoffmann* were played; Offenbach was buried in Montmartre Cemetery. The unfinished opera, orchestrated by New Orleans–born Ernest Guiraud, opened with great success at the Opéra-Comique on 10 February 1881. *See* James Harding (1980).

O'Keeffe, Georgia (1887-1986)

The century's most important American woman artist was stern, high-principled, and determined. She stood almost alone in the history of pictorial art; her paintings belong to no particular school and she was without any evident group of followers. Using thin paint and clear colors, her works evoke a mood of mystical silence.

Her chief relationships were with men widely separated from her in age. Her twenty-eight-year marriage with U.S. photographic artist Alfred Stieglitz (1864–1946) was that of a faithful, if often difficult, woman with a much older, supportive, and caring—but unfaithful—man. When his long-drawn-out affair with the young, wealthy Dorothy Norman grew unbearable to O'Keeffe in 1929 she began spending her summers away from him in New Mexico, where she had discovered the colors and shapes that entranced her. She was even reluctant to hurry to his side in New York when he collapsed in July 1946, though she did arrive in time to be with him, along with Dorothy, when he died a few days later.

O'Keeffe soon moved permanently to her adopted state and settled at remote Ghost Ranch, twelve miles north of Abiquiu, to live in a small one-story adobe house. As she aged, she retained her striking, erect appearance, her weather-beaten skin drawn taut over high cheekbones. By 1973, aged eighty-six, she was still proud and independent; though her eyesight was seriously diminished, she refused to acknowledge the fact. When a twenty-six-year-old drifter, Juan Hamilton, came by, asking for odd jobs, she took him on and in time he graduated to companion, chauffeur, and secretary. When he moved into the house the cook-housekeeper quit. "Miss O'Keeffe," said Jerrie Newsom, "I'm not going to look after your help."

The O'Keeffe-Hamilton relationship was undoubtedly one of great tenderness, even love, on both sides, though the six-decade gap in age, as well as the artist's lifelong antipathy to irregular unions, makes any sexual bond almost impossible to believe. (Indeed, in 1980 Hamilton married a young woman, Anna Marie Erskine.) His role in O'Keeffe's life made the headlines when Doris Bry, who had worked for Georgia for thirty years and claimed to be her sole agent, sued her for breach of contract and Juan for "malicious interference" after two paintings were sold in 1977 without her (Bry's) knowledge. Friends took sides during the dispute and O'Keeffe lost some of them; but many others found Hamilton to be personally charming and an essential element in the nonagenarian's life. He was given wide powers of attorney over her affairs in 1978 and the following year, after bequeathing all her paintings to museums and various charities, she made him her executor and residuary legatee.

O'Keeffe suffered a heart attack at the age of ninety-six while on a visit to Florida and she moved with the Hamiltons to a large house in Santa Fe. By then she was almost totally blind and deaf and needed continuous nursing care. Friends could still visit her, but relatives were told, mysteriously, that this was inappropriate. In August 1984 a codicil to the 1979 will transferred ownership of tens of millions of dollars worth of artworks and property to Juan Hamilton; her signature on the document wandered erratically across the page. Georgia spent most of her waking hours during the final year and a half sitting in her spacious, airy room almost silent, quite withdrawn.

Hamilton was vacationing in Mexico with his wife and their two sons when the housekeeper called to tell him O'Keeffe was sinking fast. "Call me again if things get worse," he responded, and hung up. She died that night, 6 March 1986 in St. Vincent's Hospital, Santa Fe, New Mexico. There was no funeral service; her ashes were scattered, probably near her beloved Ghost Ranch.

Probate was opposed by her relatives. A retired FBI agent was engaged to investigate, and evidence was forthcoming that, in signing the 1984 codicil, the confused, blind woman believed she was actually marrying Hamilton. In an out-of-court agreement he settled for something close to the original will; he received twenty-four paintings, the Ghost Ranch house, certain copyrights, and Georgia's letters to him. *See* Roxana Robinson (1989).

Olivier, Laurence (1907-1989)

The British actor-director became Lord Olivier in 1970, but remained "Larry" to his friends. Over Vivien Leigh, his second wife and "the love of my life," he never ceased to agonize, blaming himself for her mental instability: "it has always been impossible for me not to believe that I was somehow the cause of Vivien's disturbances."

Between 1981 and 1983, increasingly frail and dependent more and more on cuing devices to aid his failing memory, Olivier earned almost $5 million from films, television appearances, and interviews. Though most of the money went to taxes, he was able to buy a larger London home on Mulberry Walk in Chelsea, where Lady Olivier (his third wife Joan Plowright) and their children lived. (There was an unofficial separation between the couple during his final decade.) At his south-coast home near Brighton, Olivier could swim year-round in his heated pool. The house, an improved and extended malthouse, was hidden at the end of an unpaved road in the Sussex village of Steyning.

His last speaking performance was in J. B. Priestley's *Lost Empires* on Granada TV. During the taping of his small role, he fell from the stage and injured his arm, not the first accident of this kind, for dizzy spells were now frequent. He was honored on his eightieth birthday by a gala at the National Theatre, of which he had been the first director from 1963 to 1973. He appeared publicly one last time for a single day's shooting in October 1988 as a silent, wheelchair-bound old soldier outside a hospital in *War Requiem*, a series of images set to the music of Benjamin Britten's *Mass*; Olivier's voice is heard reciting Wilfred Owen's poem "Strange Meeting."

Through much of his life the actor had been plagued by illness: prostate cancer, pleurisy, appendicitis, thrombosis, and dermatomyositis (a rare muscle-wasting disease that forced his retirement from the stage in 1974). In his final year he underwent a kidney operation. During the night of 18 March 1989 he fell and shattered his hip, but recovered quickly after surgery. In June he could still enjoy being driven to the home of his old friend and agent Lawrence Evans for an afternoon of reminiscence.

By 1 July there had been a marked decline in Olivier's health and strength, and he was confined to bed. His wife, making a movie in the United States, prepared to fly home. A deathwatch began as the old actor lapsed into spells of unconsciousness, as his children and the Evanses gathered around. It was a scene powerfully evocative of Lord Marchmain's death in Evelyn Waugh's *Brideshead Revisited,* a twelve-hour TV production in 1981. In the fictional case the apostate Catholic peer, played by Olivier, returns home to die at his Yorkshire castle, making at the very last moment a sign indicating his return to the faith. In real life an Anglican priest was called to the Malthouse early on 11 July 1989. There were prayers to the accompaniment of the dying man's labored breathing. At midday a whisper, then silence.

That night, flags at the National Theatre in London flew at half-staff;

in the West End, theaters dimmed their lights. Lord Olivier's ashes were destined for burial in Westminster Abbey's Poets' Corner. Only two actors had been memorialized there before him, David Garrick and Henry Irving. the bulk of Olivier's $2 million estate was left to Joan and the children, with thoughtful mementos given to actor friends. *See* Donald Spoto (1992).

Oppenheimer, J. Robert (1904-1967)

The U.S. physicist, known to many as "the Father of the A-Bomb," directed the team of American and European scientists at Los Alamos, New Mexico, during World War II who built the first atomic bombs.

In debates over the development of a hydrogen bomb ("superbomb"), the reluctant Oppenheimer found himself at odds with many in the U.S. Atomic Energy Commission. In 1954, after four tense weeks of hearings, his government security clearance was withdrawn by a vote of two to one. He had been an open supporter of Communist causes long before the war and there were rumors of his possible disloyalty. In particular he had been inexplicably tardy in reporting advances made indirectly to him by the Soviets. The sole scientist on the investigating committee gave Oppenheimer an approving vote, pointing out that most of the current evidence had been in the AEC's hands when the physicist's services were approved seven years previously.

Though Oppenheimer's work as an AEC consultant was now terminated, he continued as director of the Institute for Advanced Study in Princeton, New Jersey. But the hearings and negative publicity had noticeably aged him and he never quite recovered his former health. There were reports of heavy drinking by Robert and Kitty Oppenheimer at their Princeton home, dubbed "Bourbon Manor."

With an incoming, more liberal, administration in Washington in 1961 the clouds of suspicion and recrimination were markedly reduced. In 1963 Oppenheimer won the annual Fermi Award; on 22 November President Kennedy announced it would be his privilege to present the prize personally, but hours later he was assassinated. It fell to President Lyndon Johnson to hand the medal and a check for $50,000 to the physicist in the Cabinet Room at the White House on 2 December 1963. The recipient, after a pregnant pause, responded, "I think it just possible, Mr. President, that it has taken some charity and some courage for you to make this award today."

After this turn in his fortunes Oppenheimer had the air of someone returned from exile—more relaxed, kinder, with a saving touch of self-deprecating humor. At a sentimental homecoming to the Los Alamos laboratory in 1964 he was met with much applause from the scientists there. Another warm reception greeted him later at the University of California, Berkeley, where he had taught physics in the 1930s. Students recalled him at the blackboard in those days with a chalk in one hand and an eternal cigarette in the other; one of them said that she often thought he would at any moment smoke the chalk and scribble with the cigarette.

Oppenheimer gave up the Princeton directorship in 1965 after a bout with pneumonia. The following year, throat cancer was diagnosed and at last he quit smoking. By June 1966 he needed a cane and a leg brace. In October he wrote to a friend, "My cancer is spreading rapidly; thus I am being radiated further, this time with electrons from a betatron." A month later, "I am much less able to speak and eat now." Finally, a few days before the end, "I am in some pain . . . my hearing and speech are very poor."

J. Robert Oppenheimer died at his Princeton home on 18 February 1967. At his funeral old colleagues delivered glowing tributes to the man and his achievements and the Juilliard String Quartet played Beethoven. Oppenheimer's ashes were flown to the Virgin Islands, a favorite vacation spot, and scattered over the ocean. *See* Peter Goodchild (1980).

Owens, Jesse (1913-1980)

The black U.S. athlete made history at the 1936 Olympic Games by winning four gold medals and making a major dent in Nazi claims of Aryan athletic superiority. (He tied the world record for the 100-meter dash, set new Olympic records in the long jump and 200-meter sprint and contributed to a new world record in the 400-meter relay.)

But he was barely literate when he flunked out of Ohio State University, and thereafter his life was a roller coaster of successes and failures. He was twice in trouble with the federal tax authorities and in 1966 narrowly escaped a prison sentence. The judge, a fellow Alabaman, imposed a small fine instead, praising Owen's well-known support for "our country and our way of life." This was an evident reference to the veteran athlete's opposition to the tactics of Martin Luther King Jr. (though he admired his principles), and even to the Kennedy-Johnson social-welfare programs, the benefits from which he regarded as "getting something for nothing." He was especially indignant at the black-gloved, clenched-fist salutes of black-activist medal winners at the Mexico City Olympics; they were pro-Negro bigots, he said. He stumped for Landon against FDR in 1936 and for Nixon against Kennedy in 1960. Through the 1970s he was in demand as an Olympic statesman, campaigning for funds to train and equip athletes on behalf of the U.S. Olympic Committee. Early in the decade he and his wife Ruth left Chicago to settle in Scottsdale, Arizona.

After a fund-raising meeting in Dallas in early November 1979 he complained of fatigue; within a week he cut short, for the same reason, the taping of an American Express commercial he was making on a New York City street. In early December he began to cough uncontrollably before a religious audience in Dayton, Ohio; next night he felt faint at the podium in St. Louis. Examined at the Michael Reese Hospital in Chicago, he was told he had adenocarcinoma of the lung, evidently the result of many years of heavy cigarette smoking. Surgery and radiation were ruled out; he had perhaps three months to live.

Back in Arizona early in 1980 more medical checks were made. His interest in the forthcoming Moscow Olympics was undiminished. At first he supported the Carter administration's boycott of the games to protest the USSR's invasion of Afghanistan, but later swung his support behind U.S. athletes, who had trained long and hard to go to Moscow. They should go as individuals, not as Americans, he wrote.

His condition turned suddenly worse on 21 March, and he was flown by helicopter to the University of Arizona Hospital in Tucson. Newly introduced drugs were tried, but to no avail. Owens slipped into a coma late on 29 March and died in the early hours of 31 March 1980.

Flags flew at half-staff across Arizona two days later while the body lay in state at the capitol in Phoenix. At the funeral service in the University of Chicago's Rockefeller Chapel, the coffin was draped with a white silk flag bearing the five-ringed Olympic emblem. Present were the U.S. Olympic Committee president, Robert Kane, and several old comrades from the 1936 games.

Burial was in the Oak Woods Cemetery, Chicago. Owens is honored by a four-foot granite monument at his birthplace, tiny Oakville, Alabama, and by a track, plaza, and sculpture at Ohio State in Columbus, Ohio. *See* William J. Baker (1986).

Palme, Olof (1927-1986)

Sweden's prime minister (1969–76, 1982–86) was educated at Kenyon College in Ohio; it was the poverty he saw while hitchhiking around the United States that, he said, was to turn him into a champion of socialism in his own country and a noted opponent of U.S. policy in Vietnam.

He was shot and fatally wounded in Stockholm by an unknown assailant on 28 February 1986 after attending a movie, *The Mozart Brothers,* at the Grand Cinema. He and his wife Lisbet had met their son Mårten and his girlfriend by arrangement at the cinema on Stockholm's main street, Sveavägen, after traveling by train from their apartment in the old part of the city. The party split up after the performance and the prime minister and Mrs. Palme crossed the street and walked toward the city center. It was 11:21 P.M. At the corner of Sveavägen and Tunnelgatan, with Palme lagging a few feet behind, a man in a dark coat with his cap pulled well down approached him from behind and shot him with a Smith & Wesson .357 Magnum revolver. The copper-tipped bullet entered the body between the shoulder blades, shattering the spine, aorta, and windpipe. Lisbet turned at the sound of the shot and the assassin fired again, grazing her back, before jogging away at an easy pace along Tunnelgatan. A taxi driver called the police by radio; an ambulance arrived at 11:35 and took the injured couple to Sabbatsberg Hospital, where Olof Palme was declared dead at 12:06 A.M. on 1 March 1986.

His largely secular funeral in the capital's Town Hall was attended by seventeen hundred official mourners, including fifteen heads of state, seventeen prime ministers, and nineteen foreign ministers. President Reagan was represented by Secretary of State George Shultz. Palme's old friend Willy Brandt, former West German chancellor, read an emotional eulogy. In a simple graveside ceremony conducted by the Bishop of Stockholm, Krister Stendahl, the body was buried in Adolf Fredrik's Churchyard, within sight of the murder scene. Lisbet Palme knelt to lay a single red rose on the coffin as it was lowered, and her three sons threw in roses after it.

On the eve of the funeral came the first arrest. Victor Gunnarsson, thirty-three, associated with a right-wing hate group founded by the American Lyndon LaRouche, was identified as the agitated man with garlic on his breath who tried to hire a cab just after the shooting and then hurried into a cinema (not the Grand) in the middle of a film. But the identification failed to hold up and Gunnarsson was released.

Four Kurdish nationalists were arrested in January 1987 but released after questioning.

On 14 December 1988, Christer Petterson, forty-one, a Stockholm drug abuser with a record of violence and a long prison record, was charged with the murder. At his trial in June 1989 eyewitnesses retracted earlier statements, but Lisbet Palme stood by the identification of Petterson she had made in a police lineup and repeated her assurance in a face-to-face confrontation before the judge. The jury verdict was guilty by a majority and Petterson received a life sentence. The conviction was overturned on appeal. In any case, no credible motive was assignable to him and the murder weapon has never been found.

Bishop Stendahl regards the failure to solve the murder as having serious implications for Palme's countrymen. "Swedes . . . have always trusted power and the authorities. They expect things to work. When they don't, as they haven't done in this case, there is a real danger of erosion of the foundations of Swedish life. This is a very frightening time for people here." Stockholm's detective force was so devastated by Petterson's release that some members required psychotherapy. The accused man himself was awarded $50,000 as compensation for his eleven months' imprisonment. *See* Chris Mosey (1991).

Parker, Dorothy (1893-1967)

Described by fellow writer Brendan Gill as one of the wittiest people in the world and one of the saddest, and by herself late in life as "just a little Jewish girl trying to be cute," U.S. poet, critic, and short-story author Dorothy Parker was a leading light at the legendary lunches of the Algonquin Round Table with George S. Kaufman, Alexander Woollcott and others. In the 1920s she shared a tiny office with humorist Robert Benchley. "An inch smaller and it would have been adultery," quipped Dorothy.

Her love life was unhappy; three times she attempted suicide. She was married twice to Alan Campbell, who died at fifty-nine. He had become a nonstop drinker and was also hooked on barbiturates, even swallowing Seconals before his afternoon nap. "He hates to toss and turn from four to six," Dorothy explained. She found him lying dead in bed of a barbiturate overdose, possibly accidental, on the afternoon of 14 June 1963 in their West Hollywood bungalow on Norma Place.

By then Dorothy herself was in poor shape, drinking and smoking heavily. Her usual cough had grown worse; as she walked her five dogs she often stumbled and once fractured her shoulder. She had failed as a teacher at Cal State in L.A., and was often late with her book column for *Esquire* magazine, the last of which appeared in December 1962.

In March 1964 she returned to New York, where she was in and out of the hospital through the rest of the year with bursitis and cardiovascular troubles which, she said, "the doctors were very brave about." She lived in the Volney Hotel at 23 East 74th Street. Persuaded to make a will, she was in no doubt about where her small estate should go: to Martin Luther King Jr. and after his death to the NAACP. She had always been emphatically left-leaning in politics, something that had caused her many difficulties during the McCarthy years. (Asked by FBI agents whether she had ever conspired to overthrow the government, she responded, "Look, I can't even get my dog to stay down. Do I *look* like someone who could overthrow the government?")

Her final magazine article was published in *Esquire*, December 1964. It ended, "As only New Yorkers know, if you can get through the twilight, you can get through the night." By then, the pains in her shoulders made typing difficult; her income was tiny and she depended on friends to pay her hospital bills. In 1965 her health for a while was improved and she was able to pay a nostalgic visit to the Algonquin Hotel for the first time in twenty years. She gave one or two interviews in which her self-deprecatory humor was still evident. She was a relic, she said, from the "long, long days ago" when she was "the toast of two continents—Australia and Greenland." But her world was shrinking; true, there were a half-dozen friends her continuous drinking had not alienated—Lillian Hellman, the S. J. Perelmans, the Zero Mostels—but there were long hours of boredom, alone, sipping Scotch and watching soap operas.

In her last months she was buoyed by plans to launch *A Dorothy Parker Portfolio* on Broadway, based on her writing and with music by Cole Porter, with Julie Harris in the lead. But on 7 June 1967 a chambermaid found her dead of a heart attack in her suite, No. 6F in the Volney Hotel. Lillian Hellman, her literary executor, refused to allow the *Portfolio* to go ahead; as in the case of Dashiell Hammett's works, her executorship was essentially negative. After King's death, Hellman fought for financial rights in the Parker properties, but the courts gave them to the NAACP, as Dorothy had decreed. "She must have been drunk when she did it," snarled Hellman.

Dorothy Parker's body was cremated at Hartsdale, New York, but there was doubt regarding the proper disposition of the ashes. After several weeks they were despatched to Hellman's attorneys, O'Dwyer and Bernstein, on Wall Street. They have been stored in a filing cabinet there for a quarter-century. *See* Marion Meade (1988).

Patton, George S. (1885-1945)

The U.S. general was widely regarded as the best of all commanders on either side in the European Theater in World War II. He was a dyslexic who had battled hard in early life to overcome his reading and writing disabilities, and this overwhelming desire to succeed was carried into his later years. But he was erratic in temperament, subject to wide swings of mood, even in a single day; this caused his superiors, notably Eisenhower as commander in chief in Europe, much concern. In Sicily in 1944 he twice slapped the faces of patients in military hospitals and cursed them for cowardice.

He had little aptitude for his postwar task of overseeing the de-Nazification program in Bavaria, viewing the true anti-Nazis recently liberated from concentration camps—Jews, labor leaders, Communists—with disfavor. In October 1945 Eisenhower moved Patton to Bad Neuheim to help with war records. On 8 December, two days before his planned departure for the United States, he was driving with his chief of staff Hobart Gay in a chauffeured limousine near Mannheim on their way to hunt pheasant. The car collided with an army truck and Patton was hurled forward against the driver's partition. His neck was broken at the third and fourth cervical vertebrae and he had skull injuries. No one else was injured in either vehicle. At Heidelberg, Patton was placed in traction. His wife Beatrice was flown over from the United States in a plane made available by Eisenhower. The patient seemed calm when visitors were present, but grew morose when alone, especially after being told he could never ride a horse again.

He lingered for thirteen days. Mrs. Patton spent the afternoon on 21 December reading to her husband. At 4:00 P.M. he dozed off and ninety minutes later, when his breathing seemed easier, she left to have dinner. A few minutes later she was summoned back to his bedside. He was dead of pulmonary edema and congestive heart failure.

Next day, Patton lay in state in an open coffin in a villa near the hospital. After a Protestant service the body was taken across town on an army half-track and then by rail to Luxembourg. At half a dozen stops Beatrice alighted to inspect a series of honor guards paying respect to the general.

General George S. ("Blood and Guts") Patton was buried in the military cemetery at Hamm in Luxembourg beneath a plain white marker. Three years later his grave was moved to the forefront of the cemetery beside the American flag, where he now lies at the head of his fallen troops.

Beatrice Patton died of an aneurysm while horseback-riding in 1953. Though her ashes were interred at South Hamilton, Massachusetts, near the family home, it is said that some of them were taken to Hamm and secretly buried in her husband's grave. *See* Martin Blumenson (1985).

Pavlova, Anna (1881-1931)

The Russian ballerina's most famous role was in *The Dying Swan,* created for her by Michel Fokine in 1905. At Ivy House, their home in Golders Green, in northwest London, she and her husband Victor Dandré raised swans so tame that they would caress her. After a five-month European tour they returned home in September 1930 for the Pavlova Company's winter season at the Golders Green Theatre.

During the season she complained of pain in her left knee and, on the advice of her Paris specialist, Dr. Zalevsky, she and Dandré traveled to southern France for treatment. She was much improved after five weeks in Cannes and Dandré returned to London in mid-January, leaving Pavlova to rehearse in Paris. On Saturday, 17 January 1931, on the train between Paris and The Hague, where the Pavlova Company was to perform, she felt ill. A doctor called to the Hotel des Indes diagnosed pleurisy in the left lung and it was surmised that she had caught a chill after becoming overheated during rehearsals.

Dr. de Jong, physician to the queen of Holland, was called in and confirmed the diagnosis. Both doctors were concerned about her heart and prescribed a little alcohol, but Pavlova disliked the idea and was disgusted even by rum concealed in hot tea. That she might be critically ill did not occur to anyone. On Monday the nineteenth she complained that she had slept badly and had difficulty in breathing; by now she was sipping warm milk continuously. Zalevsky arrived from Paris on the twenty first and expressed great anxiety. That evening the dancer discussed matters pertaining to the company with her husband; she was so clearheaded that he was reassured.

Next morning fluid was drawn from the pleural cavity and an injection of antipneumococcal serum administered. Measures were taken to improve the action of her heart, but it grew perceptibly weaker until she lost consciousness around 6:00 P.M. Oxygen was administered, but her breathing grew fainter. Around midnight she opened her eyes and raised a hand to her maid Marguerite Letienne; Marguerite bent over her to hear her mistress whisper, "Get my Swan costume ready." A few minutes later, at 12:30 A.M. on Friday, 23 January 1931, Pavlova died. Her death was ascribed to pleurisy and heart failure.

Marguerite dressed the dancer in her favorite beige lace; after she was laid in her coffin Dandré added a few sprays of lilac. He would not allow a death mask to be made. Early next morning a Russian priest of the Orthodox Church celebrated a mass for the dead, during which Dandré noticed a faint smile had appeared on her lips. The coffin was taken from the hotel to a Catholic monastery pending a decision about the place of burial. Dandré felt she would wish to be buried near her home. On the twenty-eighth the coffin was taken to St. Phillip's, the Russian Orthodox church in Buckingham Palace Road, London. One end of the polished black coffin, raised high on trestles, was draped with the Russian Imperial flag; a wreath, inscribed in English and Russian TO THE IMMORTAL PAVLOVA FROM HER COMPANY encircled the other. The air in the dark, candlelit church was heavy with the perfume of the flowers sent by countless admirers. Thousands of people filed past to pay their last respects.

On 29 January 1931, after a lengthy service, the funeral procession left the church at 2:15 P.M. and stopped briefly in front of Ivy House on the way to the Golders Green Crematorium, after which Pavlova's ashes were buried there in the Garden of Rest.

Perón, Eva (1919-1952)

The youngest of five illegitimate children of a servant and her employer, Eva Duarte, a part-time actress in Buenos Aires, caught the eye of an aspiring officer, forty-nine-year-old Colonel Juan Perón, married him secretly in October 1945 and greatly aided his election to the Argentine presidency four months later.

She fell ill toward the end of 1951 and underwent surgery for uterine cancer. The disease spread and when she died, on 26 July 1952, her weight was less than eighty pounds. Dr. Pedro Ara, a Spanish pathologist, immediately began a months-long embalming process. Elsewhere in Buenos Aires a huge crypt was begun that was to tower higher than the Statue of Liberty.

It was barely begun when Perón was overthrown by the military in September 1955.

Obsessed by the fear that Evita's corpse might become the focus of a Perónist cult, the new government moved it out of the Confederation of Labor building in turn to various locations around the city. In September 1956 it was shipped to the Argentine embassy in West Germany. In due course it arrived in Rome, identified as a certain Maria Maggi de Magistris, a widow who had died in Argentina and who wished to be buried in her native Milan. There, under a tombstone marked accordingly, it lay in Lot 86, Garden 41, in Muscocco Cemetery for fifteen years.

By 2 September 1971 a Perónista terrorist group was said to be searching Italy for the revered relic. On that day a former Argentine intelligence chief, Hector Cabanillas, in the guise of the dead woman's brother, appeared at the cemetery with the necessary papers to exhume his sister's body. The black outer coffin was badly rotted, but the zinc inner one was in excellent condition. Cabanillas sped with it in a hearse across two international boundaries to the exiled Perón and his young new wife Isobel at their suburban Madrid home. Dr. Ara was waiting there too, to see how his handiwork had survived the long years. A fingertip had become detached, and there were a few indentations where the coffin lid had pressed down on the plastic coating that covered the skin of the face; an ear was slightly bent, otherwise only a shampoo and new garments were needed to make Evita's body, regarded as a product of mortuary art, as good as new.

Perón was invited back to his country in 1972. Only in July 1974, after his death, did Evita join him in the crypt of the presidential chapel at Ovidos. Two years later the generals seized power again; a few months later Maria Eva Duarte de Peron was entombed for—possibly the last time. In the early hours of 22 October 1976 a well-armed convoy of trucks escorted her to the crowded Recoleta Cemetery, Buenos Aires, and hastily placed her, still in her glass and silver coffin, without ceremony in the black marble crypt bearing the sign FAMILIA DUARTE.

Picasso, Pablo (1881-1973)

The Spanish painter, engraver, and sculptor, the most influential artist of the twentieth century, was a compulsive worker; only during the year following his prostate surgery in November 1965 at the American Hospital in Paris did he fail to complete any paintings.

Shortly before this date, Françoise Gilot, incensed by his unfair treatment of her at the end of their eleven-year relationship, published a book about their life together that had a disastrous effect on the old man.

About the time of his secret second marriage to Jacqueline Roque in 1961 he had bought a secluded home in Mougins, north of Cannes. It was here at Mas Notre Dame de Vie that he at last began to paint again, but many of these works depict ugly, brutish, joyless sex, and they bear evidence of being slapped on canvas (and in some cases brown paper) by a frustrated, angry old man. His biographer Patrick O'Brian alludes to him as a "maimed Priapus" and reflects "upon the mutilating effect of the surgeon's knife . . . on a man whose virility was so important a part of his essence."

In the fall of 1972 hundreds of his recent paintings were displayed at Avignon, pictures much less erotic and more carefully painted than those done in the late sixties; it was difficult to believe they were the work of a nonagenarian. Later that winter a severe attack of influenza left him very weak. In the spring he began to work again in his studio, rising late but sometimes continuing to paint throughout the night. On 7 April 1973, after dinner with friends, he felt breathless; the local doctor, J. C. Rance, found a lung infection and signs of severe heart trouble. An eminent cardiologist, a friend of Picasso's, flew in from Paris early next morning. Realizing immediately there was no hope, he did what he could to make the old man comfortable. Picasso, displaying his usual lively curiosity, was fascinated by the doctor's instruments. Unaware that he was dying, he rose and shaved, saying he wanted to show the specialist his studio. But a moment later, breathless, he lay down again and could be heard talking to himself. The name of the French poet Apollinaire, an old friend long dead, was often repeated. In his final lucid moment he looked up at the specialist, a bachelor, and, taking Jacqueline's hand, said, "You are wrong not to marry. It's useful." Surrounded by a clutter of his pictures and possessions, he died of pulmonary edema at Notre Dame de Vie a little before noon on 8 April 1973.

His body was taken from Mougins to the chapel at his former home, a sixteenth-century castle at Vauvenargues, twelve miles east of Aix-en-Provence, and on 16 April he was buried privately with Catholic rites within the turreted walls. His twenty-four-year-old grandson Pablito, denied admittance at Vauvenargues, swallowed poison on 12 April and, after lingering three months, died on 11 July at La Fontanne Hospital, Antibes.

Picasso left no will; under French law his multimillion-dollar estate was divided equally between his second wife Jacqueline and his only legitimate son Paulo.

Pike, James Albert (1913-1969)

The Episcopal Bishop of California resigned in 1966, but he was still a bishop, and his outspoken rejection of the Trinity, the Virgin Birth, and the Resurrection created a scandal. His personal life was unhappy: his son shot himself in 1966 and his daughter attempted suicide in 1968; his second wife divorced him in July 1967, a month after the suicide of a woman he was involved with. He married his student Diane Kennedy in December 1968 and together they set off to Europe and Israel in August 1969.

In Jerusalem they stayed up all night reliving their three years together. In her account, *Search* (1970), Diane Kennedy writes that she was aware her husband had come to the end of the road, that "this portion of Jim's odyssey was finished . . . I would not want him back. Not now. Not physically."

They left the Intercontinental Hotel at noon on Monday, 1 September, for a short drive in the Judean wilderness. Diane drove while the bishop tried to interpret their inadequate map. When their Ford Cortina roadster got stuck on the rocky trail, they tired themselves trying to lift the back wheel out of a deep crevice. Their only liquid was two bottles of Coca-Cola.

It was 4:00 P.M., the temperature in the blazing sun around 130°F, but instead of turning back they trudged on along the dry bed of a wadi toward the Dead Sea. By 6:00 P.M., according to a 1972 U.S. Air Force study, they had each lost seventeen pounds of water by perspiration, in Diane's case a near-fatal 14 percent of her body weight. When Pike's heart began to pound, they lay down together, but, afraid their deaths might be misinterpreted as a double suicide, she got up. "Sweetheart," she said, "I'm going for help." He promised to follow her.

For ten hours the thirty-one-year-old woman, her feet protected only by thong sandals, climbed over rocks and up and down jagged cliffs by sunlight and starlight. When her thirst became all-consuming she resorted to drinking her own urine. At 4:00 A.M. her legs failed her within sight of the Dead Sea; she rolled her bruised, lacerated body down a slope and made a last desperate cry for help. Incredibly, it was overheard by two Arab road-builders asleep in a tent. They half-carried the exhausted woman to their camp nearby at Ein Fashkha.

Jeep and helicopter searches were launched by the Israelis but it was several days before any trace of Pike was found. On 6 September, his underpants were found floating in a deep pool of fresh water; he had left them there as a clue to his route. Next day his body was sighted across a deep canyon in an almost inaccessible niche halfway down a cliff; he had fallen seventy feet, probably on 2 September, while climbing out of the wadi. The only injuries observed at autopsy were three fractured ribs.

Bishop Pike was buried in St. Peter's Protestant Cemetery at Jaffa, just south of Tel Aviv, in the aluminum container used to transport the remains to the Forensic Institute. A golden rug was spread over it and it was lowered into a grave only a few yards from the shore. *See* William Stringfellow and Anthony Towne (1976).

Pliny the Elder (A.D. 23-79)

The death of the Roman polymath Gaius Plinius Secundus was directly attributable to his character, a blend of intense curiosity and a noble disregard for his own safety. He was prefect (admiral) of the fleet at Misenum (present-day Capo Miseno) west of Naples when the volcano Vesuvius erupted, for the first time in many centuries, on 24 August 79. He was working at his books after lunch when his attention was drawn to an unusual cloud, shaped like an umbrella pine, rising from a mountain to the east. Pliny climbed to a point above the house for a better look, then ordered his warships launched to aid the terrified populace along the bay. Years later the historian Tacitus asked the dead man's nephew and adopted son, Pliny the Younger, for an account of his uncle's final hours, a request happily granted, for "I know that immortal fame awaits him if his death is recorded by you."

"He hurried to the locality from which everyone else was rushing away, steering straight for the danger zone. He was quite without fear, describing each new movement and stage of the phenomenon to be noted down exactly as he observed it. Ashes were already falling, hotter and thicker as the vessels approached, followed by pumice stones and blackened rocks, charred and cracked by the flames . . ." At Stabiae (modern Castellammare di Stabia), four miles south of Pompeii, which like Herculaneum was soon to be buried, Pliny landed and attempted to hearten his panic-stricken friend Pomponianus, who hoped to escape by sea if the wind changed. "After his bath," wrote the younger Pliny, "he lay down and dined; he was quite cheerful or—what was equally splendid—with a pretense of cheerfulness . . . He then retired to rest and undoubtedly slept, for he was a stout man whose breathing was rather loud, and he could be heard by people passing his door. By this time the courtyard was full of ashes and pumice . . . and if he had stayed in his room much longer he would never have escaped."

He was roused and joined the other members of the household in debating whether it was better to stay in the shuddering building or brave the falling pumice. Dawn never came that day, 25 August 79. Through the blackness, darker than night, the party ventured with pillows tied to their heads. On the beach the waves were too wild and dangerous to allow an escape. Pliny, overcome by sulfurous fumes, lay down on a sheet. The others, increasingly nervous, soon pulled him to his feet and two slaves supported him. But after a while he "suddenly collapsed, I imagine," wrote his nephew, "because the smoke choked his breathing by blocking his wind-pipe, which was constitutionally weak and constricted and often inflamed." When daylight at last returned to the area on the twenty-sixth "his body was found intact and uninjured, still fully clothed and seeming to be asleep rather than dead."

The younger Pliny, only seventeen at the time, had stayed at Misenum with his mother, but "I have described in detail every incident which I either witnessed myself or heard about immediately after the event."

Potter, Beatrix (1866-1943)

The English writer and watercolor artist created her score of children's classics within a dozen years, beginning with *Peter Rabbit* in 1901. Dominated by her parents for much of her life, she was in her late forties when in October 1913 she married a self-effacing country lawyer, William Heelis, a few years younger than herself, who had helped her purchase Hill Top Farm in the English Lake District in 1905. The same month saw the publication of *The Tale of Pigling Bland*, "the nearest Miss Potter had approached to a conventional love story," wrote Graham Greene, and no doubt an unconscious reflection of her hopes for the future.

As Mrs. Heelis she withdrew from the world and devoted her remaining thirty years to farming, breeding Herdwick sheep, and helping the National Trust to secure neighboring lands for the enjoyment of posterity. Only one of her few books thereafter, *The Tale of Johnny Town-Mouse* (1918), comes close to capturing the earlier magic. She discouraged inquiries and kept her address secret. In her last years the rigors of wartime rationing and lack of help wore out the rosy-cheeked septuagenarian. As the bitter winter of 1943 set in she caught a cold and stayed in bed to keep warm. With her devoted William by her side, she wrote letters, questioned shepherds about the next lambing, and made sure cracker crumbs were put down for fieldmice; but slowly she lost ground. Her last writing was probably a note to a shepherd friend: "Dear Joe Moscrop . . . Still some strength in me. I write a line to shake you by the hand; our friendship has been entirely pleasant. I am very ill with bronchitis. With best wishes for the New Year . . ."

Beatrix Potter Heelis died quietly on 22 December 1943, gazing to the last through the window at her beloved frost-bound fells. Her ashes were scattered at Hill Top Farm in the field next to the wood described in *The Tale of Jemima Puddle-Duck* (1908) between the village of Sawrey and tiny Esthwaite Water.

Rebuffed four years before by "the rudest letter I have ever received in my life," the young journalist Margaret Lane, still hopeful of writing Beatrix Potter's biography, visited Heelis shortly after his wife's death and found her home, Castle Cottage in Sawrey, still haunted by the dead woman's personality. Her clothes still hung behind the door; "her muddles," writes Miss Lane, "lay unsorted at one end of the table while he took his meals at the other, even a half-eaten bar of chocolate with her teeth marks in it lay whitened and stale among the litter of letters on her writing table." Whenever the would-be biographer would ask the most innocent question—the date of her birth, the fact of their marriage—the unhappy William would look over his shoulder in alarm, as though being watched by a ghostly presence. But he died within a few months and Margaret Lane's two books about Beatrix Potter appeared in 1946 and 1978.

Pound, Ezra (1885-1972)

The influential U.S. poet made his home in London from 1908 to 1920; later, after four years in Paris, he settled permanently in Italy, from where he broadcast to American troops on behalf of the enemy. ("Every human being . . . should realize that Fascism is superior in every way to Russian Jewocracy and that Capitalism stinks.") Arrested and returned to the United States to face treason charges, he was examined by four court-appointed doctors, who reported that "his personality, for many years abnormal, has undergone further distortion to the extent that he is now suffering from a paranoid state which renders him unfit to . . . participate . . . in his own defense."

Held in St. Elizabeth's Hospital in Washington, D.C., from 1946 to 1958, he loved to talk endlessly to other inmates and to his many visitors, including his wife Dorothy Shakespear and his daughter Mary (by the concert violinist Olga Rudge). He also pushed on with his lifework, the often obscure *Cantos,* begun in the mid-1920s.

The treason indictment was dismissed in 1958 and the poet, in the custody of his wife, returned to Italy and his daughter's Alpine home, a twelfth-century castle above Merano. He had two prostate operations in 1962–63 and was given "rejuvenating" animal-cell injections at Swiss clinics. In 1969 he made a surprise two-week visit to New York and Connecticut.

In the last week of his life, Pound, now living in Venice with Olga Rudge, celebrated his eighty-seventh birthday on 30 October 1972 with a great deal of talking, as usual. He fell ill suddenly two days later and died in his sleep a few hours after admission to the Hospital of Saints John and Paul. There was a brief service at the Palladium Basilica on the island of San Gregorio. His wife, old and frail in London, was unable to come. No tributes were received from the U.S. or Italian governments. Olga, Mary, and Mary's daughter Patrizia accompanied the flower-bedecked coffin in a black and gold gondola to the *camposanto* on the burial isle of San Michele. Pound was laid to rest close to Diaghilev and Stravinsky; a simple stone, designed by the U.S. sculptor Joan Fitzgerald, reads simply, EZRA POUND. *See* C. David Heymann (1976).

Powell, William (1892-1984)

The U.S. actor, who began his career in silent movies as a villain, graduated to light comedy as Nick Charles in *The Thin Man* (1934) and *My Man Godfrey* (1936). Divorced from Carole Lombard in 1933, he was devastated by the death, at twenty-six, of Jean Harlow ("The Blonde Bombshell") (q.v.) in 1936 shortly before their planned wedding.

Powell experienced some pain during the filming of *The Baroness and the Butler* (1938); a small cancerous tumor of the rectum was discovered, and surgery, accompanied by a temporary colostomy (reversed early in 1939), was carried out in March 1938.

A month after their first meeting, the forty-seven-year-old Powell and the twenty-one-year-old actress Diana Lewis were married in January 1940. The union, his third and happiest, was to last for over forty-four years. He won his third best-actor Oscar nomination for *Life with Father* (1947). He played the cool, war-weary ship's doctor in *Mister Roberts* (1955); the filming in and around Hawaii wore him out and he made the sudden decision to retire to his Palm Springs, California, home. This meant backing out of a TV movie he'd promised to make with Myrna Loy, his costar in thirteen of his ninety-seven films, including the six *Thin Man* titles. He asked the studio to let him break the bad news to her, which he did—with five thousand red roses!

In 1968 he was deeply shocked by the suicide, at forty-three, of his only child Bill Jr. who, depressed and suffering kidney disease, stabbed himself while in the shower. Powell's old movies still drew crowds to rerun theaters throughout the sixties and seventies as the actor lived on quietly to a great age, visited occasionally by his few surviving friends, including Myrna Loy. He died quietly at home with Diana at his side on 5 March 1984, aged ninety-two. The end had come suddenly: "He was bright and alert last week," said Diana, "and doing very well." *See* Charles Francisco (1985).

Power, Tyrone (1914-1958)

As a baby in Cincinnati, the U.S. movie actor suffered from rheumatic fever; it may well have been the long-term effects of this disease on the valves of his heart that led to his early death.

In April 1958 an irregular heartbeat was discovered during a medical check in New York. He married his third wife, the divorced twenty-six-year-old Debbie Montgomery Minardos, a few weeks later. During the summer in Newport Beach, California, he enjoyed sailing his forty-two-foot ketch while studying the script of his next (and last) film, *Solomon and Sheba* (1959). It was filmed in Spain in the fall and by mid-November Power's work was more than half-completed. He was aware of discomfort in his left shoulder, but dismissed it as bursitis.

On 15 November at a Madrid location, Power (as Solomon) and George Sanders (as his elder brother Adonijah) fought a duel on a staircase landing. For an hour and a half the two actors, in heavy robes and wielding fifteen-pound swords, lunged at one another repeatedly. Sanders, an inept swordsman, used a double except when the camera was on his face. This required Power to do extra work in moving from one setup to another. One take that showed both their faces had to be reshot repeatedly after Sanders voiced dissatisfaction with the angles. Power, despite a reputation for controlling his impatience, finally—after the eighth take—threw down his sword and said, "If you can't find anything you can use, just use the closeups of me. I've had it."

Power's makeup man, Ray Sebastian, said that the actor was shaking, from either anger or exhaustion; he helped him to his trailer and made him a cup of hot tea, laced with rum. "Ty, can you hold your arms up?" Power tried, but groaned, "Boy, they hurt." Because the company doctor was nowhere to be found, the sick man was raced in costar Gina Lollobrigida's Mercedes-Benz to the U.S. Torrejon air base. A few minutes into the journey, Power cried out and fell back, lifeless. At the air base hospital, Adrenalin was injected into his heart in a vain attempt to revive him.

Debbie Power asked Sebastian to make up her husband's embalmed body, and reluctantly he agreed. He shaved off the beard the role had required and applied the makeup. "I carried on a conversation with Ty the whole time I was there," he said later. "That was the only way I could get through it." Because he couldn't find a priest, "I said my own prayer for him."

The body of Tyrone Power, who had been promoted to major in the Marine reserve a few weeks earlier, lay in state at the base until after a memorial service; it was then shipped to Los Angeles. Debbie asked the second Mrs. Power, Linda Christian, to stay away from the funeral service at the Chapel of the Palms on 21 November. (Linda and Power's two daughters celebrated mass eight blocks away.) The coffin was open, and Debbie held the dead man's hand throughout the military-style service. Six marines carried the coffin to the burial place in Hollywood Memorial Park Cemetery amid disorderly crowd scenes at which one woman fainted.

The actor's only son, Tyrone Power IV, was born two months later on 21 January 1959. The dead man's estate went to Debbie, his mother, his two daughters, and the son he never saw.

Solomon and Sheba had to be refilmed from the beginning, with Yul Brynner replacing Power. The insurance company settled with United Artists for $1,229,172, the largest movie loss of its kind to that date. *See* Hector Arce (1979).

Prokofiev, Sergei (1891-1953)

The Soviet composer was, like Shostakovich, disciplined by the Communist Party in 1948 for Western "bourgeois tendencies" but, unlike his younger colleague, held no academic positions that could be stripped from him.

Nevertheless, he submitted a written apology to the Central Committee, possibly because the status of his second wife Myra Mendelson was uncertain. (Under a retroactive Soviet law his earlier union with a Spanish-born woman was evidently, but not positively, invalid.)

Prokofiev was already a sick man. He had suffered a mild heart attack in January 1945 and fallen down a flight of stairs, and thereafter endured blinding headaches and giddiness. He moved with his wife to a dacha (country cottage) in the small village of Nikolina Gora, near Zvenigorod, some thirty-five miles west of Moscow. Under her devoted care, he was able to compose for a short period each day. A stroke in 1949 put him out of action for only a short time. In a reversal of official policy he was awarded the Stalin Prize in 1951.

By then he was spending the winters in his Moscow apartment with medical help near at hand. Though frequent spells in the hospital were needed, Myra's skilful management of his time undoubtedly lengthened his creative life. He was not well enough to orchestrate his *Seventh Symphony* in the summer of 1952; in October he attended his final public concert in Moscow's Hall of the Columns, when the symphony was conducted by Samuel Samosud. On 5 March 1953 the choreographer L. M. Lavrovsky called at Prokofiev's apartment to tell him how rehearsals of his ballet *The Stone Flower* were going at the Bolshoi. He found the composer busy revising the score and he waited while work on the adagio, "The Joy of Katerina's Meeting with Danila," was completed, for this dance was to be given a run-through that evening. Lavrovsky promised to telephone after the rehearsal.

That afternoon, Prokofiev was visited as usual by his physician, Elena Tepper, and walked back with her to her clinic to get a breath of fresh air. He promised her, with a smile, he would be a good boy and obey her orders though, he admitted, it was hard to tear himself away from his work. Two hours later she received an urgent call; her patient had suffered another stroke, and by the time she arrived at his apartment he was dead. His oppressor Stalin died the same evening.

The body was taken to the Central Composers' Home, where ceremonies on 7 March 1953 were attended by Shostakovich, Khachaturian and other musicians; David Oistrakh played movements from a Prokofiev violin sonata. The composer was buried in the cemetery of Nova-Devichy Monastery, Moscow.

Proust, Marcel (1871-1922)

The French author of the series of seven novels titled *Remembrance of Things Past* suffered his first asthma attack, a severe one, at the age of nine. As an adult he was a hypochondriac who slept during the day behind tightly closed windows in a cork-lined room crammed with notebooks and medicine bottles.

Late at night when, he believed, the air was purer, he would venture forth to the Parisian cafés, an odd figure—fragile, unnaturally pale, with huge eyes circled by dark shadows. He was a homosexual who kept a succession of handsome chauffeur-secretaries. When he visited male brothels it was usually to spy on the activities of other clients and question the owners to obtain material for future use in his writing.

Early in September 1922 Proust suffered several severe attacks of asthma. Returning from a soiree in early October he caught a bad cold and demanded round-the-clock care from his housekeeper, Céleste. On 19 October, though still feverish, he went out, only to return in a few minutes trembling with cold and racked by bouts of sneezing. He suspected pneumonia and, sure enough, that disease was diagnosed on 10 November. His doctor, finding him a difficult patient, brought his brother Robert Proust to see him. Robert wanted to move Marcel to a clinic but was met with a furious refusal. "Let me alone," he shouted. "I won't leave my bedroom. I'll have no one but Céleste; she's the only one who understands me."

On the seventeenth Proust felt much better and told Robert he intended to have a good night's sleep, but at 3:00 A.M. on the eighteenth he asked Céleste to note some alterations he wished to be made to the manuscript of his novel *Albertine Disparue*. Suddenly, utterly exhausted, he gasped, "I must stop, I can't do any more." A lung abscess had probably burst at that moment. At 6:00 A.M. he asked for milk and at 10:00 A.M. for iced beer. Though he was having great difficulty in breathing he ordered Céleste to leave him. When he detected her hiding behind a bedscreen she protested that she was afraid to leave. "Don't lie, Céleste; you know she has come." He stared in horror at the door. "She's big, very big . . . she is very big, very dark! She is all in black, she's ugly, she frightens me." The housekeeper offered to chase the apparition away, but Proust called out, "No, don't touch her, Céleste; no one must touch her! She's merciless; she's getting more horrible every moment!"

The doctors came with their orderlies, but injections and cupping were in vain. The dying man whispered. "Ah, Céleste, why did you let them?" Robert raised his brother gently and said, "I'm afraid I am hurting you." "Oh, yes, my dear Robert," replied Marcel. A little later he murmured, "Mother." With his eyes wide open, Proust died at 5:30 on the afternoon of 18 November 1922. Friends calling at the rue Hamelin to view the body in the manuscript-strewn room found the windows open for the first time in years. The funeral service was at noon on the twenty-first at the Church of Saint-Pierre-de-Chaillot and Proust was buried beside his father and mother in Père Lachaise Cemetery.

Rathbone, Basil (1892-1967)

The British actor, born in South Africa, preferred to live in the United States. A "born enthusiast" is how he described himself and "enthusiasm . . . is bad manners in England. I couldn't stand the conventional British chill." It was in one of the seven movies he made for release in 1935 that he earned his reputation as a screen villain. Yet the savage beating he had to give David (a well-padded Freddie Bartholomew) as the boy's cruel stepfather Mr. Murdstone in *David Copperfield* made the soft-hearted actor, according to the director, George Cukor, "physically ill."

Beginning with *The Hound of the Baskervilles* (1939) he played Sherlock Holmes for eight years in fourteen films, as well as on stage, radio, and television. In the minds of many, Rathbone *was* Holmes. Happy at first to have been offered the part, he later complained bitterly that the typecasting had seriously damaged his career.

Rathbone's last movie was the forgettable *Hillbillys in a Haunted House* (1967). After filming ended in June 1967 he made several appearances in his one-man show, *An Evening with Basil Rathbone,* and returned to his New York home at 135 Central Park West on 20 July. He looked "very tired," according to his widow Ouida Bergere, but his doctor next day found nothing disturbing. That evening, "Basil was very sad, as an old friend of his had died," Mrs. Rathbone reported. "We were in the living room of our apartment discussing it, when he suddenly said, 'You know, I'm not afraid to die, but I just wish it didn't have to be.' We talked a few more minutes and he seemed to cheer up a bit. Then, he went into his den, because he wanted to play a record he'd just purchased. About five minutes later, I went into the room to ask him something . . . and he was 'gone.'" The actor had suffered a heart attack and was found collapsed on the floor.

At his funeral service in St. James's Episcopal Church on Madison Avenue, Cornelia Otis Skinner read poems by Elizabeth Browning and Rupert Brooke. In his will, Rathbone had written, "I wish to be buried beside my wife—so close that, if it were possible, we might hold each other's hand." The reality was less romantic; in the decade still remaining to her, Ouida lived in straitened circumstances. Her husband's estate, divided between her and Rathbone's son Rodion from his first marriage, amounted to no more than $10,000 to $20,000. *See* Michael B. Druxman (1975).

Richard I (1157-1199)

Nicknamed "Lionheart," Richard I succeeded his father Henry II as king of England in 1189 but spent only a few months of his reign there. Earlier he had earned his reputation for boundless courage in the Third Crusade of 1191–92.

His last years were spent in a power struggle with Philip II Augustus of France over the allegiance of the French Angevin territories. In March 1199 Richard laid siege to the castle of Châlus-Chabrol, some say because the vicomte of Limoges had refused to hand over a recently unearthed golden treasure. Late on the third day, 26 March, Richard advanced with his archers and crossbowmen as sappers undermined the castle walls. Intrigued by the sight of a solitary crossbowman, by name Peter Basil or Pierre Basile, standing at the ramparts holding a fry pan as a makeshift shield, Richard ventured closer. He wore no armor but an iron headpiece, and he was a fraction late in raising his own shield as a heavy bolt struck him in the left shoulder. As he retreated to his tent he struggled to remove it, but the wooden shaft broke off. Though a surgeon was able to cut out the iron barb, infection soon set in. Despite ever-increasing pain, Richard filled his remaining twelve days with his habitual wild carousing. He died of septicemia on the evening of 7 April 1199 in the presence of his mother, Eleanor of Aquitaine.

He left his heart to the loyal citizens of Rouen, but his entrails to the treacherous people of Poitou, who had rebelled against him. His heart was buried in Rouen cathedral, where it was rediscovered in modern times within two leaden boxes near the altar. His body, bearing a crown and clothed in coronation robes, jewelled gloves and golden sandals was placed at the feet of his father, Henry II, in the abbey church of Fontevrault, where his mother joined him five years later. Effigies of mother and son still surmount the tomb, which was ransacked during the French Revolution. The bodies of all three were found in another part of the church in 1910. *See* Philip Henderson (1958).

Rilke, Rainer Maria (1875-1926)

The Prague-born German lyric poet was plagued by ill health during his last three years. His home was the thirteenth-century Château de Muzot, just north of Sierre in Switzerland. The castle lacked water and electricity, but he entertained his frequent visitors by reading aloud to them by candlelight as he stood at his desk. This pleasure was denied him after the fall of 1925, when he developed painful swellings in his mouth.

In October he made his will, imploring his friends not to permit any religious ministrations should he lapse into unconsciousness before dying and asking for burial in the old churchyard of Raron, twelve miles east of Muzot. After several months of treatment at the Valmont clinic near Montreux his illness, still undiagnosed, abated and he visited several friends during the summer of 1926. One day he was picking roses in his garden at Muzot—some say for a beautiful young Egyptian girl—when he pricked two fingers. The wounds became infected and very painful; swellings in the nose and mouth developed and the poet was also distressed by a cough, sore throat, and digestive troubles. By the end of November he was back in the Valmont clinic and acute leukemia, complicated by septicemia, was diagnosed. Though he was able to send his customary Christmas notes to friends, he was in grave discomfort from purpuric spots (small black blisters) all over his body and in his nose, mouth, and throat; these would burst open and bleed. Despite a continuous 104-degree temperature his mind remained clear until he lost consciousness at midnight on 28 December 1926. At 3:30 A.M. on the twenty-ninth he raised his head, opened his eyes wide, and fell back dead.

The coffin was first taken by sled to a small chapel nearby, then by automobile to Raron. On Sunday, 2 January 1927, while church bells chimed, four men carried the coffin up the steep, slippery footpath to the little church. A simple mass was followed by the music of Bach played on the organ and violin. Children holding wreaths surrounded the grave as Rilke was laid to rest. Inset into the church wall is a stone bearing the poet's own enigmatic inscription, ROSE, OH REINER WIDERSPRUCH, LUST, NIEMANDES

SCHLAF ZU SEIN UNTER SOVIEL LIDERN. (Rose, oh pure contradiction, desire to be nobody's sleep beneath so many lids.) The grave is also marked by a slender wooden cross engraved RMR 1875–1926.

Robert the Bruce (1274-1329)

The Scottish patriot joined in William Wallace's rebellion against English rule in 1297. He was crowned King Robert I of Scotland in 1306 and, in his greatest triumph, defeated a large English army at Bannockburn in 1314. It was not until the Treaty of Northampton in 1328 that the southern foe recognized his position as King of the Scots.

Robert was a short, muscular man whose mere presence on horseback in battle could intimidate an enemy. His final illness began in 1327, when he was described as being so feeble that "he could scarcely move anything but his tongue." He died at home in Cardross, Dunbartonshire, on 7 June 1329, and his body—all except his heart—was buried before the high altar of the abbey church of Dunfermline. A marble monument, carved in Paris, was erected above his grave.

His dying wish was that his heart be carried on a crusade. This was done by Sir James Douglas; after Douglas was killed in Spain in March 1330, the heart was laid to rest in the abbey in Melrose, Scotland.

During alterations in Dunfermline Abbey in 1819, Robert's body was exhumed. The height of the skeleton was five feet six inches; the sternum had been split to remove the heart. Four or five upper teeth were missing, but these may have been found lying loose much earlier and taken by souvenir hunters. Comparison of the skull with those of the Danish lepers of the same period indicates that they are all alike in showing erosion of the alveolar ridge opposite the upper incisors. Though most of the Danish specimens had the teeth in place, they were not held by bone. J. A. N. Rennie and W. W. Buchanan in a 1978 medical study weigh the probabilities that Robert the Bruce died of leprosy or syphilis and conclude that a diagnosis of leprosy is "highly suggestive."

Robeson, Paul (1898-1976)

The U.S.-born bass baritone, trained as a lawyer, turned to the stage when he found professional opportunities for blacks to be limited. He was especially noted for his singing of "Ol' Man River" in the musical *Showboat* (1928) and his acting in Shakespeare's *Othello* and O'Neill's *Emperor Jones*.

In June 1956 his outspoken advocacy of left-wing causes brought him before the House Un-American Activities Committee. Two years later, his passport, withheld in 1950, was returned and he was able to sing in London and Moscow. In January 1959 he was treated in a Kremlin hospital for influenza and dizzy spells. He was well enough to perform in *Othello* that spring at Stratford-on-Avon and to visit Australasia in 1960 in what was to be his last major tour. His voice, at sixty-two, was still good, but after another illness in 1961 he never sang a full concert again. For three years he was in and out of hospitals in London, Moscow, and East Germany. It was rumored that bitter disillusionment with Soviet communism had exhausted him and undermined his health.

He retired with his wife Eslanda (Essie) to Jumal Terrace in Harlem, New York, but she died of cancer in December 1965. Paul moved to Philadelphia and the spacious row house of his sister, Marion Forsythe, where he could find the help and support he needed. He was heartened by a Carnegie Hall celebration on his seventy-fifth birthday in 1973, but, apart from an occasional outing, he maintained his privacy behind drawn blinds and shutters.

One day in November 1975 Robeson dressed and came downstairs to talk about old times with a cousin, Ernestine Thomas. "His sister said he didn't do that often," said Mrs. Thomas. He was admitted to the Presbyterian University Hospital in Philadelphia on 28 December 1975 after a mild stroke. His condition worsened and he died on 23 January 1976. *See* Edwin Palmer Hoyt (1967).

Rockefeller, Nelson A. (1908-1979)

A man of wide interests and enormous energy, governor of New York (1958–74) and U.S. vice president in the Ford administration, Nelson Rockefeller after leaving public life busied himself with an accurate method of reproducing items in the enormous Rockefeller art collection and with the publishing of art books.

In December 1978 he complained to his physician, Dr. Ernest Esakof, of chest pains and was advised to lose weight. In January he looked fitter, less bloated. On Friday morning, the twenty-sixth, he arrived at his office on the fifty-sixth floor of 30 Rockefeller Plaza in midtown Manhattan to talk to Paul Anbinder about publishing a book describing the folk art collection of his late mother, Abby Rockefeller, in Colonial Williamsburg. Continually in and out of the office during the morning was his assistant, Megan Marshack, a tall and well-proportioned young woman described by Rockefeller's 1982 biographer Joseph F. Persico as being in general exuberant, brash, and uninhibited and as taking "delight in a shocking frankness." She was, writes Persico, who liked her, "an odd composite of precocious worldliness and girlish vulnerability." At twenty-two she had been Rockefeller's assistant press secretary in the last days of his vice presidency.

In the afternoon, Rockefeller went to the Buckley School on East 73rd Street, which his young sons Nelson Jr. and Mark attended, to introduce Henry Kissinger, who had agreed to talk to the students.

The sudden death of Nelson Rockefeller was announced a few hours later at 12:20 A.M. on 26 January 1979 by Dr. Esakof, who had arrived at the Lenox Hill Hospital in Manhattan shortly before. Mrs. Margaretta ("Happy") Rockefeller, the dead man's wife for fifteen years, was there; so were Mr. and Mrs. Laurance Rockefeller, his brother and sister-in-law. Standing a little apart was Megan Marshack, in tears and clutching an oxygen bottle she had been holding in the ambulance that bore her and her employer to the hospital. Over and over she kept repeating that she had done everything possible to save him. When Hugh Morrow, the family spokesman, arrived, he led Marshack away, then was heard to murmur to Happy, "Don't worry. She's not here."

Morrow, faced with a painful choice, lied to reporters when he told them Nelson Rockefeller died at his desk in Room 5600 at about 10:15 P.M. while working on a book of modern art. Stricken by a heart attack, the report continued, his bodyguard worked on him until paramedics arrived. This story was continually revised over the next two days. Finally the truth emerged. After dining with his family, Rockefeller had gone to 13 West 54th Street, his town house, which was connected to his offices on West 55th Street by a passageway and a door to which only he possessed a key. The heart attack did occur at 10:15 while he was with Marshack, but the 911 emergency call was not made until 11:16, and it was made not by Marshack but by her friend and neighbor Ponchitta Pierce, an NBC show host whom Marshack had called in desperation around 10:50 or 11:00. The call awakened her and she hurried from her apartment at 25 West 54th Street to No. 13 with an employee of her building. She found Rockefeller lying on a couch with Megan attempting mouth-to-mouth resuscitation.

Much was made in the press of the hour's delay in summoning help. Could the dead man have been saved had prompt medical attention been given? The death certificate, signed by Esakof, listed cardiopulmonary arrest, acute myocardial infarction, and arteriosclerotic cardiovascular disease. Rockefeller's four adult children issued a statement on 14 February 1979 saying they accepted the doctor's opinion that their father had died of a "single massive heart attack" and that they are "satisfied" that Megan Marshack "did her best to save him."

Nelson Rockefeller's funeral was private. His ashes were buried at the family estate in Pocantico Hills, near Tarrytown, New York. A memorial service in New York's Riverside Church was attended by twenty-two hundred, including his two wives and presidents Ford and Carter.

The bulk of his $66.5 million estate went to Happy and the two young sons; art museums were also beneficiaries. He forgave three loans, one of them of $45,000 to Megan Marshack. She went to work at the end of 1979 for Broadway producer Alexander H. Cohen. *See* Joseph E. Persico (1982).

Rogers, Will (1879-1935)

He was America's favorite folksy philosopher ("Communism is like prohibition: it's a good idea but it won't work"), an Oklahoman who was part Cherokee on both sides ("My folks didn't come over on the *Mayflower,* but they were there to meet the boat"), a man of enormous energy who turned out daily and weekly newspaper columns while constantly in demand on stage and in radio and the movies.

In 1935 he backed out of the film version of O'Neill's *Ah, Wilderness* after a clergyman declared his on-stage lines to be immoral. He thereby had time for a long-unfulfilled ambition, a visit to Alaska. His fellow-Okie, the world-circumnavigating aviator Wiley Post, had put together a hybrid craft from two crashed Lockheed planes, an Explorer and an Orion with a Pratt and Whitney engine. Will flew to Seattle to join him early in August, eager to be off. The Edo pontoons Post had ordered were delayed, so he fitted a much heavier pair from a Fokker trimotor. The combination was nose-heavy, liable to pitch forward uncontrollably at low airspeeds.

They took off from Lake Washington on 6 August. After several days' delay in Juneau because of bad weather, they roamed over the Yukon and as far as the Mackenzie River, as Will in the rear seat tapped out his columns. In Fairbanks the Alaska bush pilot advised against the pair's continuing to Barrow until their plane's instability was corrected. But Rogers was impatient to visit Charles Brower, the U.S. commissioner in Barrow, and see for himself this remote outpost at the northwest extremity of North America, a village of three hundred Eskimos and only nine whites, including a doctor and a nurse. There was also a plan to fly over into Siberia and continue via Europe. Rogers sent a telegram to his daughter Mary in Skowhegan, Maine. She was acting in summer stock there; that week her stage father was killed in a plane crash.

Post and Rogers took off from Fairbanks and roughly followed the future route of the Trans Alaska Pipeline to the coast, then turned west. For hours they flew through a heavy storm with zero visibility. Glimpsing a landlocked patch of still water, Post came down in Walakpa Lagoon, fifteen miles south of Barrow, and asked directions from a group of Eskimo seal hunters. Taking off from the lagoon, the bright red craft with its horizontal silver stripe climbed to fifty feet and banked to the right toward Barrow. Then the engine sputtered and stopped and the plane nosed steeply down into the shallow water. The fuselage split open and the right wing broke off. The horrified Eskimos heard a dull explosion and saw a flash of fire then silence. The two men were killed instantly; it was 3:18 P.M. local time on 15 August 1935.

Claire Okpeaha, who had talked to the flyers only a few moments before, began running over the swampy tundra toward Barrow and reached the village five hours later. When rescue parties arrived by sea in two launches, Will's body had been pulled clear; to reach Wiley the plane had to be dismantled. His watch had stopped at 8:18 (Oklahoma time). There was a simple service for Rogers at the Wee Kirk o' the Heather in Glendale after his body had lain in state in Forest Lawn Memorial Park. The nation's movie theaters were darkened and the radio networks went silent for half an hour. A marker of Oklahoma stone was placed near the crash site. In 1944 Will's remains were buried in his native Claremore, Oklahoma, in the sunken garden adjoining the Will Rogers Memorial Museum. His wife Betty died a month later, and she and their infant son Freddie, who had died in California in 1919, were buried beside him. In the entrance hall of the museum is a lifelike bronze statue by Jo Davidson; inscribed below it is one of his best-known sayings: I NEVER MET A MAN I DIDN'T LIKE.

The cause of the crash was predictably announced to be the instability of the aircraft, but why the engine stalled remains a mystery; maybe moisture had condensed in the carburetor during the short stop in the forty-degree air; maybe Post forgot to turn on the reserve fuel tank. Charles Brower had no doubt about what happened. In a 1963 book about his fifty years in Alaska he claims to have inspected the wreckage and to have found both tanks to be quite empty, but whether or not any remaining fuel could have evaporated or leaked away in the interim is uncertain. *See* Richard M. Ketchum (1973).

Rossetti, Dante Gabriel (1828-1882)

The British poet and artist was a central figure in the romantic Pre-Raphaelite movement. After living with a model, Elizabeth Siddal, for a decade, he married her in 1860. She was addicted to laudanum (tincture of opium) and on the night of 10 February 1862 she purposely or accidentally (probably the former) took a fatal overdose. Lizzie had retired early and Gabriel found her unconscious when he returned to their home in Chatham Place, Blackfriars, at 11:30 P.M. She had an empty vial of laudanum beside her. Despite the ministrations of three doctors, including the use of a stomach pump, Mrs. Rossetti died at 7:20 A.M. on the eleventh.

In a despairing tribute to his lost love, Gabriel placed the notebook containing his unpublished poems into her coffin before it was sealed; he tucked the book between her cheek and her red hair. Years later, hesitant to the last and fearful that the news would leak out, he encouraged a helpful acquaintance, Charles Augustus Howell, to disinter Lizzie's body and retrieve the poems. Permission was obtained and, in the dark of night on 5 October 1869, while Rossetti stayed miles away with feelings that can only be guessed, Howell and two undertakers went to Highgate Cemetery in north London and raised the coffin from the Rossetti family enclosure. The precious leatherbound notebook was gingerly removed, taken to a discreet physician in Kensington to be disinfected and returned to its shamefaced and horror-struck owner.

Lizzie had used laudanum to induce sleep; in his last days Rossetti became addicted to chloral hydrate for the same reason. In early February 1882, in worsening health, he went with the young novelist Hall Caine, Caine's twelve-year-old sister and a hired nurse to Birchington-on-Sea, four miles west of Margate on the Kentish coast, where an old friend put a bungalow at his disposal. His consumption of chloral over the years had by now affected his health irreversibly, with delusions, depression, indolence, and mental instability as the chief symptoms. He had probably suffered a stroke a decade earlier.

At Birchington Rossetti's health worsened steadily. By 1 April he declared himself, in thick, barely intelligible speech, to be dying. A few days later, hot linseed and mustard poultices were prescribed by visiting doctors to draw off the body's poisons, for they recognized marked symptoms of kidney failure. "I believe I shall die tonight," said the patient on 9 April 1882. At about 9:20 that evening he suddenly shouted out and slumped over, breathing heavily and with his mouth twitching; he died a few minutes later.

Rossetti's mental troubles and early death may not have ultimately been due to chloral addiction but to prolonged sleeplessness following Lizzie's probable suicide (there are reports that Rossetti found a note pinned to her nightgown and suppressed it). In a 1928 letter to Bernard Shaw, Hall Caine wrote, "After the death of his wife (with all that that meant to him . . .) he never slept naturally until about 4 months before his death."

Dante Gabriel Rossetti was adamant that he not be buried next to Lizzie. His grave is near the south porch of the thirteenth-century All Saints Parish Church in Birchington. Over it is a carved memorial designed by the poet's friend Ford Madox Brown. The dead man's aged mother had another friend of Rossetti's, Frederic Shields, design a two-part window for the church; on the left is Rossetti's version of Joseph and Zacharia's uniting for the Passover, on the right Shields's own portrayal of Jesus healing the blind man. *See* Brian and Judy Dobbs (1977).

Sadat, Anwar (1918-1981)

President of Egypt from 1970, Sadat restored his country's self-confidence, shattered by Israel's victory in the Six Day War of 1967, when he handled the 1973 campaign that won back parts of Sinai. He stunned the world in November 1977 by offering to go "to the end of the earth," even to the Israeli Knesset, in his search for peace. This led to the Camp David accords of September 1978 and the signing of a peace treaty with Israel in March 1979. He shared with Israeli Prime Minister Menachem Begin the Nobel Peace Prize for 1978.

Sadat did not live to see the three-year withdrawal of Israel from Sinai completed. In gaining worldwide acclaim he had lost popularity at home.

Egypt was expelled from the Arab League and Muslim fundamentalists within the country grew ever more powerful as Sadat tightened his hold on power. Even in the West criticism began to appear of his limitations on free speech. As his luster as the daring hero of peace faded and his domestic problems intensified, Sadat's emotional stability was seen to crumble. On 3 September 1981 he had ordered the arrest of three thousand students, politicians, journalists, and religious leaders. A week later, at his native village in the Nile Delta, Mit Abul-kum, he held his final press conference. He seemed, like President Richard Nixon in his last days in power, emotional, confused, and paranoic. Protesting against a reporter's question, he yelled, "I have the right to shoot you for asking such a question—but this is a democracy." It seemed that something dramatic was about to happen.

On the eighth anniversary of the historic crossing of the Suez Canal by Egyptian forces, Sadat rose early at his Giza home and put on his field marshal's uniform. It was 6 October 1981 and he joined hundreds of notables and foreign guests seated in the stands, just across from the Tomb of the Unknown Soldier in Nasser City on the outskirts of Cairo. President Sadat was flanked by the vice president and the minister of defense. A young artillery lieutenant, Khaled Ahmed Shawki al-Istanbouli, was in charge of the military parade. He was a member of a fundamentalist splinter group of the Islamic Association and a brother of a young man arrested in the recent crackdown. Shortly before 1:00 P.M. an air-display began. As low-flying aircraft passed over the spectators, everyone looked up. At that moment al-Istanbouli and his fellow conspirators charged with submachine guns and grenades, intent on wiping out Egypt's entire top brass. As the rebel soldiers opened fire, Sadat stood up and was fatally wounded. He died in a helicopter on the way to Ma'adi Hospital.

Sadat's 1985 biographer Raphael Israeli quotes the noted Egyptian psychiatrist Dr. Muhammed Sha'alan as commenting that "Sadat constantly ignored security measures . . . refused to wear his bulletproof vest" on the fatal day, "and even dismissed the guards surrounding him. When he was shot he stood up and faced the assassins rather than shy away or stoop. He chose to be a martyr and a hero rather than a despot. When a man becomes identified with a given role and faces the choice of giving up that role or dying, he often chooses death."

Anwar Sadat was buried four days later in a marble crypt below the Tomb of the Unknown Soldier after ceremonies attended by his wife Jihan, his children, Prime Minister Begin and former U.S. presidents Nixon, Ford, and Carter.

Al-Istanbouli and four coconspirators were executed for the murder in April 1982; seventeen others received prison sentences.

Sanders, George (1906-1972)

Though born in St. Petersburg of Russian parents, Sanders epitomized the suave English villain, the consummate cad, in scores of movies, including *Rebecca* (1940) and *All About Eve* (1950). For the latter role he won a supporting-actor Oscar.

His third (and happiest) marriage, to Benita Hume, widow of Ronald Colman, ended after eight years in her slow, painful death from cancer in 1967. This experience, followed within a year by the death of his mother, overwhelmed him. He had already undergone the humiliation of bankruptcy after the failure (amid allegations of fraud) of a sausage-manufacturing business in which his movie earnings were invested.

Ever since his early career as a tobacco company representative in Argentina, Sanders had been drawn to Spanish life and culture. Now, following a stroke in 1969 and haunted by fears of future helplessness, of "having someone to wipe my bum for me," he sought comfort in the company of the Mexican actress Lorraine Chanel. It was a shock to Lorraine, who spent time with Sanders in Mexico City and at his retreat in Majorca, to learn that he had, abruptly and quixotically, married Magda Gabor, sister of Zsa Zsa, his second wife, on Zsa Zsa's urging. The union, to a woman who had like himself suffered a stroke and was, moreover, aphasic, was a total disaster and ended in divorce within six weeks in January 1970.

In his final two years, Sanders found film and television roles hard to come by; producers had heard he suffered from frequent vertigo and walked with a cane. A short and unlucky liaison with a writer, Helga Moray, who persuaded him to sell his beloved house in Majorca, may have triggered his nervous breakdown early in 1972. He visited his sister Margaret in England, shocking her by his evident deterioration, then flew off to Barcelona to look for a small beach house.

He arrived alone at Castelldefels, ten miles south of Barcelona, on 23 April 1972, and checked in at the Hotel Rey Don Jaime. The weather was cold and wet. He was drinking heavily on the twenty-fourth when he asked to be wakened early next morning. He did not respond to the call; beside his dead body were found five empty tubes of Nembutal (pentobarbital), equivalent to 2,000 milligrams, quite sufficient, in combination with the vodka he used to wash down the tablets, to cause death.

In his suicide note, Sanders wrote, "Dear World, I am leaving because I am bored. I feel I have lived long enough. I am leaving you with your worries in this sweet cesspool. Good luck!" This final gesture, very much in character, was widely accepted, but those familiar with the events of his final years believe it was fear of the future that led to his death. On the night of his suicide he mailed a short message to his sister: "Dear Margoolinka, Don't be sad. I have only anticipated the inevitable by a few years." *See* Richard VanDerBeets (1990).

Sanger, Margaret (1879-1966)

The U.S. birth-control pioneer accused her father of killing his wife Anne, a devout Catholic, who died of tuberculosis at forty-nine. "Those 18 pregnancies didn't hurt you a bit," she said bitterly. "You—you'll live forever." It is said she set forth on her life-work after a tenement dweller died in her arms after an illegal, self-induced abortion.

She became addicted to meperidine (Demerol) after being prescribed the narcotic by her physician son Stuart in 1949. Thereafter she continually plagued him and other doctors for more of the drug. In her search for relief she turned to bizarre cures, such as "cosmic ray" treatment in Honolulu. In 1957 she consented to come home to Tucson, Arizona, for more conventional treatment if Stuart would keep her supplied with painkillers. Continually under the influence of Demerol and wine, she often stumbled out of her house after dark in her nightgown to appear, often bruised from falling down, at her son's home next door. He tried to care for her there, but she would fire the nurses he hired and turn up the radio so loud no one could sleep. Back next door the servants began to defraud their confused mistress. When she was discovered to have given away valuable jewelry and to be in danger of using up the $5 million left to her by her second husband, who died in 1942, measures to control her behavior became imperative.

In 1962 she was declared to be senile and taken to a nursing home, the House by the Side of the Road in Tucson. Two days before her death from leukemia on 6 September 1966, just short of her eighty-seventh birthday, friends brought delicacies. Aroused, she exclaimed joyfully, "Chicken sandwiches and champagne! A party! Let's have a party!" only to doze off again.

After funeral services at the Episcopal Church in Tucson and a memorial service at St. George's Chapel in Stuyvesant Square, New York, she was buried during a rainstorm in the family plot at Fishkill, New York. *See* Madeline Gray (1979).

Sartre, Jean-Paul (1905-1980)

The French novelist and philosopher, who was awarded but declined the 1964 Nobel Prize for literature, attempted to develop a coherent system of existentialism on the foundations laid by Kierkegaard (q.v.) a century earlier. His companion for half a century, fellow writer Simone de Beauvoir (1908–1986), had enormous influence on his writings. A stark disagreement arose between them for the first time just a few weeks before his death, over Sartre's recent dialogue with the writer "Pierre Victor" (Benni Lévi), excerpts of which were being readied for publication in the magazine *Le Nouvel Observateur*. When she read the proofs, de Beauvoir was aghast; Victor, she concluded, had grossly influenced her friend. It was, she writes in her *Adieux: A Farewell to Sartre* (1981), nothing short of a *détournement de vieillard* ("abduction of an old man"). Thus, she read that Sartre was repudiating key points in his existentialist writings: "I talked of despair, but it's nonsense . . . I've never experienced despair . . . It was Kierkegaard's influence on me." *Angst* was all the fashion then, Sartre is reported to have told Victor; as though, writes de Beauvoir, Sartre had ever paid any attention to fashion. "I let Sartre know the full extent of my disappointment," writes Simone. "It surprised him."

The second of the three excerpts had been published by 20 March 1980. On that morning, de Beauvoir at 9:00 A.M. went in to waken her friend. She found him sitting on the edge of his bed, "gasping, almost unable to speak"; he had been in this condition for four hours, too ill "to drag himself as far as my [bedroom] door and knock." He was taken from the apartment (on the Boulevard Edgar-Quinet in Paris) to Broussais Hospital, where pulmonary edema was diagnosed. He had a fever and was delirious but the prognosis was at first favorable. Then the kidneys began to fail and signs of uremia were evident. When she foresaw her friend's likely death, she "flung" herself into the arms of the physician, Dr. Housset. "Promise me he won't know he's dying, that he won't go through any mental anguish, that he won't have any pain!" To which the doctor gravely replied, "I promise you that, Madame."

The invalid was resigned. "There's just one disagreeable moment," he said, "and that is when they dress my bedsores in the morning." De Beauvoir found the sores horrifying, "great purplish-blue and reddened patches." Sartre, asking a visitor for a glass of water, remarked, "The next time we have a drink together, it'll be at my place and it'll be whisky." But to Simone next day he said, "How are you going to manage the funeral expenses?" for money worries had plagued him for years. "The next day, with closed eyes," she writes, "he took me by the wrist and said, 'I love you very much my dear Castor,' " his pet name for her.

"On April 14 he was asleep when I came; he woke and said a few words without opening his eyes, then held up his lips to me." Death did not worry him, Housset told her, only the dread of uremic poisoning undermining his brain. On the fifteenth Sartre lay in a coma; de Beauvoir stayed beside him for hours before making way for the other woman close to him in his last years, the much younger Arlette Elkaïm, Sartre's adopted daughter and executor. She called Simone at 9:00 P.M. "It's over," she said.

That night, as journalists besieged the hospital for information and photographs, the two women were joined by several other members of the Sartre circle; they gathered around the body in the hospital room, drinking whisky and recalling their years with the dead writer. "At one point," Simone writes, "I asked to be left alone with Sartre, and I made as if to lie with him under the sheet . . . A nurse stopped me . . . 'No, take care . . . the gangrene.' It was then that I understood the real nature of the bedsores. I lay on top of the sheet and I slept a little."

The president of France, Valéry Giscard d'Estaing, saying he understood Sartre's desire to avoid a state funeral, offered to pay the expenses of a private ceremony, but this was declined. The dead man had also requested not to be buried in Père Lachaise Cemetery between his mother and stepfather. There were two interments: on 19 April 1980 a crowd of fifty thousand followed the hearse through the Paris streets to Montparnasse Cemetery, where the body was laid for a few days to the left of the gate; on the twenty-third the remains were cremated at Père Lachaise and the ashes laid to rest at Montparnasse in the first alley to the right, not far from Baudelaire, about whom Sartre had written.

Simone de Beauvoir, stricken with pneumonia immediately after her friend's death and later suffering depression, writes in *Adieux*: "His death does not separate us . . . My death will not bring us together again. That is how things are . . . ."

Sayers, Dorothy L. (1893-1957)

The creator of Lord Peter Wimsey, debonair sleuth and bibliophile in eleven detective novels and many short stories, was also, by her own preference, a classical scholar and Anglo-Catholic apologist and dramatist. Her highly successful BBC radio series, *The Man Born to Be King* (1942), told Christ's story in workaday British dialects.

Wimsey was her ideal man, one whom she never succeeded in finding for herself in real life. The father of her illegitimate son John Anthony, born in 1924, was an unidentified motor mechanic unwilling to face his responsibilities as a husband and father. Dorothy's success as a detective novelist and advertising copywriter enabled her to keep the boy's existence secret even from her parents and have him cared for by a relative.

In 1926 she married "Major" Oswald Atherton Fleming (real name: ex-Captain Oswold Arthur Fleming), a divorcé twelve years her senior, who made a bare living as a part-time motoring correspondent for a London newspaper. His heavy drinking and uncertain temper were a constant trial to her. They lived on her earnings and she even supplied his ex-wife with an allowance. Though Fleming could offer her little of the intellectual companionship that was the focus of her life, they got along well enough until his death in 1950. They informally "adopted" her son in 1934, but he never lived with them.

There were no more Wimsey novels after *Busman's Honeymoon* (1937). Dorothy wrote religious dramas and essays and was much in demand as a speaker. She devoted her final thirteen years to a translation of Dante's *Divine Comedy* and to the affairs of St. Anne's House in London's Soho district, where the church's place in modern society was much discussed. After "Mac's" death she let herself go, chain-smoking cigarettes and eating excessively, so that dragging her increasing bulk to London from her cottage in Witham, Essex, grew ever more awkward.

On 11 December 1957 she was interviewed at home for a newspaper by her old friend Val Gielgud, who had produced *The Man Born to Be King*. Two days later she was in Cambridge to act as godmother to Barbara Reynolds, who was to complete the *Divine Comedy* translation and who had decided, at the age of forty-three, to be baptized.

Early the following week she visited London for the last time. Her main task was to complete her Christmas shopping, but she was also seen in a

Piccadilly gallery, looking unusually fatigued, viewing a new portrait of herself by Sir William Hutchinson. She phoned a clergyman friend from Harrod's to cancel a meeting with him because she was running late; of course, she could always stay at St. Anne's overnight, but then—who would feed her cats?

She took a taxi to Liverpool Street station and returned to Witham, the thirteenth stop on the Colchester line. There she was met by her usual cab driver, Jack Lapwood. Her home at 24 Newland Street was only half a mile away, but even without her Christmas parcels she was in no condition to walk so far. After Lapwood bade her good night at the front door she was not seen alive again. Next morning her gardener-handyman noticed that lights were on in the house. The cats had not been fed after all. Dorothy Sayers had taken off her hat and coat and then collapsed from a coronary thrombosis. Her body was found slumped near the foot of the stairs.

No recent will could be found, but a 1939 one left everything to "Mac," and in the event of his prior death to John Anthony. She left around $100,000 and of course her copyrights. Her body was cremated at Golders Green in north London and her ashes were laid below the tower of St. Anne's. *See* James Brabazon (1981).

Sterne, Laurence (1713-1768)

The author of the strange, unfinished novel *Tristram Shandy*, issued in nine parts between 1760 and 1767, was a tuberculous clergyman who lived much of his time in a state of fantasy. He traveled from Coxwold, near Thirsk in Yorkshire, where he was rector, to London and there wrote his *Journal to Eliza* and *A Sentimental Journey Through France and Italy*. The latter was published just three weeks before his death.

Early in March 1768 he retired to bed with a fever in his Old Bond Street lodging. On the fifteenth he wrote in a letter, "Your poor friend is scarce able to write—he has been at death's door this week with pleurisy— I was bled three times on Thursday, and blister'd on Friday . . . The physician says I am better . . ."

Though his room often thronged with visitors, many of them—it seems—women friends from his amorous past, none of them left a record of his dying moments. For this we must rely on a servant. On 18 March 1768, a group of Sterne's friends (among them the actor David Garrick) sitting at dinner in the Clifford Street house of John Crauford sent the footman, John Macdonald by name, to inquire about his condition. "I waited ten minutes," he reported later; "but in five he said: 'Now it is come.' He put up his hand as if to stop a blow, and died in a minute."

Sterne was laid to rest with little ceremony in the burial ground just north of Hyde Park belonging to St. George's, Hanover Square, a place haunted by the infamous "body snatchers" and shared by many unfortunates executed at Tyburn. Only four attended the funeral; the dead man's estranged wife Elizabeth and their daughter stayed away. Late the following year a headstone with an inaccurate inscription was erected, not to be corrected (by a footstone) until 1893. During World War I the stones were placed against the walls of the abandoned cemetery, which was soon taken over for vegetable gardens. In June 1969 the Laurence Sterne Trust, acting before blocks of apartments could be erected on the site, searched for the author's remains at the spot where the two stones had stood. Five skulls were found; one of them, an unusually small one, had had its top sawn off. The Trust believes that, by reason of its similarity in size and shape to Joseph Nollekens's bust of Sterne, made in Rome in 1766, this skull is the one they sought. Sterne's 1972 biographer, David Thomson, is not so sure. If the identification is correct, it gives credence to rumors that circulated shortly after the burial. According to these, body snatchers stole the body and sold it to the anatomy school at Cambridge. It was recognized during the dissection and hastily taken back to the burial ground. Sterne's skull or not, it was placed, with the two tombstones, in the churchyard at Coxwold.

Stokowski, Leopold (1882-1977)

The London-born U.S. orchestra conductor, who had a flair for self-publicity, was probably the best-known maestro of all time. He created a sensation when, as the Philadelphia Orchestra's director, he introduced Mahler's *Symphony of a Thousand* in 1916. He appeared in several films, notably Walt Disney's *Fantasia* (1940), in which his graceful hands were highlighted (he never used a baton). As he turned eighty he helped form his own group, The American Symphony Orchestra, which he directed for ten years without payment.

In June 1971 he suffered a heart attack in London but was soon back at work. A few months later friends sought out for him a quiet English retreat, a five-century-old house on two acres opposite a dairy pasture in the Hampshire village of Nether Wallop, east of Salisbury. On his ninetieth birthday, 18 April 1972, he appeared on NBC's *Today* show, being interviewed by Barbara Walters. In September, on his way by train to Prague, he fell heavily over a suitcase; only the fact that he fell on his artificial hip saved him from a dangerous fracture and allowed him to recover quickly. He conducted his final public concert in England in March 1974 with the New Philharmonia Orchestra in Walthamstow Town Hall, but appeared before an audience at the Vence Festival in southern France as late as July 1975. The ninety-three-year-old came to the hall stooped over his cane and supported on both sides, but as usual the orchestra, with all the players except the cellos standing, produced the fabulous "Stokowski sound" in five of his own Bach transcriptions for strings.

The maestro signed his final recording contract with CBS at the age of ninety-four—to run for six years instead of the more usual five, so that it would terminate on his centenary. He was actually ninety-five when he ended his career of over seventy years, comprising seven thousand concerts and countless recordings. His last recording sessions took place at EMI's Abbey Road studios in London when he conducted the so-called National Philharmonic (made up of players from the various London orchestras) in Mendelssohn's *Italian Symphony* and Bizet's *Symphony in C*. He was able to complete each recording in a single session on successive days, 31 May and 1 June 1977, amazing the critics yet again with his brisk tempos and brilliant sound.

Stokowski spent the summer at his recently built house on the French Riviera at St. Paul de Vence. Late in August he returned to his Hampshire home and studied Rachmaninov's *Second Symphony* for a recording session set for 13 September 1977. As the date approached he complained of feeling unwell, apparently from a viral infection, and the engagement was put off. It was on that very day, as he rested in his Nether Wallop home, that he died quietly of a heart attack. With him were his assistant, Charles ("Jack") Baumgarten, and his longtime companion, Natalie ("Natasha") Bender.

The five children of Stokowski's three marriages were all present at his funeral service in London's Marylebone Crematorium Chapel, where a eulogy was delivered by Edward Heath, a former British prime minister. The conductor lies near his parents in Marylebone Cemetery; his gravestone reads LEOPOLD / STOKOWSKI / 18 APRIL 1882–13 SEPTEMBER 1977 / MUSIC IS THE VOICE OF THE ALL.

As the huge container bearing Stokowski's possessions—paintings, correspondence, photographs, silverware, even carpets—was being taken to the United States, it was washed overboard in a severe Atlantic storm. It is likely that the many puzzles of the maestro's early life may now never be resolved. *See* Oliver Daniel (1982).

Surratt, Mary (1817-1865)

The only woman to be hanged for the assassination of Abraham Lincoln kept a boarding house at 541 H Street in Washington, D.C. Her son John conspired with John Wilkes Booth to kidnap the president in March 1865, but the plan failed. When Booth shot Lincoln on 14 April, John Surratt was probably in Elmira, New York. His mother was arrested on 17 April and at first occupied a cell only eight feet by two and a half. Suffering from severe menstrual bleeding, she was described by a defense lawyer as more dead than alive.

Charged with being an accessory to the murder, her chances of acquittal were never good. She was a Southern woman facing nine Union generals at the close of the bitter, divisive Civil War. Several of the conspirators had been among her transient boarders. Though one of the condemned men, Lewis Payne, repeatedly proclaimed Mrs. Surratt's innocence, Lincoln's successor as president, Andrew Johnson, commented that she had, in any event, "kept the nest that hatched the egg." When the death sentence was read on 6 July, Mrs. Surratt was reported to have "burst into a violent paroxysm of grief." Five of the nine military jurors recommended clemency, but this was denied her, though groups besieged the White House on her behalf all night.

By 11:00 A.M. on Friday, 7 July, a gallows had been erected and tested in the yard of the Old Penitentiary on the Potomac at Greenleaf Point. There was a delay of two hours, during which the crowd of onlookers grew restive in the heat. The hangman, Captain Christian Rath, said later that he "fully expected Mrs. Surratt would never hang."

At 1:00 P.M. the prisoners were led out. Just before leaving her cell Mrs. Surratt declared that God in Heaven knew she was innocent. Wearing a trailing black dress and black bonnet with a heavy black veil, she was supported by two men; her arms and ankles were shackled. Her daughter Anna's sobs were heartrending. The four prisoners were helped up the creaking stairs and seated before the nooses. One trap was employed for Payne and Mrs. Surratt, the other for George Atzerodt and David Herold. There was some delay while Mrs. Surratt's dress was tied down. Nooses were put around their necks; strips of white muslin were used to bind their arms and legs more securely and white hoods were placed over their heads. Mrs. Surratt, on the point of collapse, begged to be supported. As black-robed priests intoned the service for the dying, General W. S. Hancock, in charge of the penitentiary, ordered the execution to proceed; the soldiers knocked the props away and the traps fell with a thud. Mrs. Surratt died without a struggle; she was probably unconscious before she fell. Outside the prison a holiday air prevailed and vendors sold cake and lemonade.

The remains of the conspirators were moved to a warehouse nearby when the prison was demolished in 1867. Mrs. Surratt's remains were given to her daughter in February 1869 and her final resting place was not divulged.

In 1891 Mrs. Surratt's priest, Father Jacob A. Walter, speaking at a meeting of the Catholic Historical Society in New York, said that, although he could not divulge the secrets of the confessional, he believed she died "as innocent of that crime as a babe unborn."

In 1867 John Surratt, who had been captured in Egypt the year before, was tried before a civil court, which refused to convict him.

Teasdale, Sara (1884-1933)

The U.S. poet from St. Louis, Missouri, moved to New York on her marriage in 1914. Noted for her lyric talent, her *Love Songs* won the Pulitzer Prize in 1917. In 1919 she wrote that poems—certainly *her* poems—were written out of "a state of emotional irritation." Thus, her early poem "Alchemy" seems to have been jotted down, according to a marginal note, at 4:00 A.M. on a March day in 1913, no doubt after a sleepless night, her aim being "To change the lifeless wine of grief / To living gold."

Her husband, Ernst Filsinger, was often away on business overseas for many months at a time, and though they expressed deep love for one another their marriage was a great disappointment to her. She had expected to be able to quite "lose herself" in her lover, but she remained all too conscious of her own separate self. It was habitual with her to long for Filsinger's return, only to escape to a sanitarium or hotel in New England a day or two after he reached her in New York. She was seldom free of phantom aches and pains. Her restlessness and anguish deepened in 1928 and thoughts of divorce were her refuge. Ernst came back from a six-month overseas trip in January 1929 and left again in March after an unsatisfactory reunion. In June she wrote to him from Reno, Nevada, announcing her divorce plans; Ernst, in Johannesburg, was horror-struck but helpless. Her grounds were his long absences and total absorption in business.

After the divorce, her restlessness did not diminish. She moved from her New York hotel to another in Massachusetts and back again within a few weeks. She complained now of loneliness, but shrank from companionship when it was offered, citing illness or exhaustion. Now, thoughts of increasing poverty haunted her, though she lived luxuriously at the Bolivar Hotel on Central Park West and ordered her meals from the dining room to save herself cooking chores.

In 1931 and the following year she visited London to collect material for a book, left unfinished at her death, about the love poems of Christina Rossetti. In September 1932 she returned to New York an invalid after a bout of pneumonia and was cared for by her sister Mamie Wheless and a young admirer, Margaret Conklin. She was still bedridden when forced to move from the Bolivar to an apartment at One Fifth Avenue when her lease expired.

Oppressed by fears of a stroke and imminent poverty, she began hoarding sleeping tablets. After Christmas 1932 she fled to a friend's in Florida and back again two weeks later. By now she had hired a young English nurse, Rita Brown, as an around-the-clock companion. On Friday, 27 January 1933, the breaking of a blood vessel in her hand convinced her that the stroke she had long dreaded would come at any moment, and she asked Mamie to assume power of attorney. Margaret alerted Sara's doctor Dana Atchley that a psychiatrist should be called in, but nothing was immediately done.

It was now Saturday evening, and Sara appeared quite tranquil as she sat with Margaret, reading aloud and listening to records of Beethoven's *Fifth Symphony*. "Beethoven knew all the answers" were her last words as Margaret left.

Sometime early on Sunday morning, 29 January 1933, Sara Teasdale drew a bath, took a heavy dose of sleeping pills, and lay down in the warm water. It could have been a last despairing call for help: she may have expected to be discovered alive. But Rita Brown slept late and did not search for her until 9:00 A.M. Sara had been dead only a short time; the bathwater was still warm.

That evening, Brown, discovered dancing with friends to jazz music on Sara's Victrola, was ejected from the apartment; jewelry and other items were later found to be missing. Much to the Teasdale family's relief, the early newspaper reports indicated accidental death. The finding of a morphine and phenobarbital overdose changed the final verdict to suicide, but this was never publicized.

Sara's wish to have her ashes scattered at sea was ignored; they were interred in Bellefontaine Cemetery, St. Louis, under a marker with the name Sara Teasdale Filsinger. Ernst died in Shanghai in 1937 and his ashes were buried in the Filsinger family plot nearby, as close as possible to Sara's grave. Despite her fears of poverty, she left $83,000 mainly to Margaret and Ernst and after their deaths to Wellesley College to establish an annual poetry prize.

Tillich, Paul (1886-1965)

The German-born theologian and philosopher was forced by the Nazis from his position at the University of Frankfurt in 1933 and he later taught at New York's Union Theological Seminary, Harvard, and the University of Chicago.

In her 1973 biography, Hannah Tillich dwells on her husband's many love affairs and his preoccupation with pornography and prostitutes; the psychoanalyst Rollo May, an admirer, believes his actual infidelities to have been quite infrequent. Early in 1964, shortly after completing his trilogy *Systematic Theology,* Tillich was admitted to Chicago's Billings Hospital suffering from bronchitis and an increasingly severe cardiac condition. Even a short slow walk was now impossible without frequent rests—what he termed "inching and benching."

While spending the summer of 1965 as usual at his Long Island vacation home in East Hampton, he suffered several heart attacks. Back in Chicago he delivered a lecture at Breasted Hall and afterward enjoyed a lively argument with a group who called themselves "godless Christians." So excited did he become that Hannah prevailed on him to come home to their Windermere Hotel apartment. During the night she was awakened by tapping on the wall between their bedrooms. Finding him doubled up in pain, she had him rushed by ambulance to Billings Hospital.

"Today is dying day," Tillich told his wife on the morning of 22 October 1965, his tenth day in hospital. "Today you must not leave me at all." They talked about their beautiful East Hampton garden and he wept, knowing that he would never walk there again. But he recovered his spirits and teased the doctor at noon saying, "Today I am going to be a complete ascetic. I spent a long time yesterday figuring out the menu for today, but I'm not going to eat a thing." About seven in the evening Tillich wanted to sit up. As Hannah and a nurse helped him, a sudden spasm shook his frail body and he fell back dead.

Paul Tillich was cremated and his ashes were taken to East Hampton. Seven months later they were disinterred and brought to the Paul Tillich Park in New Harmony, Indiana, a little village on the Wabash River, twenty-nine miles west of Evansville. Trees selected many years before by Tillich himself grow there, verses from his writings are carved on the rocks, and at the end of a path that winds through a grove of fir trees is a bronze bust of the theologian sculpted by James Rosati.

Tito, Josip Broz (1892-1980)

The president of Yugoslavia (from 1953) kept together the different ethnic and religious groups that made up his nation largely by his own forceful personality. Though besieged for years by arteriosclerosis and diabetes, he had a great zest for life; he was out hunting in December 1979 when, at the age of eighty-seven, he first complained of pain in his left leg. At the Ljubljana Medical Center a dangerous blockage of the femoral and tibial arteries was found. The U.S. specialist Michael DeBakey was consulted and advocated medication. Instead, an arterial bypass was attempted; it was unsuccessful, and gangrene set in. On 20 January Tito gave reluctant permission for amputation below the knee. At first, recovery proceeded hopefully, but after three weeks the patient suffered digestive problems, cardiac weakness, and loss of kidney function.

In late February Tito was placed on a dialysis machine. Liver damage, internal hemorrhaging, pneumonia, and high fever beset the patient. An external pacemaker and a respirator were resorted to. The Yugoslav embassy in Washington requested supplies of an experimental broad-spectrum antibiotic, Moxalactam, from the manufacturers, Eli Lilly, in Indianapolis. At first, this brought about an improvement, but during April Tito sank into a coma; he died on 4 May 1980, three days before his eighty-eighth birthday.

The president's body was taken from Ljubljana to the capital, Belgrade, where it lay in state in the Federal Assembly Building. Official representatives arrived from 123 countries, including four kings, thirty-two presidents, and twenty-two prime ministers. The official news agency, Tanjug, called the gathering "The summit of mankind." Eight military officers carried the oak coffin to an open gun carriage, where it was covered with the blue, white, and red flag. Tito's third wife Jovanka followed the coffin as it was taken, in accordance with his request, to be buried in the grounds of his principal residence at 15 Uzicka Street in the hilltop suburb of Dedinje. His white marble vault bears the simple inscription in gold: JOSIP BROZ TITO 1892–1980.

Tolkien, J. R. R. (1892-1973)

The British don, Merton Professor of English at Oxford, was surprised to find himself world-famous after the publication of *The Lord of the Rings* (1954–55), a trilogy dealing with the mythical region of Middle Earth. During the 1960s the trilogy and its "prequel," *The Hobbit* (1937), gave rise to a cult that swept across U.S. campuses, where FRODO LIVES became as familiar on buttons as anti–Vietnam War slogans.

Tolkien found this fame more a burden than a pleasure. Some of his overseas readers, disregarding the time difference, would call him during the night. Admirers who rang the doorbell at his Oxford home, 76 Sandfield Road in suburban Headington, could become vituperative if the revered one was not instantly available. His dusty garage-study grew more and more disorderly, with books, letters, and manuscripts piled up everywhere, until his publishers provided him with a part-time secretary, Joy Hill.

He was rather stooped, silver-haired, and prone to rapid mumbling around the stem of his eternal tobacco pipe. "I am in fact a hobbit in all but size," he told an interviewer; more specifically, a journalist compared him to two of his characters, calling the author "a cross between Bilbo and Gandalf."

In his mid-seventies, Tolkien complained that life after retirement was "grey and grim," made more onerous by worries over his wife Edith's arthritis and migraine headaches and her lack of household help. In 1968, two years after their golden wedding anniversary, they fled Oxford and bought a bungalow in the south-coast resort of Bournemouth. There they chose a Catholic church and a suitable doctor, Denis Tolhurst, and Tolkien turned his attention to *The Silmarillion*, an unfinished work begun in 1917 and chronicling the creation of the world and the battle between elves and the power of evil. The manuscript lay around in bits and pieces, some rewritten, some not, with place and character names in various forms. After three years in Bournemouth, just as Tolkien was beginning to make real progress on the story, Edith died, following gallbladder inflammation, on 29 November 1971.

In March 1972 he moved into rooms provided at 21 Merton Street by his old Oxford college; there, a university "scout" (servant) and his wife, Charles and Mavis Carr, looked after him. He enjoyed the company of fellow dons in the Merton College common room and of townspeople in the neighborhood's senior centers, to which he made donations. The queen made him a Commander of the Order of the British Empire, an honor conferred at Buckingham Palace, and Oxford University awarded him an honorary Doctor of Letters for his philological work. But on *The Silmarillion* he made little progress.

In 1972 Tolkien suffered from "dyspepsia" and was put on a wine-free diet, which seemed to help. Daniel Grotta, in his 1978 biography, says Tolkien instructed a companion during one of their long walks in 1973 how to commune with a tree (by embracing the trunk and placing the forehead against the bark with the eyes closed). After illustrating this, Tolkien passed on the tree's message, but the companion, Lord Halsbury, declines to say what it was. Joy Hill recounts how, on one very long walk, they visited all of Tolkien's favorite trees—"All the trees in the Botanical Garden, and then we went down by the river to look at the willows. And then we came back again and did the trees all over again."

He lunched with his daughter Priscilla on 27 August and next morning was seen off, en route for a Bournemouth vacation, by Charles Carr. His hosts were the Tolhursts; on the thirtieth, Jocelyn Tolhurst's birthday, he drank a toast to her with champagne. During the night he was in pain and was taken to a private hospital in the area. An acute bleeding ulcer was diagnosed; on 1 September 1973 pneumonia set in and Tolkien died next day.

After a requiem mass in Oxford on 6 September he was buried on the outskirts of the city in the Catholic section of Wolvercote Cemetery beside his wife. There is a reminder of his then-unfinished work on their tombstone, a gray slab of Cornish granite: EDITH MARY TOLKIEN / LÚTHIEN / 1889–1971. JOHN RONALD REUEL TOLKIEN / BEREN / 1892–1973. (The tale of Lúthien Tinúviel, an immortal elf-maiden, and her lover Beren, a mortal man, was the author's favorite part of *The Silmarillion* and one with which he associated his courtship of Edith.) The entire book, edited and completed by his son Christopher, was published in September 1977 with great anticipation, enormous sales, and generally unfavorable reviews. *See* Humphrey Carpenter (1977).

Turing, Alan M. (1912-1954)

The English mathematician was only twenty-four when he described the concept of a universal machine—soon to be named the "Turing machine"—that could perform the computing activities of any machine whatever, including the human brain. He thereby laid the foundation of modern computing and advanced ideas about machine learning and artificial intelligence. In World War II he was a leader of the team at Bedford, England, that gave the Allies a critical advantage by breaking the top-secret German "Enigma" ciphers. Details of how this was done began to leak out only decades later.

From 1948, Turing worked at Manchester University on the world's first electronic stored-program computers.

Turing was a burly, athletic man with a fondness for marathon running and an eccentric manner that could be off-putting. One who discerned his true worth was a young American scientist, David Sayre, who visited him in 1950 and who wrote in 1969: "One does not expect to find in one man both the admirable intellect one had met *and* a person of the rarest human quality, but Turing was such a man, at least for me." Early in 1952 he reported a petty burglary at his suburban home on Adlington Road in Wilmslow, Cheshire, but when the police challenged his story, he freely admitted to covering up a homosexual affair with an unemployed youth he had met a few weeks earlier, nineteen-year-old Arnold Murray. It was Murray who had told Turing that the probable burglar was a disreputable friend of his. Male homosexuality, even in private, was a serious crime in Britain up to 1967 (and still is, if it involves anyone, like Murray, below the age of twenty-one). On both sides of the Atlantic gay men in 1952 were dubbed "perverts" and viewed as being on the same level as rapists. Turing's professional standing and reputation (he had been appointed a Fellow of the Royal Society in 1951) helped him avoid a prison term, but he was forced to submit to a year's administration of estrogens, sometimes referred to as "chemical castration." He took the publicity and the "therapy" in his stride; of a disconcerting side effect, he told a friend wryly, "I'm growing breasts." That he bore this reverse so well made his suicide two years later all the more bewildering.

There is some evidence that the security services were watching him and that he felt a threat to his personal movements which he was powerless to counter. In the official mind he was doubtless subject to blackmail and liable to be indiscreet about his secret wartime activities during vacations abroad. There was, for example, "the Kjell crisis" early in 1953. A young Norwegian he had met the previous year came to England to visit him. In a letter dated 11 March 1953 Turing reported, "At one stage police over the N. of England were out searching for him, especially in Wilmslow, Newcastle, etc. I will tell you all one day. He is now back in Bergen without my even seeing him!"

Alan Turing was found by his housekeeper lying dead in bed when she arrived at his Wilmslow home on 8 June 1954. He had taken several bites from half an apple that had evidently been dipped in a solution of potassium cyanide, a chemical he used in electroplating experiments. The inquest verdict was one of "suicide while the balance of his mind was disturbed." His behavior preceding his death had shown nothing unusual, his working papers were in their usual disarray, and he had several outstanding appointments.

Turing's body was cremated at Woking, Surrey, and the ashes were scattered in the crematorium garden; there is no memorial. His £11,000 estate was shared by his mother and several friends. *See* Andrew Hodges (1983).

Ward, Stephen (1912-1963)

The central figure in the Profumo sex and security scandal of 1963 was a British society osteopath whose clients included Winston Churchill, Averell Harriman, and Mahatma Gandhi. He was fond of pretty women of all social classes and some of them from time to time made his London apartment their home. It was there that the Minister for War, John Profumo, would meet a call girl, Christine Keeler, who numbered among her clientele the Soviet agent Yevgeny Ivanov. When Profumo admitted to lying to the House of Commons about the affair, the resulting scandal threatened Harold Macmillan's administration.

Ward's trial on charges that he had lived on Keeler's immoral earnings was seen in retrospect as a blot on British justice. After Ward's death Keeler and others admitted they had given false evidence under police pressure. The accused man's high-placed friends abandoned him. Information—that he had warned the security services about the Keeler-Profumo-Ivanov triangle and had even been an MI5 agent during the affair—was withheld from the jury.

A guilty verdict on two counts was brought in at the Old Bailey on 31 July 1963, but by then Ward was dying. He had lost hope during the judge's summing-up on the thirtieth. As he left the court he said bitterly, "This is a political revenge trial. Someone had to be sacrificed and that someone was me." Much of the evening was spent with his girlfriend Julie Gulliver as he wrote numerous letters in a friend's Chelsea apartment, where he was staying. At 9:00 P.M. he cooked Julie a meal, then drove her home. His host Noel Howard-Jones heard him return at midnight. Soon after, Ward evidently swallowed several Nembutal (pentobarbital) capsules and wrote one more letter, to Howard-Jones: "It is really more than I can stand—the horror, day after day at the courts and in the streets . . . Incidently, it [suicide] was surprisingly easy and required no guts . . . Delay resuscitation as long as possible." At this point the pen and his cigarette fell from his hands and he collapsed onto his mattress on the floor.

Awakened by a phone call at 8:30 A.M., Howard-Jones found his friend purple-faced, foaming at the lips and breathing only about twice a minute. At St. Stephen's Hospital on Fulham Road he lingered for three days. The experimental drug "619" (later named Doxapram) was given in an effort to revive him, but he died at 3:50 P.M. on 3 August 1963 without regaining consciousness.

At the Mortlake Crematorium six days later there were only two wreaths. One was from Ward's family; the other, from several playwrights and critics, including Kenneth Tynan and John Osborne, was inscribed, TO STEPHEN WARD, VICTIM OF HYPOCRISY. See Phillip Knightley and Caroline Kennedy (1987).

Warhol, Andy (1928-1987)

The U.S. pop artist with a flair for self-publicity was best known for his silk-screen prints of multiple images of soup cans, Coca-Cola bottles, and Marilyn Monroe. He was shot and critically wounded on 3 June 1968 by a deranged radical feminist, Valerie Solanas, a hanger-on at his "Factory" in Manhattan, where his creations were turned out en masse. He was hospitalized for six weeks and his punctured spleen was removed.

By the time of the first showing of his gigantic paintings of *The Last Supper* in Milan, Italy, in January 1987, he was in considerable pain. He had been repeatedly warned his gallbladder must eventually be removed, but hospitals terrified him. Whenever he was driven past one, he would block out the view with his hands. As for death, he called it the most *embarrassing* thing that could happen to anyone, with other people making all the very personal decisions about the treatment and disposal of one's body. Back in New York he ran out of a restaurant on 5 February and headed for home, complaining to fellow diners of pain in his right side. But he continued to avoid seeing his regular physician, visiting instead his dermatologist, who injected collagen under his skin to fill the wrinkles, and a chiropractor-nutritionist, who massaged his side. He had great faith, too, in a "crystal doctor," who would pass amethyst and quartz pieces over his body; but now crystals seemed to have lost their power. On 17 February he stood in a cold dressing room, enduring great pain while waiting to model menswear. That night he took Seconal, Valium, and aspirin to find temporary oblivion, and next day finally saw his orthodox physician, Dr. Denton Cox.

A sonogram showed the need for immediate surgery; Warhol called in a surgeon and a third doctor, but their advice was the same as Cox's. Nevertheless, he must first hide his "stuff": an incredible assemblage of valuable jewelry mixed with miscellanea of dubious value, mostly stacked in a pile of shopping bags, just as he had brought it home from innumerable buying expeditions. (It was later discovered in various nooks and crannies of his Manhattan apartment.) Only then was he ready to tell a close associate obliquely that he was going to "that place" to have "it"; most friends were told nothing.

When he checked into New York Hospital–Cornell Medical Center on 20 February under the name "Bob Robert" he seemed in good spirits. Next day his badly infected gallbladder was removed in a routine three-hour operation. What happened between the time he was brought back to his room in mid-afternoon until 6:31 P.M. next day, Sunday, 22 February 1987, when he was pronounced dead, became the subject of much speculation. He died in his sleep of cardiac arrhythmia while in the care of a young Korean woman, Min Chou, a private nurse. Ten days later, after a review of the case, she was barred from further hospital duties.

In early April the New York State Department of Health charged that Warhol had been given inadequate care throughout his stay at New York Hospital. The hospital denied the allegations and the Manhattan district attorney found insufficient evidence to bring criminal charges. Health officials began disciplinary proceedings in December 1987 and the Warhol estate filed suit for malpractice and wrongful death against the Hospital and eleven doctors and nurses.

Andy Warhol's body was taken to a funeral home in his native Pittsburgh, Pennsylvania. For his final public appearance he lay in a white-lined coffin dressed in a black suit and paisley tie; he wore a favorite platinum wig and sunglasses and held a prayer book and a red rose. After a service in the Holy Ghost Byzantine Rite Catholic Church he was buried twenty-five miles away in St. John the Baptist's Cemetery, Bethel Park. A memorial service in St. Patrick's Cathedral, New York, was attended by more than two thousand. On the first day of a ten-day auction of Warhol's collection at Sotheby's, $5.3 million was bid; his cookie jars alone brought in almost $248,000. *See* Bob Colacello (1990).

Warren, Leonard (1911-1960)

The U.S. baritone won the Opera Auditions of the Air in 1938 and began his career at the Metropolitan Opera Company in New York City on 27 November of that year. He was a large man with a phenomenal voice that could fill a hall of any size. During his Met career he sang 636 performances in twenty-two roles.

The audience on Friday evening, 4 March 1960, had the feeling of a gala performance. The opera was Verdi's *La Forza del Destino*. Renata Tebaldi, in superb voice, was making her first appearance of the season; in the third-act duet "Solenne in quest' ora," Warren, in the role of Don Carlo, and the tenor Richard Tucker (Don Alvaro) revealed that both were singing as beautifully as ever. Warren, with the perfection his audience was accustomed to expect, then sang the solo aria, "Urna fatale del mio destino." He ended it with his arms outspread—his habitual gesture of triumph—and was greeted by thunderous applause from the packed house. He responded to the news, given by the surgeon (Roald Reitan), that an injured comrade's life had been saved with the sung words, "Oh, gioia, Oh gioia!"; he then turned to make his exit, looking at a portrait he held of his sister Leonora (Tebaldi). The portrait slipped from his fingers and a moment later he pitched forward on his face and lay motionless. Reitan hurried to his side. The conductor, Thomas Schippers, stopped the orchestra. Reitan bent over Warren, then threw a despairing glance toward the conductor. At that point the curtain came down. Tucker, a longtime friend of the stricken baritone, rushed forward, crying "Lennie, Lennie!" The house physician, Dr. Adrian W. Zorgniotti, ran up an aisle and onto the stage. He examined Warren and called for oxygen. Several people attempted to give him mouth-to-mouth resuscitation until oxygen from the first-aid room could be administered.

Mrs. Agathe Warren left her box and hurried backstage. She later said that she had detected something peculiar in her husband's face just before he fell and, unlike some members of the audience, never believed that he had simply tripped. Monseigneur Edwin Broderick of St. Patrick's Cathedral, who had been in the audience, also went behind to administer the last rites. (Born a Jew, Warren had converted eighteen years before.)

At 10:30 P.M., nearly half an hour after the singer had collapsed, a grim-faced Rudolf Bing, general manager of the Met, came before the curtains. "This," he said, "is one of the saddest nights in the history of the Metropolitan." There were cries of "No, no," from the audience; women sobbed openly and men dabbed their eyes. Bing continued, "May I ask you all to rise in memory of one of our greatest performers who died in the middle of one of his greatest performances." He added, "I am sure you will agree with me that it would not be possible to continue with the performance."

Zorgniotti said that the apparent cause of death was a massive cerebral vascular hemorrhage. He thought that death had occurred at 10:03 P.M., though he did not pronounce Warren dead until 10:20 and oxygen was administered until 10:35.

Three thousand people filed past the singer's bier at the Abbey Funeral Home. His body was dressed in the white robe, embroidered in gold, of a Knight Commander of the Equestrian Order of the Holy Sepulchre in Jerusalem. The funeral service, a low Requiem Mass without music by request of Mrs. Warren, was held on 7 March at St. Vincent Ferrer's Roman Catholic Church at Lexington Avenue and 66th Street in New York. Warren was buried at St. Mary's Cemetery, Greenwich, Connecticut, after a brief graveside service.

Washington, Booker T. (1856-1915)

The most powerful black American of his time, a leader in Negro educational and economic advancement, founded Tuskegee Institute in Alabama's Black Belt in 1881. He was accused by more radical black activists of an over-conciliatory approach to the white power structure and to the white philanthropists upon whom he largely depended.

In private he was an earnest, obsessive worker who, says his 1983 biographer Louis R. Harlan, "never learned to play." In 1899 and again four years later only the rest afforded him by ocean voyages saved him from physical collapse. He suffered from chronic indigestion, for which he sought relief in papaya extracts.

In 1901, after the deaths of two wives, he married again. He was upright in family matters, but there was a suspicious incident in November 1911 when, after arriving in New York, he traveled by subway to an apartment building on West 63rd Street in a disreputable white neighborhood. Why he went there and haunted the vestibule for over an hour was never convincingly explained. A resident, Henry A. Ulrich, suspicious of the loiterer's intentions, struck Washington repeatedly with a heavy cane as he chased him, bleeding, along the street. The knowledge that even he, a distinguished, nationally known black man, was lynchable caused him to speak out thereafter in stronger terms against racial segregation.

His Tuskegee secretary described him in his final months as being "wasted by disease and suffering almost constant pain." In October 1915 he made plans to visit the Mayo Clinic in Minnesota but postponed his trip. His doctor, George C. Hall, reported "three severe attacks of kidney trouble" and "extremely high blood pressure."

The news that Washington was seriously ill broke into the headlines on 10 November. He had checked into St. Luke's Hospital in New York after making two speeches at Yale. Walter A. Bastedo, a specialist in abdominal medicine, told the Tuskegee Institute trustees that the director had "pretty serious kidney trouble and a blood pressure of 215." He also revealed to reporters that his patient was "worn out" and "aging rapidly." The indiscreet physician continued, "There is a noticeable hardening of the arteries and he is extremely nervous. Racial characteristics are, I think, in part responsible for Dr. Washington's breakdown. He is prone to worry under the strain of work, and while there is nothing to indicate that he is mentally unbalanced he is in no shape to go back to Tuskegee." The "racial characteristics" remark gave particular offense to Hall, who said it "means a 'syphilitic history' when applied to Colored people." Bastedo never repeated the phrase; after Washington's death he said the educationist "was completely worn out [and] suffering from nervous exhaustion and arteriosclerosis."

Washington was determined to die at home. "I was born in the South," he said, "I have lived and labored in the South, and I expect to die and be buried in the South." At Pennsylvania Station he spurned an awaiting wheelchair. At Chehaw, Alabama, the train was met by ambulances. Barely alive on arrival at his Tuskegee home, he died a few hours later at 4:15 A.M. on Sunday, 14 November 1915, surrounded by his family.

Booker T. Washington's body lay in state in the chapel of his institute for a day preceding his simple funeral, attended by large crowds. He was buried in the shadow of the large boulder that dominates the campus grave-yard. In Washington, D.C., every school flag was lowered during the cer-emony and teachers told their classes about the great man's career.

Wayne, John (1907-1979)

The U.S. actor had been appearing in movies for thirty-five years (as a star, since his first big success in John Ford's *Stagecoach*, for twenty-four) when he felt really ill for the first time in 1964. X rays disclosed "something as big as a golf ball" on his left lung. After surgery at Good Samaritan Hospital, Los Angeles, he didn't mind talking about it. "It was a rough operation," he said. The surgeon entered his chest from behind and removed the lower half of the affected lung. "He also took a rib, moved my diaphragm up and my stomach over," said Wayne. He wanted the public to know that "The Big C," as he called it, had to be caught early. "I don't want people to feel having cancer is like leprosy. This is something you can beat." Formerly a five-packs-a-day man, Wayne quit smoking and recovered to resume his career. He won an Oscar at last for his role in *True Grit* (1969).

During the filming of *The Shootist* (1976), Wayne noticed a developing hoarseness in his voice. A heart murmur was detected and at age seventy the actor underwent open-heart surgery at Massachusetts General Hospital in Boston on 3 April 1978, when a valve from a pig's heart was inserted. He went back home to Newport Beach, California, where he lived with his secretary Pat Stacy (he had separated from his Peruvian-born third wife, Pilar Palette, some years before).

In January 1979 he entered UCLA Medical Center, Los Angeles, for a gallbladder operation, but when a malignancy was discovered, his stomach was removed in a nine-and-a-half-hour procedure. A week later involve-ment of the gastric lymph nodes was detected—an ominous sign. Down by forty pounds, he appeared at the Oscar ceremonies on 10 April. When the lengthy ovation had subsided he said: "That's the only medicine a fella'd ever really need. Believe me when I tell you I'm mighty pleased that I can amble down here tonight."

Six of the Duke's seven children were at his bedside in the UCLA Medical Center when he sank into unconsciousness and died at 5:23 P.M. on 11 June 1979. He had been admitted on 2 May with an intestinal ob-struction and, though he was in considerable pain during his last hours, refused to take more than the bare minimum of narcotics; he wished to remain conscious as long as possible. According to Bernard Strohm, administrator of the medical center, "Sometimes his vital signs would stabilize and he would look over and call, often in a loud voice, for his children. When they would appear, he would lapse into a coma. It was the damndest thing. I have been around teaching hospitals for 20 years and I've never seen anything like the love in that family."

Despite his gruff-macho image, in private he was warm, well-mannered, and considerate of others. He hated to inflict his funeral on his friends. "When I go, just shove me in an oven somewhere, burn me and toss the ashes wherever it's convenient." But Wayne, a Catholic, was not cremated. After services at Our Lady Queen of Angels Catholic Church, Corona del Mar, California, on 15 June 1979, he was buried at Pacific View Memorial Park on a hill overlooking the ocean.

Webern, Anton (1883-1945)

The Austrian composer who refined Schoenberg's atonal twelve-note technique to produce incredibly spare, concentrated pieces died in a mysterious shooting incident in the Tyrol. After Hitler's invasion of his country in 1938, Webern's works were outlawed as degenerate and he was reduced to working as a proofreader for a music publisher in Vienna. Early in 1945 he was shaken by the death of his only son Peter on the Yugoslav front and at Easter he and his wife Wilhelmine (Mina) traveled west to take refuge from advancing Russian troops with his second daughter, Maria Halbich, at their home in Mittersill, south of Salzburg. When U.S. forces occupied the province, Webern raised his hands and fervently exclaimed, "Thanks be to God; now this horrible murdering has found its end . . ."

On the evening of 15 September 1945 the Weberns walked through the village to the house "am Markt 101" where they were to dine with their youngest daughter, Christine Mattel, and her family. After dinner, around 9:45, the composer lighted an American cigar—a rare treat procured for him by his son-in-law Benno—and moved to step outside the house so that the smoke would not disturb his sleeping grandchildren. Benno Mattel himself had gone across the hallway to the kitchen to meet two U.S. soldiers, Sergeant Andrew W. Murray and Private First Class Raymond N. Bell, an army cook from Mount Olive, North Carolina, who was serving with the 242nd Infantry Regiment of the U.S. 42nd Division. Their aim, following complaints that Mattel was engaging in black-market activities, was to entrap him into buying groceries and then to arrest him. In this they succeeded. He was standing with his hands above his head when his father-in-law, all unconscious of the state of affairs, went out through the hallway. Murray kept Mattel covered while Bell hurried out to fetch a military policeman. In the darkness the cook evidently bumped into Webern and, in a panic, shot him three times, through the abdomen, stomach, and chest, before hurrying on his way. The bullet holes in the house were still visible years later, two to the left, one to the right of the front door, all at waist height. The victim staggered into the house; "I was shot," he gasped, as his startled wife and daughter laid him on a mattress; and, as he lost consciousness he murmured, "It is over." He died a few minutes later; after his body was released by the authorities it was buried in Mittersill churchyard, where his wife joined him in 1949. Mattel was sentenced to a year in prison; later, he and his family settled in Argentina.

Bell, a tall, well-built man, successfully pleaded self-defense; the slightly built, sixty-one-year-old composer (110 pounds, five feet four inches) had attacked him with an iron bar, he claimed. After the war the killing preyed on his mind and he drank heavily. "I wish I hadn't killed that man," he would sometimes admit to his wife. The memory of the incident probably accelerated his death from alcoholism in 1955 at the age of forty-one. *See* Hans Moldenhauer (1961).

Welles, Orson (1915-1985)

The U.S. film actor-writer-director achieved fame with his 1941 movie *Citizen Kane* (which he claimed never to have watched after its release) and, three years earlier, with his and John Houseman's radio version of H. G. Wells's *War of the Worlds*, which drove thousands in panic from their homes in the belief that Martians had landed in New Jersey.

In his last years Welles led a much-diminished life, being often reduced to doing voice-overs for children's programs and appearing on television talk shows. He commuted between Sedona, south of Flagstaff, Arizona, where his wife Paola Mori and his youngest daughter Beatrice lived, and Los Angeles, where his companion was the Yugoslav actress Olga Palinkas, whom he had renamed Oja Kodar. In 1981, warned to diet, he eschewed his previous daily twenty cups of coffee, four or five portions of caviar and tumblerfuls of vodka, and vowed to lose 125 pounds. His major unfulfilled ambition was to stage *King Lear* with the help of French film and television interests. With his lifetime total of only a dozen films, he disappointed many who had foreseen a brilliant career for the boy wonder.

He played himself in the movie *Someone to Love*, writing for the part the words: "We're born alone, we live alone, we die alone. Only through love and friendship can we create the illusion for the moment that we're not alone."

During his final weekend he worked on the autobiography of Joseph Cotten, having promised his fellow actor to help him with the manuscript. He also labored on the script of another projected movie, *The Magic Show*. On Tuesday, 8 October 1985, he lunched with Burt Reynolds at Ma Maison. Next day he was chauffeured to the *Merv Griffin Show*, where his recent biographer Barbara Leaming would also appear. He performed a card trick on the show. That evening he dined with Leaming and Alessandro Tasco, his friend and production manager; they noticed he seemed to be in great pain as he rose from the table.

Late that night, 9 October 1985, Orson Welles died while sitting at his desk in his bathrobe. He had been overcome by a massive heart attack at the typewriter while inserting stage directions and camera movements in the script of *The Magic Show*. His chauffeur discovered his body next morning. His doctor Thomas Daily said he had been treating Welles for diabetes and a heart ailment. The funeral was private. The dead man had wished his ashes to be taken to Spain. On what would have been his seventy-second birthday his daughter Beatrice took them to a favorite spot, the country house of retired bull fighter Antonio Ordonez in Ronda, Spain, where Welles had often vacationed. She placed the blue urn in a small brick well, which was then sealed; there is no distinguishing mark.

In his 1982 will, Welles left $10,000 to each of his three daughters, Christopher, Rebecca, and Beatrice. His wife Paola was to receive his Las Vegas house and the remainder of the estate, except for the Los Angeles house and its contents, which were bequeathed to Oja Kodar. Moreover, Kodar, not the children, would inherit the estate if Paola died. Paola contested the will, but two days before she was to meet Oja to attempt an amicable settlement she was killed in a Las Vegas automobile accident. *See* Frank Brady (1989).

Wesley, John (1703-1791)

The English preacher was a High Church Anglican until he experienced a "conversion" in 1738 after his return from a mission to the United States. Thereafter he preached the gospel throughout Great Britain, traveling on horseback over four thousand miles a year in all weathers. His forty thousand sermons formed the basis of the Wesleyan Methodist Church.

He was unmarried until 1771, when he wed Mary Vazeille, a shrewish widow with four children. In his later years he gratefully traded horseback for a coach, and toward the end needed physical support in the pulpit.

One day in mid-February 1791 he rose as usual at 4:00 A.M. and traveled to Kingstone House at Leatherhead in Surrey to console an old friend on the death of his wife. There he preached his final sermon. He returned to his tall, narrow house, to the right of the forecourt of his Foundery Chapel in City Road, London, and with great difficulty climbed the steep stairs to his room. His anxious friends realized that he was dying, but Wesley disagreed. If they would just leave him alone for a while he would, he was sure, be better. When he expressed a wish to lie down they summoned a physician. He asked that he be buried in nothing but woolens and cheerfully sang hymns until he became too weak to continue. To his friends he murmured, "Farewell, farewell." Presently he roused himself to say with great eagerness, "Give my sermon on the love of God to everybody." To rally the spirits of his unhappy friends the dying man raised his arm and cried out, "The best of all is, *God is with us*." Throughout the night he murmured, "I'll praise, I'll praise," until, at about ten o'clock next morning, 2 March 1791, he passed away quietly.

By that date Wesley had been joined by three hundred other itinerant preachers; the Wesleyan movement had seventy-two thousand members in Britain and almost as many overseas, especially in America, where it was spreading rapidly. In spite of this, its founder never ceased to regard himself as a loyal Anglican priest.

Ten thousand people came to pay their last respects to the indomitable old preacher. For fear of an unmanageable crowd he was buried by lantern light at 5:00 A.M. in the small cemetery behind Foundery Chapel. The hundreds who attended the funeral were each given an effigy of Wesley, arrayed in canonicals and adorned with a halo and crown, beautifully stamped on bisque ware and enclosed in an envelope.

Whistler, James McNeill (1834-1903)

The U.S.-born artist settled permanently in London in 1889. His mistress for many years was the redheaded model Joanna (Jo) Heffernan, who also cared for his son by another model. His 1888 marriage to Beatrice Philip, a widow, ended with her death from cancer eight years later.

In his last years Whistler had trouble keeping warm. He consistently suffered from colds and feverish sore throats and his doctor worried about his heart, which had been damaged by childhood attacks of rheumatic fever in Russia. Traveling in Holland in 1902 with the Detroit millionaire Charles L. Freer he fell ill and returned to his London house at 74 Cheyne Walk in Chelsea. A bedroom was prepared for him on the ground floor next to his studio. Most days he spent dozing in an armchair, a calico cat on his lap. No longer the dandy of earlier years, he shuffled around wearing an old fur-lined overcoat on top of his nightshirt. Yet, one afternoon in May 1903, he completed a portrait in less than two hours of the redheaded model Dorothy Seton holding an apple. Named *The Daughter of Eve*, it was the finest of his late small studies.

In June pneumonia worsened his heart condition and on the afternoon of 17 July 1903 Freer arrived too late to take him for a carriage ride: Whistler was dead. Freer was asked to remain with the coffin to receive visitors; he recognized one woman when she raised her veil: it was Jo. Fewer than fifty people attended Whistler's funeral service in the Old Chelsea Church on the twenty-second. He was buried near his wife in Chiswick churchyard. The sculptor Rodin tried to raise $10,000 for a memorial depicting Venus leaning over Whistler as if to protect him. The plan had little attraction for the people of Chelsea and the opposition of fellow artist John Singer Sargent (on the grounds that Whistler would have hated the idea) brought the matter to a close.

White, Ryan (1971-1990)

The teenage victim of the acquired immune deficiency syndrome aroused the nation's sympathy in 1985 after his school in Kokomo, Indiana, invoking a 1949 Indiana statute applicable to communicable-disease sufferers, barred him from attending classes. Family members were shunned by neighbors and even by their Methodist church. Garbage was piled on their lawn and a bullet fired through their window. Ryan won an exhausting legal fight early in 1986 and, escorted by his stepfather, went back to school, but the harassment continued.

Ryan's AIDS-related pneumonia was diagnosed in December 1984 and he was given a probable survival time of only three to six months. Because he was a hemophiliac, he had been receiving twice-weekly infusions of blood extracts containing an essential clotting factor, and it was from this source that he was infected with the AIDS virus, HIV, at some date in the past. During his fight with the Kokomo school he was plagued by other AIDS-related illnesses, including thrush (a fungus infection of the mouth) and herpes.

Celebrities—singers Michael Jackson and Elton John, talk-show host Phil Donahue and Olympic diving champion Greg Louganis among others—supported Ryan and his mother Jeanne in his fight. In 1987 the Whites moved to Cicero, Indiana, and Ryan was welcomed to a more sympathetic high school, where the students were educated about AIDS before he arrived.

But the disease continued its remorseless assault and by the fall of 1989 Ryan's body was clearly wearing out; just taking a shower exhausted him. "He got shingles," his mother Jeanne recalled, "and sores on his legs that wouldn't heal. Often his throat was so sore he could barely whisper."

The end came in April 1990. A week before Ryan died, he was hooked up to a respirator. "I explained everything to him, why I felt it necessary," said the doctor, "and he said, 'Go for it.'" Ryan soon sank into a coma as infections spread through his body, his kidneys shut down and internal bleeding sapped his remaining strength. As poisons accumulated, his skin turned yellow and his flesh puffed up.

Jeanne White, exhausted and close to collapse, sat in a rocking chair at his bedside as Elton John came and went, helping tidy up coffee cups and tissues, making telephone calls for the family, bringing toys for the other young patients. In the early hours of Palm Sunday, 8 April 1990, Ryan's blood pressure sank ominously, and the doctor told Jeanne the end had come. "Just let go, Ryan," she whispered as she kissed his cheek. "It's time, sweetheart. It's time to go." The readings on the monitor dropped to zero; the eighteen-year-old's chest was still. The nurses were weeping as they removed masks, goggles, and rubber gloves. The dead boy's grandparents, his sister Andrea, the Whites' pastor Raymond Probasco and several friends came in to say good-bye.

Ryan White had, months before, chosen for himself a cemetery near

Cicero; it looked so peaceful, he said to his mother as they drove by. His funeral service in the Second Presbyterian Church, Indianapolis, was attended by First Lady Barbara Bush. Donahue and Elton John were pallbearers and the singer performed his own "Skyline Pigeon." Flags flew at half-staff across Indiana.

After her son's death, Jeanne White continued his crusade to help AIDS victims, and she appeared before Congress on behalf of the Ryan White Comprehensive AIDS Resources Emergency Act, which was passed to help cities heavily impacted by the disease.

There is little doubt that Ryan White's ordeal helped transform the public's perception of AIDS sufferers.

Williams, Tennessee (1911-1983)

The U.S. playwright's first success came in 1944 with *The Glass Menagerie;* a play that grew, he said, out of the intensity of his emotions while watching the mental decline of his sister Rose. His own sanity was always precarious; he had nervous breakdowns twice in his teen years, and often felt he was going out of his mind. In 1969, after years of depression, he spent over three months in a St. Louis hospital, recovering from overuse of Seconal and half a dozen other prescription drugs. As an escape from homosexual cravings and utter loneliness he wrote all the time, one play after another, regardless of their chances of production.

Williams's last Broadway play, *Clothes for a Summer Hotel;* opened to disastrous reviews in March 1981 and ran for only fourteen performances. To cheer him up, friends threw him a party in a seventh-floor New York apartment, but were dismayed when he ran out of the room and tried to jump from the balcony.

His longtime loving relationships were now far in the past. At seventy, sex was less important. "It's not appropriate to a gentleman my age," he said wryly to his close friend and 1985 biographer Dotson Rader. "I just want to touch. I get lonely, you know." He relied on a series of paid companions, hoping he would not die alone.

Late in the evening of 24 February 1983 he retired to bed in his two-room suite at the Hotel Éiysée in Manhattan, leaving his current companion, Jon Uker, an unemployed actor, in the sitting room. Scattered on the nightstand, as usual, were his various pills, spilled out of their vials to eliminate trouble unscrewing their lids. In among them was the small plastic cap from a bottle of eyedrops, used to help his glaucoma. Groping for Seconal around 11:00 P.M. to help himself sleep, he slipped the bottle cap into his mouth. His gag reflex may have been temporarily weakened by drugs or alcohol. The cap stuck in his throat and he began to choke. He toppled out of bed and knocked the nightstand over. Uker heard the crash but failed to investigate; he found the playwright at 10:45 next morning lying dead on the bedroom floor.

In a 1972 codicil to his will, the dead playwright asked that he be buried at sea, as near as possible to the spot where the U.S. poet Hart Crane had leaped to his death in the Caribbean in 1932. But Tennessee's brother Dakin elected to have him buried in St. Louis, next to his mother, Edwina, who had died in 1980. The Williams estate, valued at $10 million, was left to Harvard and to the University of the South in Sewanee, Tennessee.

Wilson, Woodrow (1856-1924)

The twenty-eighth president of the United States endured a catalogue of illnesses and incapacities, including dyslexia, frequent colds, digestive disorders, and phlebitis, but most serious were his strokes, the first of which he suffered in 1896 at the early age of thirty-nine while a Princeton professor. A second stroke deprived him of sight in the left eye while president of the university; there is little doubt that weakness of the right hand thereafter, attributed to "neuritis," was also due to cerebral thrombosis.

After the signing, in June 1919, of the Treaty of Versailles, incorporating at Wilson's urging the covenant of the League of Nations, he traveled the United States, urging for the treaty's ratification in thirty-four major speeches. Even as he set out he was beset by double vision and breathing difficulties. In Pueblo, Colorado, on 25 September he found his left side paralyzed and was rushed back to Washington.

On 2 October he collapsed in the bathroom. It seems likely that Edith Bolling Galt Wilson, his second wife, wished to hide the fact that he had fallen from the toilet seat and struck his head on a bathtub fixture. Only after she had somehow got him to bed and cleaned up his facial cuts did she call the doctor. The president was immobile, unable to speak or swallow, and, because of an enlarged prostate, had for several hours a complete urinary blockage. In his *Woodrow Wilson: A Medical and Psychological Biography* (1981), Dr. Edwin A. Weinstein diagnoses this latest stroke as "an occlusion of the right middle cerebral artery," causing "complete paralysis of the left side of his body . . . and a left homonymous hemianopia—a loss of vision in the left half fields of both eyes." (The 1906 stroke had already deprived Wilson of *central* vision in the left eye.) Weinstein also asserts that the president "developed manifestations of anosognosia—literally, lack of knowledge of disease"; he would refer to himself simply as "lame," but denied he was incapacitated—indeed, for a while he contemplated a third term. His physician Dr. Cary T. Grayson and Mrs. Wilson encouraged this denial. Grayson told the cabinet that the president was suffering from "a nervous breakdown, indigestion, and a depleted nervous system," and must not be bothered. At a bedside meeting in December his political foe Republican Senator Albert B. Fall assured him, "We have been praying for you Mr. President." "Which way?" quipped Wilson. When the invalid obstinately refused to accept GOP reservations, ratification of the treaty was doomed to defeat. By April 1920 he was able to walk a few steps with the aid of a cane but had to be wheeled into the room for a cabinet discussion; once there, he could be seen to have difficulty focusing his mind. In the final months of his administration he was heartened by the award of the 1920 Nobel Peace Prize.

Wilson lived on for four years more with Edith in a three-story house at 2340 S Street in Washington, along with his brother-in-law (who served as his secretary), two nurses and two servants. For a while he was nominal partner in a law firm, but because he viewed any business to do with government as a conflict of interest and turned it away, no profits were generated. Over 3 million listeners, the largest radio audience to that date, tuned in to hear his Armistice Day message in 1923. Next day, the actual holiday, he addressed a large crowd from his porch. Swaying slightly on his feet, he assured his audience that the principles he had stood for, though for a while delayed, would triumph at last. "That we shall prevail is as sure as that God reigns. Thank you."

Woodrow Wilson bade bon voyage to Grayson on 26 January 1924 while secretly wishing, as he confided to Edith, that the doctor would postpone his vacation. A few days later Mrs. Wilson recalled him; her husband was slowly weakening, and his daughters were summoned from New York, Los Angeles, and Bangkok. On Friday, 1 February, Grayson and two other physicians came in to examine the patient, who smiled and whispered, "Too many cooks spoil the broth." That night, Grayson told Woodrow Wilson that he was dying, to which the enfeebled man murmured, "I am a broken piece of machinery. When the machinery is broken . . ." Then silence, followed by, "I am ready."

Crowds began to gather in the street, ambassadors and government dignitaries left their cards at the door. But still the dying man held on. Margaret had arrived from New York; Nellie was on the *California Limited,* speeding east; Jessie had not yet left Siam. Once, when Mrs. Wilson briefly left the room, the dying man spoke his last word: "Edith!" A little later with daughter and wife holding his hands, Wilson opened his now sightless eyes for the final time; after ten minutes they closed again. At 11:15 A.M. on 3 February 1924 Grayson felt the last beat of the pulse.

A day of mourning was proclaimed by President Coolidge, who was one of four hundred invited guests at the private funeral on 6 February in the Bethlehem Chapel of the unfinished Washington Cathedral. After the guests had departed, Woodrow Wilson's coffin was lowered into the crypt. Years later his remains were moved to the crypt below St. John's Chapel. After Edith's death on Woodrow's 105th birthday, 28 December 1961, at the age of eighty-nine, she joined him there in a limestone sepulchre.

Windsor, Duke of (1894-1972)

The eldest son of George V (q.v.), king of Great Britain, Northern Ireland and the British dominions, succeeded him as Edward VIII on 20 January 1936 but abdicated within a year, on 11 December, in order to marry the Baltimore-born, twice-divorced Bessie Wallis Warfield Simpson. He was created Duke of Windsor by his successor, his brother George VI (q.v.). During World War II the duke was governor of the Bahamas, but, idle and bored, the Windsors lived out the rest of their lives in France. The duchess was never granted the title of "Royal Highness," something that never ceased to rankle in her husband. But then, for a man not noted for singleness of purpose, his unwavering devotion to his often difficult wife was a saving grace.

From 1953 they lived with a large staff in a white mansion in Paris, 4 Route de Champ de l'Entraînement, set in two acres of grounds on the Neuilly side of the Bois de Boulogne. By 1970 the duke was slowing down, barely able to finish a round of golf, but he never eased up on his heavy smoking, and in the fall of 1971 a biopsy indicated an inoperable cancer of the larynx. "I *told* him to stop smoking all those cigarettes," said the duchess. Cobalt treatment was begun but by March 1972 his weight was down to around one hundred pounds.

In May he insisted, despite a recent hemorrhage, on getting up to greet his niece Queen Elizabeth, who, with Prince Philip and their son Charles, was making her one and only visit. He was seated in a bedside chair when they arrived, the intravenous tube which sustained him hidden by his clothing. "My dear Lilibet, it's lovely to see you again," he greeted her, and they chatted for a few minutes.

Nine days later, after another hemorrhage, the Duke of Windsor died; it was 2:25 A.M. on 28 May 1972. According to one version of events, Wallis was asleep at the time and was awakened to hear the sad news; according to another, the duchess was dozing in a chair and was brought to the dying man's bedside; as she held him, he looked up at her and slipped peacefully away.

The duke's body lay in state in St. George's Chapel at Windsor as 57,000 mourners filed past. The funeral service was private, with only the royal family, government representatives, and special guests present. The coffin was then taken across Windsor Park to the royal burial ground at Frogmore and interred beneath the lawn close to the dead man's brother, the Duke of Kent, and not far from the Victoria and Albert mausoleum. The Duchess of Windsor, who was present, felt bitter at the proper but cool treatment she received. "After the burial," she told a friend, "I stood looking at the place next to him where I will be buried . . . My tiny piece of earth was just a sliver. I turned to the Archbishop of Canterbury . . . and said, 'I realize I am very thin, but I do not think that even I could fit into that miserable little narrow piece of ground.' [He] replied, 'I don't think there's much we can do. You'll fit all right.' " In the event a hedge was later moved and all was well.

The duchess lived on in her Paris mansion, secluded and in worsening health, for fourteen long, unhappy years. She died, aged ninety, on 24 April 1986; after another private service in St. George's Chapel attended by the royal family, she was buried beside her beloved husband.

Repeated attempts were made over the fourteen years, by Lord Louis Mountbatten and others, to have the Windsors' estate returned to Britain, but the duke left everything to Wallis, and she bequeathed the bulk of her fortune to the Pasteur Institute in Paris.

Wood, Natalie (1938-1981)

The U.S. actress, child of Russian parents, made her first movie at the age of five and grew up to star in *West Side Story* (1961) and *Bob and Carol and Ted and Alice* (1969). The first of her two marriages to fellow actor

Robert Wagner ("R.J.") ended after her involvement with Warren Beatty, her costar in *Splendor in the Grass* (1961). After an intervening marriage to British agent-producer Richard Gregson she again wed R.J., who was by then divorced from actress Marion Marshall, in 1972 aboard a borrowed yacht off Malibu, California.

On 27 November 1981, the Wagners set off from Marina del Rey, California, for a weekend cruise aboard their sixty-foot yacht *Splendour*. Their guest was Christopher Walken, Natalie's leading man in *Brainstorm,* then in production; the skipper-cook-bodyguard was bearded Dennis Davern. Ashore at Avalon on Santa Catalina Island, Natalie was reported to have grown tipsy and argumentative in a restaurant after several margaritas. Back on board, arguments between her and R.J. continued, and she went ashore again in a temper, asking Davern to take her in the dinghy *Valiant* and stay with her at an Avalon hotel overnight for protection.

The party sailed next day to Isthmus Cove, near the northwest tip of the island. Natalie and Walken spent several hours at a bar in the small community of Two Harbors, drinking and talking. R.J., by this time said to be very tense, came ashore and joined them for dinner. His wife, evidently drunk, flirted ostentatiously with Walken, snuggling up to him and caressing his shoulder. Nevertheless, they all sounded in good spirits as they climbed aboard the *Splendour* around 11:00 P.M.

At 1:15 A.M. on Sunday, 29 November 1981, Wagner reported by radio that "we may have someone missing in an eleven-foot rubber dinghy." A search was begun, and at 7:44 A.M. the body of Natalie Wood was spotted by a helicopter, floating facedown near Blue Cavern Point. She was wearing a red down-filled bed jacket, a blue flannel nightgown, and knee-length socks. The *Valiant* was beached one hundred yards away; its oars were tied down and the ignition switch was in the off position. The chief medical examiner of Los Angeles County, Thomas Noguchi, reported on Monday that the dead woman had evidently slipped and fallen into the water as she tried to climb aboard the dinghy. Ruling out foul play, the examiner said a scrape found on her left cheek was consistent with her having struck the edge of the dinghy as she fell. She was "slightly intoxicated," with a .14 percent blood-alcohol content; equivalent to a recent consumption of seven or eight glasses of wine.

Those who knew of Wood's dread of deep water were relieved to learn she had drowned quickly. (As a child, playing Bette Davis's daughter in *The Star* (1952), she had screamed so loudly when asked to dive from a yacht that Davis, overhearing her in her trailer, rushed to the scene and demanded that a stunt double be brought in.) But later, Noguchi was persuaded by a specialist in ocean currents that the position of the *Valiant* so near to the body almost certainly meant that Natalie, prevented from climbing aboard the dinghy by the forty-pound deadweight of her sodden jacket, had propelled the craft for a mile by kicking and one-handed paddling until hypothermia had overcome her. "She did not give up," Noguchi recalled two years later. "Instead, she began to perform a feat that was both unique and gallant. And she almost achieved a miracle."

Why did she want to leave the *Splendour* in the middle of the night? Davern's account was published in a tabloid in 1983. According to this, she continued to flirt with Walken after the party's return to the yacht. At last, Wagner, enraged, smashed a bottle on the table in front of them and shouted at the actor, "What are you trying to do? Seduce my wife?" Upon which, Walken jumped to his feet, confronted Wagner for a second, then shrugged and walked away. Natalie, furious, ran off to the master cabin, shouting, "R.J., I won't stand for this!"

Davern thought Wagner's reaction exaggerated, but maybe the apprehensive husband dreaded a replay of the Beatty infatuation. Around midnight, R.J. and Davern broke off their conversation and retired. Whether husband and wife saw one another again before Natalie left the boat Davern doesn't know. A woman on a neighboring yacht said she had heard a woman calling for help from 11:45 P.M. until 12:10 A.M. and a man's voice responding, "We're coming to get you."

Natalie Wood was buried in Westwood Memorial Park, Los Angeles, after a brief Russian Orthodox service at which a balalaika furnished the music. Many Hollywood celebrities attended; Lord Olivier flew over from England, and Queen Elizabeth II sent condolences. The considerable estate went mainly to eleven-year-old Natasha, Natalie's daughter by Gregson, and seven-year-old Courtney, daughter of the second Wood-Wagner marriage, with 10 percent for R.J.'s seventeen-year-old daughter Kate. *See* Warren G. Harris (1988).